Neutrophilic Dermatoses

Editor

STANISLAV N. TOLKACHJOV

DERMATOLOGIC CLINICS

www.derm.theclinics.com

Consulting Editor
BRUCE H. THIERS

April 2024 • Volume 42 • Number 2

ELSEVIER

1600 John F. Kennedy Boulevard ● Suite 1800 ● Philadelphia, Pennsylvania, 19103-2899

http://www.theclinics.com

DERMATOLOGIC CLINICS Volume 42, Number 2
April 2024 ISSN 0733-8635, ISBN-13: 978-0-443-18392-8

Editor: Stacy Eastman
Developmental Editor: Nitesh Barthwal

Dermatologic Clinics (ISSN 0733-8635) is published quarterly by Elsevier Inc., 360 Park Avenue South, New York, NY 10010-1710. Months of publication are January, April, July, and October. Business and editorial offices: 1600 John F. Kennedy Blvd., Suite 1800, Philadelphia, PA 19103-2899. Customer service office: 11830 Westline Drive, St. Louis, MO 63146. Periodicals postage paid at New York, NY, and additional mailing offices. Subscription prices are USD 447.00 per year for US individuals, USD 478.00 per year for Canadian individuals, USD 547.00 per year for international individuals, USD 100.00 per year for US students/residents, USD 100.00 per year for Canadian students/residents, and USD 240 per year for international students/residents. For institutional access pricing please contact Customer Service via the contact information below. International air speed delivery is included in all *Clinics* subscription prices. All prices are subject to change without notice. **POSTMASTER:** Send address changes to *Dermatologic Clinics*, Elsevier Health Sciences Division, Subscription Customer Service, 3251 Riverport Lane, Maryland Heights, MO 63043. **Customer Service: 1-800-654-2452 (U.S. and Canada); 314-447-8871 (outside U.S. and Canada). Fax: 314-447-8029. E-mail: journalscustomerservice-usa@elsevier.com (for print support); journalsonlinesupport-usa@elsevier.com (for online support).**

Reprints. For copies of 100 or more, of articles in this publication, please contact the Commercial Reprints Department, Elsevier Inc., 360 Park Avenue South, New York, New York 10010-1710. Tel.: 212-633-3874; Fax: 212-633-3820; Email: reprints@elsevier.com.

The *Dermatologic Clinics* is covered in *MEDLINE/PubMed (Index Medicus), Current Contents/Clinical Medicine, Excerpta Medica, Chemical Abstracts,* and *ISI/BIOMED.*

Contributors

CONSULTING EDITOR

BRUCE H. THIERS, MD
Professor and Chairman Emeritus, Department of Dermatology and Dermatologic Surgery, Medical University of South Carolina, Charleston, South Carolina

EDITOR

STANISLAV N. TOLKACHJOV, MD, FAAD, FACMS
Director, Mohs Micrographic and Reconstructive Surgery, Epiphany Dermatology; Clinical Associate Professor, Texas A&M School of Medicine; Clinical Assistant Professor, Department of Dermatology, University of Texas at Southwestern; Core Clinical Faculty, Division of Dermatology, Baylor University Medical Center; Clinical Faculty, Section of Dermatology, Veterans Affairs Medical Center, Dallas, Texas, USA

AUTHORS

AFSANEH ALAVI, MD
Professor, Dermatologist, Department of Dermatology, Mayo Clinic, Rochester, Minnesota, USA

FARAH ALMHANA, BA
Medical Student, The Ohio State University College of Medicine, Columbus, Ohio, USA

MAXIME BATTISTELLA, MD, PhD
Professor, Pathology Department, APHP Nord, Hopital Saint-Louis, Université Paris Cité, INSERM U976 "Human Immunology, Pathophysiology, and Immunotherapy", Paris, France

JEAN-DAVID BOUAZIZ, MD, PhD
Dermatology Department, Saint Louis Hospital, APHP Nord Université Paris Cité and INSERM u976 "Human Immunology, Pathophysiology and Immunotherapy", Paris, France

JEREMY BRAY, MD
Resident Dermatologist, Department of Dermatology, Mayo Clinic, Jacksonville, Florida, USA

JEFFREY P. CALLEN, MD, FACP, FAAD, MACR
Professor of Medicine, Department of Dermatology, University of Louisville, Louisville, Kentucky, USA

MICHAEL J. CAMILLERI, MD
Associate Professor, Departments of Dermatology and Laboratory Medicine and Pathology, Mayo Clinic, Rochester, Minnesota, USA

ANNE COAKLEY, MD
Dermatology Resident, Department of
Dermatology, Mayo Clinic, Rochester,
Minnesota, USA

NNEKA COMFERE, MD
Dermatologist and Dermatopathologist,
Professor, Departments of Dermatology and
Laboratory Medicine and Pathology, Mayo
Clinic, Rochester, Minnesota, USA

MARK D.P. DAVIS, MD
Dermatologist, Department of Dermatology,
Mayo Clinic, Rochester, Minnesota,
USA

JÉRÉMIE DELALEU, MD
Dermatology Department, Saint Louis
Hospital, APHP Nord Université Paris Cité and
INSERM u976 "Human Immunology,
Pathophysiology and Immunotherapy", Paris,
France

RONI DODIUK-GAD, MD
Head and Associate Professor, Department of
Dermatology, Emek Medical Center, Bruce
Rappaport Faculty of Medicine, Technion
Institute of Technology, Haifa, Israel; Division
of Dermatology, Department of Medicine,
University of Toronto, Toronto, Ontario,
Canada

ELISABETH GÖSSINGER, MD
Dermatologist, Department of Dermatology,
University Hospital of Basel, Basel, Switzerland

ASHLEY N. GRAY, MD
Resident Physician, Department of
Dermatology, The Ohio State University
Wexner Medical Center, The Ohio State
University College of Medicine, Columbus,
Ohio, USA

SAMANTHA GREGOIRE, BS
Department of Dermatology, Brigham and
Women's Hospital, Boston, Massachusetts,
USA

MATTHEW L. HRIN, MD
Resident Physician (Dermatology), Department
of Dermatology, Wake Forest School
of Medicine, Winston-Salem, North
Carolina, USA

WILLIAM W. HUANG, MD, MPH
Professor, Department of Dermatology, Wake
Forest School of Medicine, Winston-Salem,
North Carolina, USA

JOURDAN HYDOL-SMITH, BA
Texas A&M University School of Medicine,
Bryan, Texas, USA

BENJAMIN H. KAFFENBERGER, MD, MS
Assistant Professor, Director of Dermatology
Inpatient Consultation Service, Department of
Dermatology, The Ohio State University
Wexner Medical Center, Columbus, Ohio,
USA

KANIKA KAMAL, BA
Department of Dermatology, Brigham and
Women's Hospital, Boston, Massachusetts,
USA

THÉODORA KIPERS, JD, MS
School of Medicine, Texas A&M University
School of Medicine, Dallas, Texas, USA

SOPHIA LY, BA
Department of Dermatology, Brigham and
Women's Hospital, Boston, Massachusetts,
USA

BEDA MÜHLEISEN, MD
Dermatologist, Department of Dermatology,
University Hospital of Basel, Basel,
Switzerland

GANESH B. MANIAM, MD, MBA
Dermatology Resident, Department of
Dermatology, Mayo Clinic, Rochester,
Minnesota, USA

PRIYA MANJALY, BA
Department of Dermatology, Brigham and
Women's Hospital, Boston University School
of Medicine, Boston, Massachusetts, USA

CARLO ALBERTO MARONESE, MD
Dermatologist, Department of Pathophysiology
and Transplantation, Università degli Studi di
Milano; Dermatology Unit, Fondazione IRCCS
Ca' Granda Ospedale Maggiore Policlinico,
Milan, Italy

ANGELO VALERIO MARZANO, MD
Full Professor and Head of the Dermatology
Unit, Department of Pathophysiology and
Transplantation, Università degli Studi di

Milano; Dermatology Unit, Fondazione IRCCS Ca' Granda Ospedale Maggiore Policlinico, Milan, Italy

JULIA-TATJANA MAUL, MD
Senior Physician, Department of Dermatology, University Hospital of Zurich, Zurich, Switzerland

ABENA MINTA, BS
Medical Student, Department of Dermatology, The Ohio State University Wexner Medical Center, The Ohio State University College of Medicine, Columbus, Ohio, USA

ROHAN MITAL, BS
Medical Student, Department of Dermatology, The Ohio State University Wexner Medical Center, The Ohio State University College of Medicine, Columbus, Ohio, USA

CHIARA MOLTRASIO, PhD
Research Assistant, Dermatology Unit, Fondazione IRCCS Ca' Granda Ospedale Maggiore Policlinico, Milan, Italy

ESTER MORENO-ARTERO, MD
Dermatologist, Department of Dermatology, Hospital de Galdácano-Usansolo, Vizcaya, Bilbao, Spain

ARASH MOSTAGHIMI, MD, MPH, MPA
Assistant Professor, Department of Dermatology, Brigham and Women's Hospital, Boston, Massachusetts, USA

ALEXANDER A. NAVARINI, MD, PhD
Chairman, Department of Dermatology, University Hospital of Basel, Basel, Switzerland; Departments of Biomedical Research, Biomedical Engineering and Clinical Research, University of Basel, Allschwil, Switzerland

GIANG HUONG NGUYEN, MD, DPhil
Assistant Professor, Dermatologist, Department of Dermatology, Mayo Clinic, Rochester, Minnesota, USA

CHOON CHIAT OH, MD
Consultant and Adjunct Instructor, Department of Dermatology, Singapore General Hospital, Singapore; Duke-NUS Medical School, Singapore, Singapore

HAZEL H. OON, MD
Head of Department, Department of Dermatology, Emek Medical Center, Bruce Rappaport Faculty of Medicine, Technion Institute of Technology, Haifa, Israel; National Skin Centre and Skin Research Institute of Singapore (SRIS), Singapore, Singapore

AMARACHI ORAKWUE, BS
Medical Student, University of Minnesota Medical School, Minneapolis, Minnesota, USA

KATHERINE SANCHEZ, BS
Department of Dermatology, Brigham and Women's Hospital, Boston, Massachusetts, USA

COURTNEY R. SCHADT, MD, FAAD
Associate Professor of Medicine, Department of Dermatology, University of Louisville, Louisville, Kentucky, USA

OLAYEMI SOKUMBI, MD
Dermatologist and Dermatopathologist, Associate Professor, Departments of Dermatology and Laboratory Medicine and Pathology, Mayo Clinic, Jacksonville, Florida, USA

MARCUS G. TAN, MD, FAAD, FRCPC
Adjunct Professor, Division of Dermatology, University of Ottawa, Richardson, Texas, USA

STANISLAV N. TOLKACHJOV, MD, FAAD, FACMS
Director, Mohs Micrographic and Reconstructive Surgery, Epiphany Dermatology; Clinical Associate Professor, Texas A&M School of Medicine; Clinical Assistant Professor, Department of Dermatology, University of Texas at Southwestern; Core Clinical Faculty, Division of Dermatology, Baylor University Medical Center; Clinical Faculty, Section of Dermatology, Veterans Affairs Medical Center, Dallas, Texas, USA

ANTONIO TORRELO, MD
Head of Department, Department of Dermatology, Hospital Infantil Universitario Niño Jesús, Madrid, Spain

MARIE-DOMINIQUE VIGNON-PENNAMEN, MD
Pathology Department, APHP Nord, Hopital Saint-Louis, Université Paris Cité, Paris, France

DANIEL WALLACH, MD
Senior Lecturer and Physician (Hon.), Department of Dermatology, Paris Hospitals, France

MARGO WATERS, BS
Medical Student, The Ohio State University College of Medicine, Columbus, Ohio, USA

DAVID A. WETTER, MD
Professor, Department of Dermatology, Mayo Clinic, Rochester, Minnesota, USA

MIKA YAMANAKA-TAKAICHI, MD, PhD
Research Fellow, Department of Dermatology, Mayo Clinic, Rochester, Minnesota, USA

MALLORY L. ZAINO, MD
Resident Physician, Department of Dermatology, University of Louisville, Louisville, Kentucky, USA

Contents

Daniel Wallach

Acute febrile neutrophilic dermatosis, or Sweet syndrome, has been described in 1964 and is now considered as a prototypical condition of the group of the neutrophilic dermatoses. Since this time, many clinical conditions have been included in this group and a clinical-pathological classification in 3 subgroups has been proposed. Neutrophilic infiltrates can localize in all internal organs. This defines the neutrophilic disease, which induces difficult diagnostic and therapeutic problems. Autoinflammation is the main pathophysiological mechanism of the neutrophilic dermatoses. There is a special link between myeloid malignancies (leukemia and myelodysplasia) and the neutrophilic dermatoses.

Jérémie Delaleu and Jean-David Bouaziz

Neutrophilic dermatoses are a group of inflammatory skin conditions characterized by a neutrophilic infiltrate on histopathology with no evidence of infection. These conditions present with a wide range of clinical manifestations, including pustules, bullae, abscesses, papules, nodules, plaques, and ulcers. The classification of neutrophilic dermatoses is based on the localization of neutrophils in the skin. The pathogenic mechanisms of neutrophilic dermatoses involve autoinflammation, neutrophilic dysfunction, clonal somatic mutation and differentiation of the myeloid precursors as encountered in myeloid neoplasm.

Mallory L. Zaino, Courtney R. Schadt, and Jeffrey P. Callen

Pyoderma gangrenosum (PG) is an inflammatory neutrophilic dermatosis with variable clinical features. The classic presentation is an ulceration with an erythematous to violaceous undermined border. Extracutaneous manifestations may occur. Associated systemic diseases include inflammatory bowel disease, inflammatory arthritides, and hematologic disorders. The pathophysiologic mechanism of disease is not completely known but likely related to the cumulative impact of inflammation, immune-mediated neutrophilic dysfunction, and genetic predisposition. Incidence is between 3 and 10 people per million but may be greater due to under recognition. In this article, we will discuss the diagnostic criteria, disease subtypes, systemic associations, and workup.

that is histopathologically characterized by a perivascular and interstitial neutrophilic infiltrate with intense leukocytoclasia and without vasculitis or dermal edema. NUD clinically presents as a chronic or recurrent eruption that consists of nonpruritic macules, papules, or plaques that are pink to reddish and that resolve within 24 hours without residual pigmentation. NUD is often associated with systemic diseases such as Schnitzler syndrome, lupus erythematosus, adult-onset Still's disease, and cryopyrin-associated periodic syndromes.

Neutrophilic dermatoses are a broadly heterogeneous group of inflammatory skin disorders. This article reviews 5 conditions: amicrobial pustulosis of the folds, aseptic abscess syndrome, Behçet disease, neutrophilic eccrine hidradenitis, and pyostomatitis vegetans—pyodermatitis vegetans.The authors include up-to-date information about their epidemiology, pathogenesis, clinicopathologic features, diagnosis, and management.

Hidradenitis suppurativa (HS) is an autoinflammatory skin disorder of the terminal hair follicle, which can present in sporadic, familial, or syndromic form. A classification has been proposed for the latter, distinguishing cases associated with a known genetic condition, with follicular keratinization disorders or with autoinflammatory diseases. This review focuses on the clinical and genetic features of those entities (ie, pyoderma gangrenosum [PG], acne and HS [PASH]; pyogenic arthritis, PG, acne, and HS [PAPASH]; psoriatic arthritis, PG, acne and HS [PsAPASH]; synovitis, acne, pustulosis, hyperostosis, osteitis [SAPHO]; and so forth) for which the collective term HS-related autoinflammatory syndromes is proposed.

The term neutrophilic dermatosis encompasses a heterogeneous group of diseases, often associated with an underlying internal noninfectious disease, with an overlapping histopathologic background characterized by perivascular and diffuse neutrophilic infiltrates in one or more layers of the skin; extracutaneous neutrophilic infiltrates may be associated. Neutrophilic dermatoses are not frequent in children and, when they appear in this age group, represent a diagnostic and therapeutic challenge. Apart from the classic neutrophilic dermatoses such as pyoderma gangrenosum, Sweet syndrome, and Behçet disease, a neutrophilic dermatosis can be the presentation of rare genetic diseases of the innate immune system, such as autoinflammatory diseases.

Neutrophilic panniculitides are a heterogeneous group of inflammatory disorders encompassing many different entities. This review article focuses on the epidemiology, pathogenesis, clinicopathological features, diagnosis, and treatment of selected diseases. Patients often seek care due to systemic involvement, but the variable presentation of panniculitides can present a diagnostic challenge. Most therapeutic modalities for neutrophilic disorders are anecdotal at best with a notable lack of standardization of the responses to medications. There is an urgent need for a larger multi-institutional collaboration to address the unmet needs of these challenging, yet rare conditions.

Neutrophilic dermatosis is a heterogeneous group of inflammatory skin diseases characterized by the presence of a sterile neutrophilic infiltrate on histopathology. Three specific types of neutrophilic dermatoses are reviewed in this article: palisaded neutrophilic granulomatous dermatitis, bowel-associated dermatosis–arthritis syndrome, and rheumatoid neutrophilic dermatitis. The authors review the literature and highlight the clinical and histopathological features, disease pathogenesis, and the association of these conditions with various systemic diseases such as rheumatoid arthritis, inflammatory bowel disease, and others. A multidisciplinary approach is necessary for the diagnosis and management of these inflammatory skin conditions.

Sneddon–Wilkinson disease (SWD), IgA pemphigus, and bullous systemic lupus erythematosus (BSLE) are superficial and bullous neutrophilic dermatoses. They are all characterized by sterile neutrophilic infiltrate but differ in the level of skin affected and presence of autoantibodies. Both SWD and IgA pemphigus present with grouped flaccid pustules and have epidermal involvement; it is unclear whether they are distinct or exist on a spectrum of the same disease. IgA pemphigus is distinguished from SWD by positive direct immunofluorescence showing intercellular IgA deposition. BSLE presents with tense bullae, dermal neutrophilic infiltrate, and direct immunofluorescence showing linear IgG deposition along the dermal–epidermal junction.

Generalized pustular rashes have various etiologies and can be challenging to diagnose and manage at first presentation. The authors provide an in-depth analysis of common pustular skin eruptions including generalized pustular psoriasis (GPP) and acute generalized exanthematous pustulosis, focusing on their pathophysiology, triggers, clinical presentation, diagnostic challenges, and management strategies. The article also highlights recent advances in genetic research and biologic therapies for GPP and the future directions in personalized medicine and prevention strategies.

Neutrophilic dermatoses (NDs) encompass a wide range of cutaneous and extracutaneous manifestations, many of which impair quality of life (QoL) and are difficult to treat. Although NDs are transient and mild, others are chronic, severely debilitating conditions with profound impacts on QoL, including pain, mental health, occupational limitations, and sexual health implications. Current literature lacks attention to these unique care challenges to the ND patient population. The authors aim to summarize what is currently known about QoL in NDs and identify which diseases would benefit from additional research and disease-specific QoL assessment.

DERMATOLOGIC CLINICS

SERIES OF RELATED INTEREST

Medical Clinics
https://www.medical.theclinics.com/
Immunology and Allergy Clinics
https://www.immunology.theclinics.com/
Clinics in Plastic Surgery
https://www.plasticsurgery.theclinics.com/
Otolaryngologic Clinics
https://www.oto.theclinics.com/

Preface

Neutrophilic Dermatoses: A Medley of Inflammatory Cutaneous and Systemic Disorders

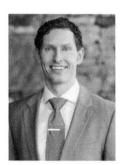

Stanislav N. Tolkachjov, MD, FAAD, FACMS
Editor

Before coining of the term "neutrophilic dermatosis" by a British dermatologist Dr Robert Sweet[1] in 1964, inflammatory cutaneous conditions with heterogenous presentations, often having systemic associations, were reported. Over time, due to the aseptic infiltration of neutrophils in the skin, subcutaneous tissue, and other organs, this grouping of disorders as neutrophilic dermatoses (NDs) became commonly accepted. Dr Louis Brocq[2,3] of France first described a form of cutaneous ulceration that we now call pyoderma gangrenosum (PG) as "geometric phagedenism." Dr Thomas Cullen[4] from Johns Hopkins reported a form of progressive postoperative "gangrene" of the skin in 1924 that was later termed postoperative or postsurgical PG, while Drs Louis Brunsting, William Goeckerman, and Paul Oleary[5] from the Mayo Clinic coined the term "pyoderma (ecthyma) gangrenosum" in 1930.

The evolution of the nomenclature of NDs can only be matched by the discoveries of multiple types of inflammatory and autoinflammatory conditions of the skin with a neutrophilic infiltration, many of which are unique presentations, while others may lie along a disease continuum. With the help of histopathology, pustular disorders, such as certain drug reactions and pustular

psoriasis, have also had an overlap with NDs. With increasing use of genetic testing, autoinflammatory conditions with neutrophilic pathology were also added to NDs. And as overlaps of autoinflammatory syndromes with acne, arthritis, and hidradenitis suppurativa with NDs like PG were reported, we gained a better understanding of these multifactorial disease states and their relationships. This potential for a systemic association and the act of solving a medical puzzle from cutaneous findings is what interests many of us who study NDs.

As evident by the history of NDs, the interest in these disorders spans across the globe. In this issue, I aimed to bring together an international group of experts in the field of NDs and related disorders and asked them to give an expert perspective on current understanding of specific NDs. In addition, several giants in the field of NDs contributed some historical perspective to give context to the evolving understanding of this group of disorders. Each ND is discussed in appropriate detail with some grouped as part of an overview. Adult and pediatric NDs are presented as well as overlapping disorders that should be mentioned with these inflammatory NDs. Last, quality-of-life indices are discussed, as patient care and the

Dermatol Clin 42 (2024) xiii–xiv
https://doi.org/10.1016/j.det.2024.01.002
0733-8635/24/© 2024 Published by Elsevier Inc.

patient experience should be at the center of our focus.

Understanding of NDs and their systemic associations will continue to evolve. This issue of *Dermatologic Clinics* brings together international experts to provide a comprehensive review of the past, present, and future of these disorders and outlines how we can best use our knowledge to provide excellent patient care.

Stanislav N. Tolkachjov, MD, FAAD, FACMS
Mohs Micrographic &
Reconstructive Surgery
Epiphany Dermatology
1640 FM 544, Suite 100
Lewisville, TX 75056, USA

E-mail address:
stan.tolkachjov@gmail.com

REFERENCES

1. Sweet RD. An acute febrile neutrophilic dermatosis. Br J Dermatol 1964;76:349–56 PMID: 14201182.
2. Brocq L, Simon CL. Contribution a l'etude du phagedenisme. Bull Soc Med Hosp 1908;25:290–307.
3. Brocq LA. New contribution to the study of geometric phagedenism. Ann Dermatol Syphligr (Paris) 1916;9: 1–39.
4. Cullen TS. A progressively enlarging ulcer of the abdominal wall involving the skin and fat, following drainage of an abdominal abscess apparently of appendiceal origin. Surg Gynecol Obstet 1924;38(5): 579–82.
5. Brunsting LA, Goeckerman WH, Oleary PA. Pyoderma (ecthyma) gangrenosum: clinical and experimental observations in five cases occurring in adults. Archderm Syphilol 1930;22(4):655–80.

The Neutrophilic Dermatoses, or the Cutaneous Expressions of Neutrophilic Inflammation

Daniel Wallach, MD

KEYWORDS

• Neutrophilic dermatoses • Autoinflammation • Sweet syndrome • Pyoderma gangrenosum

KEY POINTS

• Sweet syndrome and pyoderma gangrenosum are the prototypic conditions of the group of the neutrophilic dermatoses.
• Aseptic neutrophilic infiltrates can involve not only the skin but also all internal organs, defining the neutrophilic disease.
• The neutrophilic disease is linked with multisystemic disorders and has a special link with myeloid dyscrasias.
• These nonhereditary neutrophilic inflammations may be included in the group of autoinflammatory diseases.

INTRODUCTION

The goal of this article is to present an updated review of the understanding of the skin conditions referred to as "neutrophilic dermatoses.". This review can be divided in 7 chapters, starting in 1964 and leading to today's acquisitions and uncertainties. Table 1 lists the main stages of the current conception of the neutrophilic dermatoses.

CHAPTER 1: AN ACUTE FEBRILE NEUTROPHILIC DERMATOSIS

The term "neutrophilic dermatosis" appeared in the medical literature in 1964, coined by a British dermatologist, Robert Douglas Sweet (1917–2001).[1] Dr Sweet described the condition of 8 women, aged 32 to 55 years, which he had seen during a 15-year period. Their "distinctive and fairly severe illness" had 4 cardinal features.

• Fever
• Neutrophilic hyperleukocytosis (neutrophilia) of the blood

• Raised painful plaques, "somewhat resembling erythema multiforme" but clinically distinctive
• A dense dermal infiltration with neutrophils

These patients with fever and hyperleukocytosis were fully investigated but no evidence of infection was found. The noninfectious nature of this syndrome was again proven by the rapid and complete response to corticosteroids, another important feature of this dermatosis.

The condition described by RD Sweet was rapidly and universally called "Sweet syndrome" (SS), an eponymous tribute that Sweet modestly attributed to his monosyllabic name.[2] He always favored the title he had chosen, "acute febrile neutrophilic dermatosis (AFND)."

RD Sweet was right when he indicated that the disease he described was distinctive and had not been reported before. Hence, his article contains no bibliographic reference. Similar conditions might have existed, however, probably considered as variants of erythema multiforme. It has also been suggested that some leukemids,

Department of Dermatology, Paris Hospitals, France
E-mail address: dr.danielwallach@gmail.com

Dermatol Clin 42 (2024) 139–146
https://doi.org/10.1016/j.det.2023.08.001
0733-8635/24/© 2023 Elsevier Inc. All rights reserved.

Table 1
Timeline of advances on neutrophilic dermatoses during twentieth to twenty-first centuries
1908　Brocq and Simon: Geometric Phagedenism[11]
1930　Brunsting, Goeckerman, O'Leary: Pyoderma gangrenosum[10]
1964　Sweet: Acute febrile neutrophilic dermatosis[1]
1983　Caughman, Stern, Haynes: Neutrophilic dermatosis of myeloproliferative disorders[9]
1991　Wallach: Neutrophilic dermatoses spectrum[14]
1991　Vignon-Pennamen and Wallach: Neutrophilic disease[18]
2006　Wallach and Vignon-Pennamen: Classification of the neutrophilic dermatoses[15]
2016　Satoh, Mellett, Contassot, French: The neutrophilic dermatoses are autoinflammatory disorders[30]
2022　Calvo: A spectrum of myeloid dermatoses[44]

nonleukemic skin lesions in leukemia patients, might be true AFND. Such a patient had been reported by Costello and colleagues in 1955.[3]

Rapidly after Sweet's publication, many observations of SS were reported. In 1973, Matta and colleagues[4] reported 5 cases. Two of these patients suffered from acute myeloid leukemia, and this could not be considered coincidental. Following this report, many authors insisted on the fact that a significant proportion of patients with SS suffer from a malignant disease, solid cancer, or more often, blood malignancy. The most frequent of these malignancies are acute myelogenous leukemia and myelodysplastic syndromes. Although poorly understood, the link between SS and the neutrophil lineage was therefore obvious since the initial descriptions: blood neutrophilia, dermal neutrophilia, clinical resemblance with leukemids, and possible association with myeloid malignancy.

It was also highlighted that patients with SS could suffer from neutrophilic infiltrates in internal organs. This important finding had been mentioned by Matta and colleagues[4] and will be detailed below.

Due in part to the link with internal medicine and malignancies, many reports of patients with SS have been published, as well as excellent reviews.[5,6]

Another article of this issue of *Dermatologic Clinics* is committed to a detailed account of SS.

Almost 6 decades after its description, SS may be considered as the beacon of the neutrophilic dermatoses.[7] Important data have been developed on clinical variants, associated diseases, internal involvement, pathogenesis, and therapy.

CHAPTER 2: A NEUTROPHILIC DERMATOSIS OF MYELOPROLIFERATIVE DISORDERS

In the 1970s, the frequency of malignancies in patients with SS attracted much attention. About 20% of patients with SS were considered paraneoplastic, the most frequent of these malignancies being myeloid leukemias and myelodysplastic syndromes. In reviewing cases of SS and myeloproliferative disorders, Cooper and colleagues[8] recommend searching for these blood abnormalities in all patients with SS.

Patients with a blood malignancy-associated SS may have typical papular-nodular lesions. However, in a significant number of cases, they present with atypical SS, featuring bullous, ulcerated lesions.

In 1983, Caughman and colleagues[9] reported the case of a patient with myeloid metaplasia, who presented with skin lesions, which were diagnosed as both atypical, bullous SS and atypical, bullous pyoderma gangrenosum (PG). They reviewed similar cases published between 1972 and 1982 and proposed that this SS-PG overlap be named "Neutrophilic dermatosis of myeloproliferative disorders."

This proposal could be considered as a surprise. Indeed, ulcerative PG is obviously different from papular SS, and typical PG and SS do not overlap; however, atypical forms do.

PG had been named in 1930 by Brunsting and colleagues.[10] It is a severe ulcerative disease, with distinctive typical clinical features, also called geometric phagedenism, accurately described by Brocq and Simon in 1908.[11] In addition to the typical ulcerative form, clinical variants have been described[7]: bullous PG, pustular PG, vegetative PG, and pathergic PG. Comprehensive reviews have been published,[12] and other articles of this issue are dedicated to many aspects of PG.

Recently, diagnostic criteria have been proposed,[13] which indicate that histopathology is important for ulcerative PG diagnosis.

CHAPTER 3: THE NEUTROPHILIC DERMATOSES SPECTRUM

Having observed many patients with typical and also atypical pustular, papular, nodular, ulcerated aseptic neutrophilic dermatoses, and reviewed the relevant literature, I proposed in 1991 to gather these neutrophilic dermatoses together in a unique spectrum.[14]

The arguments, or criteria, to include clinically dissimilar conditions in this group were stated as follows:

- Skin disorders characterized by an infiltrate of the skin by normal neutrophils;
- No infectious cause;
- Diverse cutaneous features (pustules, plaques, nodules, and ulcerations) defining typical forms as well as associations, overlaps, and transitional atypical forms;
- Possible presence of extracutaneous symptoms, due to neutrophilic infiltrates in internal organs;
- Significant association with multisystemic disorders. These are mainly blood disorders but also inflammatory diseases of the digestive tract and of the joints;
- Sensitivity to steroids and other anti-inflammatory drugs.

At this time, 4 conditions were included in the neutrophilic dermatoses group: SS, PG, subcorneal pustular dermatosis (Sneddon-Wilkinson disease), and erythema elevatum diutinum.

These criteria have not been scientifically validated. Moreover, some well-defined entities, such as pustular psoriasis, severe acne, erythema nodosum, dermatitis herpetiformis, and Behçet disease could be considered as ND. However, the fact that they had a different pathologic profile and were almost never associated with other entities of the ND group, seemed sufficient at this time not to include them.

In the following years, other conditions were added to the ND group, and in 2006, it was thought necessary to propose a classification. The most logical approach was the clinical-pathological one, and we proposed to classify the neutrophilic dermatoses according to the main localization of the cutaneous neutrophilic infiltrate.[15]

Three ND subgroups can be defined.

- The superficial group, where the infiltrate is primarily epidermal, and the main lesions are pustular; the prototypic conditions here are the subcorneal pustular dermatosis and its variant IgA pemphigus[16] and the aseptic pustulosis of the folds.[17]
- The intermediate group, where the infiltrate predominates in the superficial dermis, and the lesions are papular; prototypes here are SS, erythema elevatum diutinum, and urticarial neutrophilic dermatoses.

- The deep group, where the infiltrate involves the deep dermis and the hypodermis. Prototypes are PG, the PAPA group syndromes, and aseptic abscesses.

Table 2 indicates the many conditions currently included in the ND spectrum. This list must be seen as provisional. As new research investigates the pathophysiology of inflammatory skin conditions, it will be subject to changes.

Many ND patients present with a typical form of one of the diseases listed in Table 2. However, other patients present with an atypical condition, which cannot be clearly classified in one of these well-defined entities but rather belongs to a continuous spectrum. For these transitional or overlapping complex presentations, one can propose the diagnosis of "neutrophilic dermatosis" without any additional specificity.

CHAPTER 4: THE NEUTROPHILIC DISEASE

An important feature of the abovementioned neutrophilic dermatoses: the frequency of systemic symptoms, and the possible involvement of internal organs.

Many patients suffer from flu-like initial symptoms, fever, arthralgias, myalgias, and general malaise. More importantly, in some patients with well-defined ND entities and also with atypical overlapping forms, sterile neutrophilic infiltrates can be located in internal organs. The resulting symptoms are nonspecific and highly variable, giving rise to difficult diagnostic problems and possible inappropriate management. We reported some of these patients and proposed to denominate "neutrophilic disease" this multisystemic condition with cutaneous and internal aseptic neutrophilic infiltrates.[18]

All internal organs may be involved in the neutrophilic disease.[19] The most frequent of these neutrophilic internal inflammations hit the lungs, the bones, the joints, the central nervous system, the liver, the spleen, the lymph nodes, and the eye. When these internal disorders are isolated, the diagnosis can be extremely difficult. All clinicians, including surgeons, should be aware of this possibility of extracutaneous aseptic neutrophilic disease.

The internal neutrophilic disease must be differentiated from the multisystemic conditions possibly associated with the neutrophilic dermatoses (inflammatory bowel diseases, joint inflammations, and others).

CHAPTER 5: NEUTROPHILIC DERMATOSES IN AUTOINFLAMMATORY SYNDROMES

Neutrophils, the cell population which define the neutrophilic disease, are the main effector cells

Table 2
Classification of the neutrophilic dermatoses

Superficial (Epidermal, Pustular) ND	Sneddon-Wilkinson disease (Subcorneal pustular dermatosis)
	IgA pemphigus
	Amicrobial pustulosis of the folds
	Pustular vasculitis
	Bowel-associated dermatosis-arthritis syndrome
	Pyodermatitis/Pyostomatitis vegetans
	Pustular psoriasis
	Palmoplantar pustuloses
	SAPHO syndrome
	Behçet disease
	Acne fulminans
	Acute generalized exanthematous pustulosis and other drug-induced pustuloses
	Infantile acropustulosis
Dermal (en plaques) ND	SS (Acute febrile neutrophilic dermatosis)
	Neutrophilic dermatosis of the dorsal hands
	Neutrophilic eccrine hidradenitis
	Erythema elevatum diutinum
	Vegetative pyoderma gangrenosum
	Neutrophilic urticarial dermatosis
	Schnitzler syndrome
	Neutrophilic lupus erythematosus
Deep ND	Pyoderma gangrenosum
	PAPA and related syndromes (Syndromic PG)
	Neutrophilic panniculitis
	Aseptic abscesses
	Hidradenitis suppurativa

Adapted from Ref.[47]

of innate immunity. As a front line of defense against bacterial infections, their main role is to induce an inflammation, which destroys invading pathogens.

It is interesting to mention here that the neutrophilic inflammation secondary to a cutaneous bacterial infection can be superficial, as in folliculitis or impetigo, or involve the superficial dermis as in erysipelas, or the hypodermis as in necrotizing fasciitis or abscesses (**Table 3**). These conditions are the main differentials of the aseptic neutrophilic dermatoses, and this may pose difficult diagnostic problems for many patients.

Our understanding of the aseptic neutrophilic inflammations changed in 1999 when Michael F Mc Dermott, Daniel L Kastner, and their coworkers coined the terms "autoinflammation" and "autoinflammatory syndromes" to name self-directed inflammation provoked by an activation of the innate immune system. This inflammation is not induced by infectious or other exogenous agents and is independent from adaptive immune responses, which are responsible for autoimmunity.[20]

The first identified autoinflammatory diseases were hereditary recurrent fevers, familial Mediterranean fever (FMF), and TNF-receptor-associated periodic fever syndrome (TRAPS). During the last 20 years, many monogenic diseases have been included in this group. Excellent reviews have been published on autoinflammatory diseases.[21–23] It is beyond the scope of this study to further describe the important genetic and immunologic acquisitions in this field.

I would like, however, to stress the importance of the description of the PAPA syndrome by Lindor and colleagues in 1997.[24] PAPA means pyogenic arthritis, PG, and severe cystic acne. This autosomal dominant autoinflammatory syndrome is due to mutations in the CD2BP1 gene, also called PSTPIP1.[25] This was the first indication of a genetic cause for PG and also of a link between PG and acne. In the following years, the description of closely related autoinflammatory syndromes led to the concept of syndromic PG[26] and the link to acne was extended to hidradenitis suppurativa, sometimes called acne inversa.

The substantial group of autoinflammatory diseases can be categorized in more than one way (**Table 4**). The initial classification is a clinical one[27]: the main classes of autoinflammatory diseases are hereditary recurrent fevers, idiopathic febrile syndromes, pyogenic disorders, granulomatous diseases, disorders of the skin and bone, metabolic disorders, and vasculitis.

Another classification of the autoinflammatory diseases is based on the genetic, or molecular mechanism of inflammation.[28] Inflammasomopathies are due to disorders in the activation of interleukin-1 (IL-1) beta. The main diseases in this group are CAPS, FMF, PAPA, and DIRA. The fact that mutations in the IL-1 pathway are involved in many autoinflammatory diseases with a prominent cutaneous component indicates an important role of this pathway in the pathophysiology of nonmonogenic neutrophilic dermatoses. It is interesting to remember that this had been suggested as early as 1987.[29]

Other autoinflammatory diseases involve NF-kB activation, protein folding, complement activation, cytokine signaling, and macrophage activation.

Table 3
Skin conditions secondary to an activation of neutrophils (only prototypic conditions are indicated), very similar clinical lesions can be created by neutrophilic inflammation, whether bacterial (cutaneous infections), aseptic monogenic (autoinflammatory diseases), or aseptic polygenic (neutrophilic dermatoses)

		Cause of the Neutrophils Activation		
		Infectious	Auto-inflammatory, Monogenic	Auto-inflammatory, Polygenic
Localization of the neutrophilic infiltrate	Superficial	Bullous impetigo	DIRA DITRA	Subcorneal pustular dermatosis
	Intermediate	Erysipelas, cellulitis	FMF	Sweet syndrome
	Deep	Abscess, ecthyma	PAPA syndrome	Pyoderma gangrenosum

In view of the importance of the cutaneous manifestations of the hereditary autoinflammatory diseases, it seems relevant, from the point of view of clinical dermatologists and their patients, to also propose a cutaneous classification of these monogenic diseases. One may adopt the same clinical-pathological pattern proposed for the neutrophilic dermatoses spectrum.

- Superficial ND (pustules) are present in DIRA syndrome, DITRA syndrome, and PAPA syndrome;
- Dermal ND are present in FMF (so-called erysipelas-like plaques) and in NLRP12-AID (urticaria);
- Hypodermal ND are present in PAPA group syndromes (PG).

This proposal for a dermatologic classification of autoinflammatory hereditary disorders is shown on **Table 4**.

Transitions and overlaps are a hallmark of the neutrophilic dermatoses spectrum. Accordingly, atypical neutrophilic cutaneous lesions have been found in many autoinflammatory diseases. Some authors even use the diagnostic term "neutrophilic dermatosis" alone. This could become popular among nondermatologists dealing with such complex skin manifestations.[22]

CHAPTER 6: AUTOINFLAMMATION IN NONHEREDITARY NEUTROPHILIC DERMATOSES

The concept of autoinflammation provides a solid basis for the pathophysiology of the neutrophilic dermatoses. The criteria for autoinflammation, that is, absence of infection, of autoantibodies, and of T-cell involvement, are fulfilled by the neutrophilic dermatoses.[30] Both neutrophilic dermatoses and autoinflammatory diseases can be included in the same group of innate immune disorders.[31] Indeed, many studies have shown that the main cytokines of autoinflammation, IL-1 beta, TNF-alpha, and others, are elevated in the serum and the skin of patients with nonhereditary neutrophilic dermatoses.[32] Anti-IL-1 therapy proved beneficial in many of these situations. Specific anticytokine therapy may represent the best treatment of the neutrophilic dermatoses.[33]

CHAPTER 7: THE MYELOID DERMATOSES

The neutrophilic dermatoses are defined by an autoinflammation mainly mediated by cells of the neutrophil lineage. When it became obvious that malignancy was an important comorbidity of SS and other neutrophilic dermatoses,[34] hematologic disorders, and specifically myeloid neoplasms, were identified as the most frequent of these associations.[35]

As soon as 2007, Magro and colleagues, using an X-inactivation assay, found that clonality was frequent in the cutaneous neutrophilic infiltrates of patients with SS or PG, whether they were suffering from an associated myeloid dyscrasia (leukemia or Myelodysplastic syndromes [MDS]) or not.[36] The clonal link between the blood malignancy and the dermal infiltrate was further investigated by Sujobert and colleagues[37] using fluorescent in situ hybridization and Passet and colleagues,[38] from the same group, using next-generation sequencing. Their studies indicate that the malignant blood cells and the mature dermal neutrophils in myeloid neoplasms-associated ND are clonally related.

In 2005, Requena and his coworkers described a histopathological variant of SS in

Table 4
Classifications of « classic » autoinflammatory diseases (only prototypic conditions are indicated)

The « classic » autoinflammatory diseases.
A clinical classification
(abridged and adapted from Kastner and colleagues[36])

Hereditary recurrent fevers
    FMF, TRAPS, CAPS

Idiopathic febrile syndromes
    Still disease, Schnitzler syndrome

Pyogenic disorders
    PAPA and related syndromes

Granulomatous diseases
    Crohn's disease, Blau syndrome

Autoinflammatory disorders of skin and bone
    DIRA, DITRA
    CRMO, SAPHO

Vasculitis
    Behcet's disease

The « classic » autoinflammatory diseases.
A molecular/genetic classification
(abridged and adapted from Masters and colleagues[37])

IL-1 beta activation disorders (inflammasomopathies)
    CAPS, FMF, PAPA, DIRA, ...

NF-kB activation disorders
    Crohn's disease ....

Protein folding disorders of the innate immune system
    TRAPS

Complement disorders
    Cytokine signaling disorders
    Macrophage activation

A clinical/dermatologic classification of the cutaneous lesions found in the « classic » monogenic
    autoinflammatory diseases

Pustules (epidermal infiltrates)
    DIRA
    DITRA

Erythematous papules and plaques (infiltrates of the superficial dermis)
    FMF
    CAPS syndrome (FCAS, MWS, NOMID)
    TRAPS

Ulcerations and deep lesions (deep dermal and hypodermal infiltrates)
    PAPA Syndrome
    PASH, PAPASH, ... syndromes
    Others

which the infiltrating cells were morphologically similar to histiocytes but were in fact immature myeloid cells.[39] In 2006, Vignon-Pennamen and her coworkers similarly reported on patients with a SS with an initially predominant lymphocytic infiltration and suggested that this atypical SS could represent a marker of myelodysplasia.[40]

Other studies confirmed that these SS variants are strongly associated with hematological malignancies, especially with MDS.[41] The finding of the MDS molecular alteration in the dermal infiltrate of these atypical SS led to the concept of myelodysplasia cutis.[42]

Myelodysplasia cutis may be considered as intermediate between the mature cells of classic SS and leukemia cutis.[43] For KR Calvo,[44] there is a spectrum of myeloid dermatoses including SS with mature neutrophils, histiocytoid SS and myelodysplasia cutis with immature myeloid cells, and leukemia cutis with blastic myeloid cells.

Genetic studies may provide a more precise definition of these autoinflammatory myeloid dermatoses: the recently individualized Vacuoles, E1 enzyme, X-linked, autoinflammatory, somatic (VEXAS) syndrome[45] is a good example of the contribution of the modern genetic approach to the understanding of the neutrophilic dermatoses.[46,47]

SUMMARY

Since 1964, significant progress has been made in the understanding of the neutrophilic dermatoses. Many clinical conditions have been included in this group. The prototypic ND conditions, SS and PG, can be considered as only points on a continuous spectrum of diseases characterized by the noxious accumulation in the skin of neutrophils, without any infection or other exogenous cause.

Similar neutrophilic infiltrates can localize in all internal organs. This defines the neutrophilic disease, which induces difficult diagnostic and therapeutic problems.

Autoinflammation is the main mechanism of the neutrophilic dermatoses. The group of autoinflammatory diseases includes monogenic hereditary syndromes and the nonhereditary neutrophilic dermatoses. In both cases, similar skin lesions can be found. They can be categorized as superficial (epidermal), intermediate (dermal), and deep (hypodermal).

There is a special link between myeloid malignancies (leukemia and myelodysplasia) and the neutrophilic dermatoses.

Until recently, nonspecific anti-inflammatory drugs, such as corticosteroids, were the mainstay of therapy for the ND. Following investigations on the mechanisms of autoinflammation, it seems that specific anticytokine therapy is efficient in many situations.

DISCLOSURE

Commercial or financial interest: none.

FUNDING SOURCE

None.

REFERENCES

1. Sweet RD. An acute febrile neutrophilic dermatosis. Br J Dermatol 1964;76:349–56.
2. Sweet RD. Acute febrile neutrophilic dermatosis–1978. Br J Dermatol 1979;100:93–9.
3. Costello MJ, Canizares O, Montague M, et al. Cutaneous manifestations of myelogenous leukemia. AMA Arch Derm 1955;71:605–14.
4. Matta M, Malak J, Tabet E, et al. Sweet's syndrome : systemic associations. Cutis 1973;12:561–5.
5. Vignon-Pennamen MD. Sweet's syndrome. In: Wallach D, Vignon-Pennamen MD, Marzano A-V, editors. Neutrophilic dermatoses. London, UK: Springer; 2018. p. 13–35.
6. Heath MS, Ortega-Loayza AG. Insights into the pathogenesis of sweet's syndrome. Front Immunol 2019 12;10:414.
7. Wallach D, Vignon-Pennamen MD. Pyoderma gangrenosum and sweet syndrome: the prototypic neutrophilic dermatoses. Br J Dermatol 2018;178:595–602.
8. Cooper PH, Innes DJ Jr, Greer KE. Acute febrile neutrophilic dermatosis (Sweet's syndrome) and myeloproliferative disorders. Cancer 1983;51:1518–26.
9. Caughman W, Stern R, Haynes H. Neutrophilic dermatosis of myeloproliferative disorders. Atypical forms of pyoderma gangrenosum and Sweet's syndrome associated with myeloproliferative disorders. J Am Acad Dermatol 1983;9:751–8.
10. Brunsting LA, Goeckerman WH, O'Leary PA. Pyoderma (ecthyma) gangrenosum. Arch Dermatol Syphilol 1930;22:655–80.
11. Brocq L, Simon CI. Contribution à l'étude du phagédénisme. Bull. Soc méd. Hôp. Paris 3eme série 1908;25:290–307.
12. Wallach D. Pyoderma gangrenosum. In: Wallach D, Vignon-Pennamen MD, Marzano A-V, editors. Neutrophilic dermatoses. London, UK: Springer; 2018. p. 55–83.
13. Maverakis E, Ma C, Shinkai K, et al. Diagnostic Criteria of Ulcerative Pyoderma Gangrenosum: A Delphi Consensus of International Experts. JAMA Dermatol 2018;154:461–6.
14. Wallach D. Les dermatoses neutrophiliques [Neutrophilic dermatoses]. Presse Med 1991;20:105–7.
15. Wallach D, Vignon-Pennamen MD. From acute febrile neutrophilic dermatosis to neutrophilic disease: forty years of clinical research. J Am Acad Dermatol 2006;55:1066–71.
16. Wallach D. Intraepidermal IgA pustulosis. J Am Acad Dermatol 1992;27:993–1000.
17. Marzano AV, Ramoni S, Caputo R. Amicrobial pustulosis of the folds. Report of 6 cases and a literature review. Dermatology 2008;216:305–11.
18. Vignon-Pennamen MD, Wallach D. Cutaneous manifestations of neutrophilic disease. A study of seven cases. Dermatol 1991;183:255–64.
19. Vignon-Pennamen MD. The extracutaneous involvement in the neutrophilic dermatoses. Clin Dermatol 2000;18:339–47.
20. McDermott MF, Aksentijevich I, Galon J, et al. Germline mutations in the extracellular domains of the 55 kDa TNF receptor, TNFR1, define a family of dominantly inherited autoinflammatory syndromes. Cell 1999;97:133–44.
21. Farasat S, Aksentijevich I, Toro JR. Autoinflammatory diseases: clinical and genetic advances. Arch Dermatol 2008;144:392–402.

22. Georgin-Lavialle S, Fayand A, Rodrigues F, et al. Autoinflammatory diseases: State of the art. Presse Med 2019;48:e25–48.

23. Goldbach-Mansky R. Immunology in clinic review series; focus on autoinflammatory diseases: update on monogenic autoinflammatory diseases: the role of interleukin (IL)-1 and an emerging role for cytokines beyond IL-1. Clin Exp Immunol 2012;167:391–404.

24. Lindor NM, Arsenault TM, Solomon H, et al. A new autosomal dominant disorder of pyogenic sterile arthritis, pyoderma gangrenosum, and acne: PAPA syndrome. Mayo Clin Proc 1997;72:611–5.

25. Wise CA, Gillum JD, Seidman CE, et al. Mutations in CD2BP1 disrupt binding to PTP PEST and are responsible for PAPA syndrome, an autoinflammatory disorder. Hum Mol Genet 2002;11:961–9.

26. Marzano AV, Borghi A, Meroni PL, et al. Pyoderma gangrenosum and its syndromic forms: evidence for a link with autoinflammation. Br J Dermatol 2016;175:882–91.

27. Kastner DL, Aksentijevich I, Goldbach-Mansky R. Autoinflammatory disease reloaded: a clinical perspective. Cell 2010;140:784–90.

28. Masters SL, Simon A, Aksentijevich I, et al. Horror autoinflammaticus: the molecular pathophysiology of autoinflammatory disease. Annu Rev Immuno 2009;27:621–68.

29. Going JJ. Is the pathogenesis of Sweet's syndrome mediated by interleukin-1? Br J Dermatol 1987;116:282–3.

30. Satoh TK, Mellett M, Contassot E, et al. Are neutrophilic dermatoses autoinflammatory disorders? Br J Dermatol 2018;178:603–13.

31. Navarini AA, Satoh TK, French LE. Neutrophilic dermatoses and autoinflammatory diseases with skin involvement–innate immune disorders. Semin Immunopathol 2016;38:45–56.

32. Marzano AV, Damiani G, Ceccherini I, et al. Autoinflammation in pyoderma gangrenosum and its syndromic form (pyoderma gangrenosum, acne and suppurative hidradenitis). Br J Dermatol 2017;176:1588–98.

33. Marzano AV, Ortega-Loayza AG, Heath M, et al. Mechanisms of Inflammation in Neutrophil-Mediated Skin Diseases. Front Immunol 2019;10:1059.

34. Cohen PR. Neutrophilic dermatoses occurring in oncology patients. Int J Dermatol 2007;46:106–11.

35. Hensley CD, Caughman SW. Neutrophilic dermatoses associated with hematologic disorders. Clin Dermatol 2000;18:355–67.

36. Magro CM, Kiani B, Li J, et al. Clonality in the setting of Sweet's syndrome and pyoderma gangrenosum is not limited to underlying myeloproliferative disease. J Cutan Pathol 2007;34:526–34.

37. Sujobert P, Cuccuini W, Vignon-Pennamen D, et al. Evidence of differentiation in myeloid malignancies associated neutrophilic dermatosis: a fluorescent in situ hybridization study of 14 patients. J Invest Dermatol 2013;133:1111–4.

38. Passet M, Lepelletier C, Vignon-Pennamen MD, et al. Next-Generation Sequencing in Myeloid Neoplasm-Associated Sweet's Syndrome Demonstrates Clonal Relation between Malignant Cells and Skin-Infiltrating Neutrophils. J Invest Dermatol 2020;140:1873–6.

39. Requena L, Kutzner H, Palmedo G, et al. Histiocytoid Sweet syndrome: a dermal infiltration of immature neutrophilic granulocytes. Arch Dermatol 2005;141:834–42.

40. Vignon-Pennamen MD, Juillard C, Rybojad M, et al. Chronic recurrent lymphocytic Sweet syndrome as a predictive marker of myelodysplasia: a report of 9 cases. Arch Dermatol 2006;142:1170–6.

41. Ghoufi L, Ortonne N, Ingen-Housz-Oro S, et al. Histiocytoid Sweet Syndrome Is More Frequently Associated With Myelodysplastic Syndromes Than the Classical Neutrophilic Variant: A Comparative Series of 62 Patients. Medicine (Baltim) 2016;95:e3033.

42. Osio A, Battistella M, Feugeas JP, et al. Myelodysplasia Cutis Versus Leukemia Cutis. J Invest Dermatol 2015;135:2321–4.

43. Delaleu J, Kim R, Zhao LP, et al. Clinical, pathological, and molecular features of myelodysplasia cutis. Blood 2022;139:1251–3.

44. Calvo KR. Skin in the game: the emergence of myelodysplasia cutis. Blood 2022;139:1132–4.

45. Beck DB, Ferrada MA, Sikora KA, et al. Somatic Mutations in UBA1 and Severe Adult-Onset Autoinflammatory Disease. N Engl J Med 2020;383:2628–38.

46. Zakine E, Schell B, Battistella M, et al. UBA1 Variations in Neutrophilic Dermatosis Skin Lesions of Patients With VEXAS Syndrome. JAMA Dermatol 2021;157:1349–54.

47. Wallach D. Neutrophilic dermatoses: an overview. In: Wallach D, Vignon-Pennamen MD, Marzano A-V, editors. Neutrophilic dermatoses. London, UK: Springer; 2018. p. 5–9.

Overview of Neutrophilic Biology, Pathophysiology, and Classification of Neutrophilic Dermatoses

Jérémie Delaleu, MD, Jean-David Bouaziz, MD, PhD*

KEYWORDS

- Neutrophilic dermatoses neutrophils • Autoinflammation • Myeloid neoplasm

KEY POINTS

- Neutrophilic dermatoses (NDs) are a heterogeneous group of inflammatory skin conditions characterized by a primitive infiltrate of the skin by neutrophils without evidence of infection.
- The most well-defined NDs include pyoderma gangrenosum, Sweet's syndrome, subcorneal pustular dermatosis, neutrophilic eccrine hidradenitis, amicrobial pustulosis of the folds, generalized pustular psoriasis, and neutrophilic urticarial dermatosis.
- The pathogenic mechanisms of the various NDs involves autoinflammation, neutrophilic dysfunction and clonal somatic mutation and differentiation of the myeloid cells as encountered in myeloid neoplasm.

INTRODUCTION

Neutrophilic dermatoses (NDs) are a heterogeneous group of inflammatory skin conditions characterized by a primitive infiltrate of the skin by neutrophils without evidence of infection.[1,2] Clinical presentations of ND are polymorphic, including pustules, bullae, abscesses, papules, nodules, plaques, and ulcers, and almost any organ system can be involved, giving rise to the term of "neutrophilic disease."[3] The most well-defined NDs include pyoderma gangrenosum (PG), Sweet's syndrome (SS), subcorneal pustular dermatosis (SPD), neutrophilic eccrine hidradenitis (NEH), amicrobial pustulosis of the folds (APF), generalized pustular psoriasis, and neutrophilic urticarial dermatosis (NUD).[1,2] Although each entity may present within an overlapping clinically and/or pathologically spectrum, making diagnosis and management difficult.

Nowadays, NDs are classified based on the localization of neutrophils within the skin and clinical features.[3] The pathogenic mechanisms of the various NDs are not well understood, and studies on ND pathophysiology in humans are limited. However, the discoveries on the innate immune system such as the inflammasome physiology or neutrophilic diversity, and the emergence of the concept of autoinflammation in humans allowed us to understand those diseases better.[4,5]

Indeed, ND's clinical and pathophysiological features have significant overlap with disorders included within the spectrum of autoinflammatory diseases that manifest as relapsing periods of sterile tissue inflammation including the skin.[2,6,7]

Also, a great number of patients with ND suffer from another underlying condition such as hematological malignancies, autoinflammatory diseases, inflammatory bowel disease, and connective tissue diseases.[2,8–10] As the skin is not the only organ targeted by the activated neutrophils, and as many organs may be involved by a similar sterile inflammation, the term "neutrophilic disease" has

Dermatology Department, Saint Louis Hospital, APHP Nord Université Paris Cité and INSERM u976 "Human Immunology, Pathophysiology and Immunotherapy", Paris, France
* Corresponding author. Service de Dermatologie – Hôpital Saint Louis, 1 Avenue Claude, Vellefaux, Paris 75010, France.
E-mail address: jean-david.bouaziz@aphp.fr

Dermatol Clin 42 (2024) 147–156
https://doi.org/10.1016/j.det.2023.08.002

been proposed.[3] Recent findings suggest that NDs are due to 2 main mechanisms: (i) a polyclonal hereditary activation of the innate immune system (polygenic or monogenic) and (ii) a clonal somatic activation of myeloid precursor cells as encountered in myeloid.[1,7,11,12]

First, we will provide an overview of neutrophilic biology, then explain the latest findings in the pathophysiology of ND, and finally we will present a classification of these diseases.

OVERVIEW OF NEUTROPHILIC BIOLOGY

Neutrophils are key players of innate immunity; they are the most abundant type of white blood cells in the circulation and are produced in the bone marrow.[13] Once released into the bloodstream, they circulate until they are needed to fight infection or respond to tissue damage. Once within the tissue, neutrophils are activated to perform multiple innate immune responses including phagocytosis, release a variety of proinflammatory mediators, including cytokines, chemokines, and reactive oxygen species.[14,15] These mediators promote the recruitment of other immune cells, such as monocytes and lymphocytes, and contribute to the destruction of pathogens. Neutrophils can also release neutrophil extracellular traps (NETs) – a web-like structures composed of DNA, histones, and antimicrobial proteins that play a role in trapping and clearing infectious agents.[16]

Neutrophils are primarily known for their role in the immune response, they also play a role in maintaining the health of the skin at steady state by clearance of apoptotic cells and debris and promote cell proliferation and wound healing.[17]

Neutrophils are short-lived cells, with a lifespan of only a few days. After they have performed their function, they undergo apoptosis, which is a programmed cell death.[18] Once they have undergone apoptosis, they are phagocytosed by other immune cells, such as macrophages, and are eliminated from the body promoting anti-inflammatory immune responses due to retention of granular and cytoplasmic components intracellularly.[18]

PATHOPHYSIOLOGY OF NEUTROPHILIC DERMATOSIS
Immune Dysregulation in Neutrophilic Dermatoses

Studies have revealed complex gene expression profiles in the skin of patients with ND suggesting activation of inflammasomes (interleukin [IL]-1β), dysregulation of the innate immune system (IL-17, IL-23, IL-36, TNFα, INF-γ), and recruitment and activation of neutrophils (IL-8, IL-17, granulocyte colony-stimulating factor [G-CSF]).

- The lesional skin of PG has showed overexpression of IL1β, IL-8, IL-17, IL-23, IL-36, and TNFα.[19,20]
- IL-1β, IL-6, and IL-8, IL-17, and TNFα are also elevated in the lesional skin of other NDs such as SS and APF.[19,21,22]
- Serum of patients with SS have significantly elevated IL-1 and INF-γ.[23]
- A role for G-CSF – a hormone cytokine that stimulates neutrophils' survival, proliferation, and differentiation – has been highly suggested in SS. Indeed G-CSF drugs, used in neutropenia, are a common cause of drug-induced SS and higher serum levels of G-CSF have been described in patients with active SS compared with SS patients with nonactive disease.[24]
- Matrix metalloproteinases (MMP)-2 and MMP-9 are overexpressed in inflammatory infiltrate of PG and may lead to tissue damage.[25]

NEUTROPHILIC DYSFUNCTION IN NEUTROPHILIC DERMATOSES

Although neutrophils play a crucial role in the immune response to infection and inflammation, they can also contribute to tissue damage in certain conditions including ND. In normal condition, after they have performed their function, neutrophils undergo apoptosis, promoting immunosuppressive response in the phagocyte and anti-inflammatory regulation: IL10 and TGFβ increase whereas TNFα, IL6, G-CSF, IL8, and IL17 downregulate recruitment and activation of neutrophils. The anti-inflammatory response relies on a long-lasting presence of apoptotic neutrophils.[26]

Certain infectious or inflammatory diseases including ND can trigger lytic forms of neutrophil death, which allows the release of proinflammatory cytokines and granular proteins that may worsen local tissue injury and sustain the inflammation.[18] Abnormal NETs release and NETosis – a form of lytic, proinflammatory death related to NETs release – has been showed to increase into the skin of patients with ND.[27]

- Increased in NET release has been demonstrated in SS, PG, SPD, hidradenitis suppurativa (HS), and NUD compared with control skin.[28–30]
- NETotic neutrophils are present in HS lesions, particularly in the lesional tunnel, and the degree of NETs and the severity of HS are positively correlated.[31]

- A study showed that more than 50% of neutrophils infiltrating the skin in the setting of PG exhibit NET formations.[28–30]
- Circulating neutrophils from PG and HS patients spontaneously undergo NETosis.[28,31]
- The sera of patients with HS are unable to degrade NETs induced in healthy neutrophils.
- Autoantibodies against citrullinated proteins derived from NET components have been detected in patients with HS.[31]
- There is a colocalization of IL-1 and TNFα in NETs of SS and PG.[28–30]

NEUTROPHILIC DERMATOSES AND AUTOINFLAMATION

ND-related syndromic diseases belong to systemic autoinflammatory diseases: a family of genetic disorders characterized by aberrant antigenic-independent activation of the innate immune system pathways.[5] Several NDs occur as clinical manifestations of autoinflammatory diseases (**Table 1**), for example,

- SS is seen in chronic atypical neutrophilic dermatosis with lipodystrophy and elevated temperature syndrome and SS-like (erysipelas-like skin lesion) in patients with familial Mediterranean fever;[32,33]
- PG occurred in the context of autoinflammatory syndromes induced by mutation of the *proline-serine-threonine phosphatase interacting protein 1* (*PSTPIP1*) gene such as PAPA (pyogenic arthritis, PG, and acne), as well as in the context of pyrin-associated autoinflammation with ND caused by mutations in exon 2 of *MEFV* and A20 haploinsufficiency (*TNFAIP3*).[34,35]
- NUD occurred in cryopyrin-associated periodic syndrome (a monogenic autoinflammatory diseases related to *NLRP3* inflammasome) and Schnitzler syndrome or Still's disease (polygenic acquired diseases that probably primarily involve autoinflammatory pathways).[36]
- Deficiency of IL-1 receptor antagonist (IL1RN, deficiency of interleukin-1 receptor antagonist) and deficiency of the IL-36 receptor antagonist (IL-36RN/IL1F5 deficiency of IL-36 receptor antagonist) are monogenic diseases with skin pustular phenotypes.[37,38]

By extension some authors propose that ND by themselves should be considered as autoinflammatory diseases as they both share common clinical manifestations (such as fever or arthralgias), dermatopathological features (intense infiltration by neutrophils within the skin), cytokine profiles, and therapeutic approaches.[1,6,7]

PATHERGY

Eventually, NDs share the pathergy phenomenon, a skin condition in which a trauma such as surgical incisions leads to the development of skin lesions or ulcers that may be resistant to healing. This condition is well known in Behçet's disease, but it may also be seen in SS, PG, or neutrophilic necrotizing cellulitis.[39–41] Thus, postoperative PG is often misdiagnosed as wound infection, and pathergy may complicate wound debridement.[42,43]

Trauma and skin injuries release cytokines like IL36 and IL8 and dangers signals promoting innate immune response and may drive ND.[44]

SOMATIC MUTATION, AUTOINFLAMMATION

Recently, somatic mosaic *NLRP3* variations have been described in patients who presented with reminiscent late-onset urticaria with NUD. Whereas patients were refractory to antihistaminic drugs, steroids, and colchicine, they dramatically responded to IL-1β antagonist anakinra.[45,46] A new syndrome named Vacuoles, E1 enzyme, X-linked, autoinflammatory, somatic (VEXAS) syndrome, was recently described. VEXAS is due to myeloid-restricted, somatic missense mutation in codon 41 of *UBA1 gene*, an X-linked gene that encodes the enzyme that initiates ubiquitination.[47] These mutations in *UBA1 gene* led to production of catalytically deficient cytoplasmic UBA1 and activation of multiple innate immune pathways. This syndrome includes SS, relapsing polychondritis, polyarteritis nodosa, giant-cell arteritis, MDS, and multiple myeloma.[47] Moreover, a lot of polygenic and multifactorial diseases included in the spectrum of autoinflammation, are associated with ND such as inflammatory bowel disease or spondylarthritis.[9,42,48] In addition, *MEFV* variation has been detected in 2 patients with MDS and SS.[49]

LEUKEMIC CELLS AND NEUTROPHILIC DERMATOSIS

Leukemic cells, under various stimuli, are able to differentiate into clonally restricted well-differentiated cells.[50] For example, preleukemic cells HL-60 can differentiate in vitro into granulocytes after stimulation with retinoic acid.[51] In clinical hematology, this phenomenon is responsible of the differentiation syndrome, a potentially fatal complication of treatment inducing maturation of myeloid blast in the setting of acute myeloid leukemia (AML), such as all-trans retinoic acid or

Table 1
Autoinflammatory disease and associated neutrophilic skin conditions

Diseases	Protein and Related Gene	Mode of Inheritance	Type of Neutrophilic Dermatosis
Autoinflammatory diseases caused by excessive interleukin-1 signaling, production, and secretion			
Familial Mediterranean fever Pyrin-associated autoinflammation with neutrophilic dermatosis	*MEFV* Pyrin MEFV (exon 4) Pyrin	Autosomal recessive (AR)	Erysipelas-like skin lesion "Sweet-like" Acne, aseptic abscesses, pyoderma gangrenosum
Tumor necrosis factor receptor-1 associated periodic syndrome (TRAPS)	*TNFRSF1A* TNF receptor-1A	Autosomal dominant (AD)	Migratory edematous rash "Sweet-like"
Hyperimmunoglobulin D syndrome (HIDS)	*MVK* Mevalonate kinase	AR	Erythematous macules and edematous papules (neutrophilic urticaria), aphthous ulcers
Cryopyrin-associated periodic syndromes — Neonatal-onset multisystem inflammatory disease — Muckle–Wells syndrome — Familial cold autoinflammatory syndrome (FCAS)	*NLRP3* Cryopyrin	AD	Urticarial papules and plaques (neutrophilic urticarial dermatosis); aphthous ulcers; Urticarial papules and plaque (neutrophilic urticarial dermatosis); Cold-induced urticarial papules and plaques (neutrophilic urticarial dermatosis)
FCAS type 2	*NLRP12* Monarch-1	AD	Neutrophilic urticarial dermatosis
Deficiency of interleukin-1 receptor antagonist	*IL1RN* IL-1 receptor antagonist	AR	Pustules within areas of erythema – appearance similar to pustular psoriasis, pyoderma gangrenosum
Pyogenic arthritis, PG, and acne (PAPA) PG, acne, and HS (PASH) syndrome PAPASH (PAPA + PASH) syndrome	*PSTPIP1* Proline-serinethreonine phosphatasesinteracting protein-1	AD	Pyoderma gangrenosum Acne Hidradenitis suppurativa Aseptic abscesses Pathergy

Disease	Gene / Protein	Inheritance	Clinical features
Majeed syndrome	LPIN2 Lipin 2	AR	Pustular dermatitis
Autoinflammation with infantile enterocolitis	NLRC4 NLRC4 inflammasome	AR	Neutrophilic urticarial dermatosis, aphthous ulcers
Interferon mediated autoinflammatory diseases			
Chronic atypical neutrophilic dermatosis with lipodystrophy and elevated temperature syndrome or proteosome-associated autoinflammatory syndrome	PSMB8 Proteosome subunit, beta type 8	AR	Sweet syndrome, neutrophilic panniculitis
Autoinflammatory diseases caused by nuclear factor kappa B (NF-κB) dysregulation			
CAMPS (CARD14 mediated pustular psoriasis)	CARD14 gene Caspase recruitment domain-containing protein 14	AD	Generalized pustular psoriasis
Deficiency of IL-36 receptor antagonist	IL36RN IL-36 receptor antagonist	AR	Pustules within areas of erythema – resembles generalized pustular psoriasis
OTULIN-related autoinflammatory syndrome	OTULIN M1-specific deubiquitinase OTULIN	AR	Nodular panniculitis and lipodystrophy, pustular and scarring rash
VEXAS syndrome	UBA1 Ubiquitin-activating enzyme (E1)	Myeloid-restricted, somatic missense mutation	Sweet syndrome
A20 haploinsufficiency	TNFAIP3 A20	AD	Oral ulcers, genital ulcers, erythematous papules, folliculitis, pathergy
Famillial necrotizing neutrophilic cellulitis	NFKB1 (p.R157X)	AR	Neutrophilic necrotizing cellulitis
Autoinflammatory diseases caused by enzymatic defects in innate and adaptive immune cell-signaling pathways			
PLCG2-associated antibody deficiency and immune dysregulation Autoinflammation and PLCG2 associated antibody deficiency and immune dysregulation	PLCG2 Phospholipase C, γ2	AD	Erysipelas-like skin lesion "Sweet-like", neutrophilic urticaria

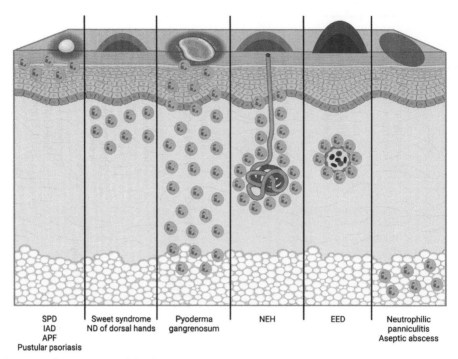

Fig. 1. Schematic of main neutrophilic dermatoses in accordance with neutrophils localization within the skin. APF, aseptic pustulosis of the folds; EED, erythema elevatum diutinum; IAD, intercellular IgA dermatoses; ND, neutrophilic dermatosis; NEH, neutrophilic eccrine hidradenitis; SPD, superficial pustular dermatoses. (Created with BioRender.com.)

inhibitor of FLT3. In the setting of myeloid neoplasm, historically, NDs were classified as "nonspecific"/paraneoplastic disorder whereas leukemia cutis (skin infiltration of AML blast cells) was classified as specific. This dichotomic classification has been questioned because: (i) ND occurs under different treatments inducing myeloid cell differentiation; (ii) ND as well as leukemia cutis predominate in AML with prominent monocytic component; (iii) several cases of mixtures of tumoral myeloid cells and mature neutrophils have been reported.[52] Since then, cytogenetic and molecular investigations have demonstrated that SS neutrophils and AML blast cells have a common precursor, suggesting a differentiation of tumoral cells into neutrophils within the skin in AML-associated SS.[11,53,54] Considering these findings, a disease spectrum from leukemia cutis to AML-associated SS might be suspected. Likewise, patients with MDS may develop skin involvement by immature myeloid dysplastic cell as myelodysplasia cutis, or infiltration by more mature clonal cells leading to mature SS neutrophils.[11,54,55] This also suggests in MDS a disease spectrum ranging from myelodysplasia cutis to MDS-associated classical SS.[55]

Moreover, Zakine and colleagues showed, in a case series study of 8 men with VEXAS syndrome,

that skin infiltrates were made of a mixture of neutrophils and immature myeloid cells and that the *UBA1* mutation was found in cutaneous lesions in those patients, suggesting that the inflammatory skin manifestations found in VEXAS syndrome might be a direct consequence of the clonal infiltration of the skin rather than just a proinflammatory activation state.[12] The differentiation of myeloid cells into skin infiltrating neutrophils may be due to a specific skin immunologic environment that allows cell maturation.[56]

CLASSIFICATION OF NEUTROPHILIC DERMATOSIS

In 2006, Vignon-Pennamen and Wallach proposed a classification of the numerous NDs based on the localization of neutrophils within the skin (**Fig. 1**).[3] There are associations, transitions, and overlap of forms between these entities.

Epidermal/Superficial Neutrophilic Dermatoses: Pustulosis

- *Superficial neutrophilic dermatoses: SPD and intercellular IgA dermatoses (IAD):* The SPD is characterized by subcorneal, nonfollicular, unilocular pustules filled with neutrophils. There is no epidermal spongiosis in SPD

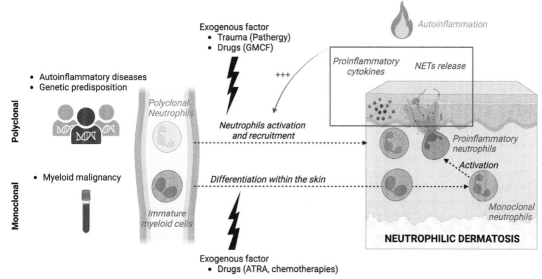

Fig. 2. Schematic of neutrophilic pathophysiology. There are 2 main mechanisms: (i) a polyclonal hereditary activation of the innate immune system: (a) polygenic like in inflammatory bowel diseases and (b) monogenic like in CAPS. (ii) Clonal somatic activation of myeloid cells as encountered in myelodysplastic syndromes. Once the proinflammatory neutrophils are within the skin, they release neutrophil extracellular traps, proinflammatory cytokines, and die by NETosis promoting inflammation of the skin, more neutrophils recruitment and activation, and skin tissue damage. In the setting of myeloid neoplasms, neutrophilic dermatoses are a direct consequence of clonal infiltration of the skin due to the ability of myeloid cells to differentiate. Those monoclonal neutrophils may bear proinflammatory mutations inducing inflammation and tissue damage. (Created with BioRender.com.)

unlike in pustular psoriasis. Acantholysis may be present in older lesions as a secondary change. Direct immunofluorescence studies for IAD staining should be performed to distinguish antibody-mediated subtype of SPD or variants of pemphigus.

- *Aseptic pustulosis of the folds:* Histologic examination reveals subcorneal or intraepidermal spongiform pustules with primarily periadnexal and perivascular neutrophilic infiltration of the dermis and no evidence of infection or vasculitis.[57] Direct immunofluo-rescence is usually negative.
- *Pustular psoriasis:* Pathology shows neutrophilic collections occurring in the stratum corneum and associated with spongiosis.

Dermal Neutrophilic Dermatoses: en Plaque

- *Sweet syndrome:* The characteristic histologic features of SS include prominent edema in the superficial dermis, dense and diffuse infiltrate of neutrophils in the upper and mid-dermis sparing the epidermis, leukocytoclasia, and endothelial swelling without vasculitis. Risk for malignancy may be elevated in patients with the histiocytoid variant of SS.[58] In this histologic variant, the infiltrate is composed

of immature myeloid cells mixed with few mature neutrophils.

- *Neutrophilic eccrine hidradenitis:* NEH pathology shows neutrophils surrounding and infiltrating the eccrine gland with occasional intraductal abscess formation.[59] Syringosquamous metaplasia of sweat glands and fibrosis of adjacent dermis may occur. A variable degree of necrosis of the epithelial cells is usually present.
- *Palmoplantar NEH:* Relationship to physical activity and hyperhidrosis is speculated, potentially resulting in eccrine duct obstruction and rupture leading to inflammation. Differential diagnoses of palmoplantar NEH are plantar urticaria, plantar erythema nodosum, erythema multiforme, SS, chilblains, and pool palms.
- *Erythema elevatum diutinum:* The pathologic findings in erythema elevatum diutinum (EED) correlate with the age of the lesion at the time of biopsy. Early lesions show leukocytoclastic vasculitis.[60] Middle age lesions show a diffuse dermal infiltrate composed of histiocytes, lymphocytes, aggregates of neutrophils, and vasculitis. Lastly, old age lesion is characterized by a storiform fibrosis, sometimes with foci of neutrophils, neutrophilic vasculitis, and macrophage infiltration.

Deep Neutrophilic Dermatoses: Abscess and Ulceration

- *Pyoderma gangrenosum:* Earliest lesions of PG show perifollicular inflammation and intra-dermal abscess formation. Then the lesions progress to ulceration, pathology shows epidermal and superficial dermal necrosis with an underlying neutrophilic infiltrate and abscess formation.[61]
- *Neutrophilic panniculitis:* Neutrophilic panni-culitis (NP) is a rare condition that belongs to the group of ND and the lobular panniculitis. In this condition, there is a subcutaneous fat lobules accumulation of mature neutrophils. NP has been reported to be significantly asso-ciated with MDS[62] and other myeloid malignancies.[63]

SUMMARY

Neutrophils play a central role in ND as the main characteristic of ND is a dense skin infiltrate by neutrophils without infection.[1] Even a great clinical and pathologic diversity, their classification has been made simple by a pathologic classification based on the localization of the neutrophils within the skin. Although not fully understood, patho-genic mechanisms of the various NDs are thought to be multifactorial, with neutrophilic dysfunction (NETs release and NETosis), auto-inflammation, and genetic predisposition each playing a role (Fig. 2).[11,30] It has also been suggested that a part of ND found in the setting of myeloid neoplasm might be a direct consequence of the clonal infiltration of the skin rather than just a proin-flammatory activation state, due to the myeloid cells ability to differentiation. Eventually recent research into the neutrophil biology has increased appreciation of neutrophils' heterogeneity with an ongoing categorization of neutrophils subsets, which might be involved in several inflammatory diseases.[64]

CLINICS CARE POINTS

- ND are a spectrum of inflammatory skin con-ditions characterized by polymorphous cuta-neous lesions resulting from a sterile neutrophil-rich inflammatory infiltrate.

- A great number of patients with ND suffer from an underlying condition (such as hema-tological malignancy, inflammatory bowel disease, connective tissue diseases).

- Pathogenic mechanisms of the various ND are thought to be multifactorial, with neutrophilic dysfunction, auto-inflammation, and genetic predisposition each playing a role.

- ND are diagnoses of exclusion and physicians should always consider differential diagno-ses, particularly skin infections.

CONFLICT OF INTEREST

None to declare.

FUNDING

None.

REFERENCES

1. Marzano AV, Borghi A, Wallach D, et al. A Comprehensive Review of Neutrophilic Diseases. Clin Rev Allergy Immunol 2018;54(1):114–30.
2. Delaleu J, Lepelletier C, Calugareanu A, et al. Neutrophilic dermatoses. Rev Med Interne 2022; 43(12):727–38.
3. Wallach D, Vignon-Pennamen MD. From acute febrile neutrophilic dermatosis to neutrophilic dis-ease: forty years of clinical research. J Am Acad Dermatol 2006;55(6):1066–71.
4. Bernard NJ. Inflammation: New classification criteria for autoinflammatory periodic fevers. Nat Rev Rheu-matol 2015;11(3):125.
5. Broderick L. Hereditary Autoinflammatory Disorders: Recognition and Treatment. Immunol Allergy Clin 2019;39(1):13–29.
6. Satoh TK, Mellett M, Contassot E, et al. Are neutro-philic dermatoses autoinflammatory disorders? Br J Dermatol 2018;178(3):603–13.
7. Marzano AV, Damiani G, Genovese G, et al. A dermatologic perspective on autoinflammatory dis-eases. Clin Exp Rheumatol 2018;36(Suppl 110):32–8.
8. Lepelletier C, Bouaziz JD, Rybojad M, et al. Neutro-philic Dermatoses Associated with Myeloid Malig-nancies. Am J Clin Dermatol 2019;20(3):325–33.
9. Marzano AV, Ishak RS, Saibeni S, et al. Autoinflam-matory skin disorders in inflammatory bowel dis-eases, pyoderma gangrenosum and Sweet's syndrome: a comprehensive review and disease classification criteria. Clin Rev Allergy Immunol 2013;45(2):202–10.
10. Hau E, Vignon Pennamen MD, Battistella M, et al. Neutrophilic skin lesions in autoimmune connective tissue diseases: nine cases and a literature review. Medicine (Baltim) 2014;93(29):e346.
11. Passet M, Lepelletier C, Vignon-Pennamen MD, et al. Next-Generation Sequencing in Myeloid Neoplasm-Associated Sweet's Syndrome Demon-strates Clonal Relation between Malignant Cells

and Skin-Infiltrating Neutrophils. J Invest Dermatol 2020. https://doi.org/10.1016/j.jid.2019.12.040.

12. Zakine E, Schell B, Battistella M, et al. UBA1 Variations in Neutrophilic Dermatosis Skin Lesions of Patients With VEXAS Syndrome. JAMA Dermatol 2021; 157(11):1349–54.

13. Berliner N, Coates TD. Introduction to a review series on human neutrophils. Blood 2019;133(20): 2111–2.

14. Cowland JB, Borregaard N. Granulopoiesis and granules of human neutrophils. Immunol Rev 2016; 273(1):11–28.

15. Nauseef WM. How human neutrophils kill and degrade microbes: an integrated view. Immunol Rev 2007;219:88–102.

16. Papayannopoulos V. Neutrophil extracellular traps in immunity and disease. Nat Rev Immunol 2018;18(2): 134–47.

17. Jones HR, Robb CT, Perretti M, et al. The role of neutrophils in inflammation resolution. Semin Immunol 2016;28(2):137–45.

18. Pérez-Figueroa E, Álvarez-Carrasco P, Ortega E, et al. Many Ways to Die. Front Immunol 2021;12: 631821.

19. Marzano AV, Fanoni D, Antiga E, et al. Expression of cytokines, chemokines and other effector molecules in two prototypic autoinflammatory skin diseases, pyoderma gangrenosum and Sweet's syndrome. Clin Exp Immunol 2014;178(1):48–56.

20. Marzano AV, Damiani G, Ceccherini I, et al. Autoinflammation in pyoderma gangrenosum and its syndromic form (pyoderma gangrenosum, acne and suppurative hidradenitis). Br J Dermatol 2017; 176(6):1588–98.

21. Marzano AV, Tavecchio S, Berti E, et al. Cytokine and Chemokine Profile in Amicrobial Pustulosis of the Folds. Medicine (Baltim) 2015;94(50):e2301.

22. Amazan E, Ezzedine K, Mossalayi MD, et al. Expression of interleukin-1 alpha in amicrobial pustulosis of the skin folds with complete response to anakinra. J Am Acad Dermatol 2014;71(2):e53–6.

23. Kawakami T, Ohashi S, Kawa Y, et al. Elevated serum granulocyte colony-stimulating factor levels in patients with active phase of sweet syndrome and patients with active behcet disease: implication in neutrophil apoptosis dysfunction. Arch Dermatol 2004;140(5):570–4.

24. White JML, Mufti GJ, Salisbury JR, et al. Cutaneous manifestations of granulocyte colony-stimulating factor. Clin Exp Dermatol 2006;31(2):206–7.

25. Marzano AV, Cugno M, Trevisan V, et al. Role of inflammatory cells, cytokines and matrix metalloproteinases in neutrophil-mediated skin diseases. Clin Exp Immunol 2010;162(1):100–7.

26. Brostjan C, Oehler R. The role of neutrophil death in chronic inflammation and cancer. Cell Death Dis 2020;6(1):1–8.

27. Ogawa Y, Muto Y, Kinoshita M, et al. Neutrophil Extracellular Traps in Skin Diseases. Biomedicines 2021;9(12):1888.

28. Croia C, Dini V, Loggini B, et al. Evaluation of neutrophil extracellular trap deregulated formation in pyoderma gangrenosum. Exp Dermatol 2021;30(9): 1340–4.

29. Eid E, Safi R, El Hasbani G, et al. Characterizing the presence of neutrophil extracellular traps in neutrophilic dermatoses. Exp Dermatol 2021;30(7):988–94.

30. Bonnekoh H, Scheffel J, Wu J, et al. Skin and Systemic Inflammation in Schnitzler's Syndrome Are Associated With Neutrophil Extracellular Trap Formation. Front Immunol 2019;10:546.

31. Byrd AS, Carmona-Rivera C, O'Neil LJ, et al. Neutrophil extracellular traps, B cells, and type I interferons contribute to immune dysregulation in hidradenitis suppurativa. Sci Transl Med 2019;11(508):eaav5908.

32. Drenth JP, van der Meer JW. Hereditary periodic fever. N Engl J Med 2001;345(24):1748–57.

33. Kitamura A, Maekawa Y, Uehara H, et al. A mutation in the immunoproteasome subunit PSMB8 causes autoinflammation and lipodystrophy in humans. J Clin Invest 2011;121(10):4150–60.

34. Cugno M, Borghi A, Marzano AV. PAPA, PASH and PA-PASH Syndromes: Pathophysiology, Presentation and Treatment. Am J Clin Dermatol 2017;18(4):555–62.

35. Moghaddas F, Llamas R, De Nardo D, et al. A novel Pyrin-Associated Autoinflammation with Neutrophilic Dermatosis mutation further defines 14-3-3 binding of pyrin and distinction to Familial Mediterranean Fever. Ann Rheum Dis 2017;76(12):2085–94.

36. Gusdorf L, Lipsker D. Neutrophilic urticarial dermatosis: A review. Ann Dermatol Venereol 2018;145(12): 735–40.

37. Cowen EW, Goldbach-Mansky RDIRA. DITRA, and new insights into pathways of skin inflammation: what's in a name? Arch Dermatol 2012;148(3):381–4.

38. Aksentijevich I, Masters SL, Ferguson PJ, et al. An autoinflammatory disease with deficiency of the interleukin-1-receptor antagonist. N Engl J Med 2009;360(23):2426–37.

39. Camargo CM dos S, Brotas AM, Ramos-e-Silva M, et al. Isomorphic phenomenon of Koebner: facts and controversies. Clin Dermatol 2013;31(6):741–9.

40. Kaustio M, Haapaniemi E, Göös H, et al. Damaging heterozygous mutations in NFKB1 lead to diverse immunologic phenotypes. J Allergy Clin Immunol 2017;140(3):782–96.

41. Moon JH, Huynh J. Pathergy in Neutrophilic Dermatosis. N Engl J Med 2021;384(3):271.

42. Tolkachjov SN, Fahy AS, Wetter DA, et al. Postoperative pyoderma gangrenosum (PG): the Mayo Clinic experience of 20 years from 1994 through 2014. J Am Acad Dermatol 2015;73(4):615–22.

43. Ehrl DC, Heidekrueger PI, Broer PN. Pyoderma gangrenosum after breast surgery: A systematic review.

J Plast Reconstr Aesthetic Surg JPRAS 2018;71(7): 1023–32.

44. Maverakis E, Marzano AV, Le ST, et al. Pyoderma gangrenosum. Nat Rev Dis Prim 2020;6(1):1–19.

45. Assrawi E, Louvrier C, Lepelletier C, et al. Somatic Mosaic NLRP3 Mutations and Inflammasome Activation in Late-Onset Chronic Urticaria. J Invest Dermatol 2019. https://doi.org/10.1016/j.jid.2019.06.153.

46. Louvrier C, Assrawi E, El Khouri E, et al. NLRP3-associated autoinflammatory diseases: Phenotypic and molecular characteristics of germline versus somatic mutations. J Allergy Clin Immunol 2020;145(4): 1254–61.

47. Beck DB, Ferrada MA, Sikora KA, et al. Somatic Mutations in UBA1 and Severe Adult-Onset Autoinflammatory Disease. N Engl J Med 2020. https://doi.org/10.1056/NEJMoa2026834.

48. Cugno M, Gualtierotti R, Meroni PL, et al. Inflammatory Joint Disorders and Neutrophilic Dermatoses: a Comprehensive Review. Clin Rev Allergy Immunol 2018;54(2):269–81.

49. Jo T, Horio K, Migita K. Sweet's syndrome in patients with MDS and MEFV mutations. N Engl J Med 2015; 372(7):686–8.

50. Wei C, Yu P, Cheng L. Hematopoietic Reprogramming Entangles with Hematopoiesis. Trends Cell Biol 2020;30(10):752–63.

51. Collins SJ. The HL-60 promyelocytic leukemia cell line: proliferation, differentiation, and cellular oncogene expression. Blood 1987;70(5):1233–44.

52. Park CJ, Bae YD, Choi JY, et al. Sweet's syndrome during the treatment of acute promyelocytic leukemia with all-trans retinoic acid. Korean J Intern Med 2001;16(3):218–21.

53. Sujobert P, Cuccuini W, Vignon-Pennamen D, et al. Evidence of differentiation in myeloid malignancies associated neutrophilic dermatosis: a fluorescent in situ hybridization study of 14 patients. J Invest Dermatol 2013;133(4):1111–4.

54. Delaleu J, Battistella M, Rathana K, et al. Identification of Clonal Skin Myeloid Cells by Next Generation Sequencing in Myelodysplasia Cutis. Br J Dermatol 2020.

55. Delaleu J, Kim R, Zhao LP, et al. Clinical, pathological, and molecular features of myelodysplasia cutis. Blood 2022;139(8):1251–3.

56. Mo W, Wang X, Wang Y, et al. Clonal neutrophil infiltrates in concurrent Sweet's syndrome and acute myeloid leukemia: A case report and literature review. Cancer Genet 2018;226-227:11–6.

57. Marzano AV, Ramoni S, Caputo R. Amicrobial pustulosis of the folds. Report of 6 cases and a literature review. Dermatol Basel Switz 2008;216(4):305–11.

58. Haber R, Feghali J, El Gemayel M. Risk of malignancy in histiocytoid Sweet syndrome: A systematic review and reappraisal. J Am Acad Dermatol 2020; 83(2):661–3.

59. Harrist TJ, Fine JD, Berman RS, et al. Neutrophilic eccrine hidradenitis. A distinctive type of neutrophilic dermatosis associated with myelogenous leukemia and chemotherapy. Arch Dermatol 1982; 118(4):263–6.

60. Doktor V, Hadi A, Hadi A, et al. Erythema elevatum diutinum: a case report and review of literature. Int J Dermatol 2019;58(4):408–15.

61. Binus AM, Qureshi AA, Li VW, et al. Pyoderma gangrenosum: a retrospective review of patient characteristics, comorbidities and therapy in 103 patients. Br J Dermatol 2011;165(6):1244–50.

62. Sutra-Loubet C, Carlotti A, Guillemette J, et al. Neutrophilic panniculitis. J Am Acad Dermatol 2004;50(2):280–5.

63. de Masson A, Bouvresse S, Clérici T, et al. [Recurrent neutrophilic panniculitis in a patient with chronic myelogenous leukaemia treated with imatinib mesilate and dasatinib]. Ann Dermatol Venereol 2011; 138(2):135–9.

64. Chatfield SM, Thieblemont N, Witko-Sarsat V. Expanding Neutrophil Horizons: New Concepts in Inflammation. J Innate Immun 2018;10(5–6):422–31.

Pyoderma Gangrenosum
Diagnostic Criteria, Subtypes, Systemic Associations, and Workup

Mallory L. Zaino, MD*, Courtney R. Schadt, MD, FAAD,
Jeffrey P. Callen, MD, FACP, FAAD, MACR

KEYWORDS

- Pyoderma gangrenosum • Neutrophilic dermatoses • Necrotizing neutrophilic dermatosis

KEY POINTS

- Pyoderma gangrenosum (PG) is an inflammatory neutrophilic dermatosis with variable clinical features.
- Associated systemic diseases include inflammatory bowel disease, inflammatory arthritides, and hematologic disorders.
- Women are affected more often than men, and the disease most often occurs between the second to fifth decade of life.
- Incidence is between 3 and 10 people per million but may be greater due to underrecognition.

INTRODUCTION

Pyoderma gangrenosum (PG) is an inflammatory neutrophilic dermatosis with variable clinical features.[1] The classic presentation is an ulceration with an erythematous to violaceous undermined border (**Fig. 1**).[2] The lesion may present de novo or in response to minimal trauma, also known as pathergy.[2] Extracutaneous manifestations may occur, most frequently involving the lungs.[3] Associated systemic diseases include inflammatory bowel disease (IBD), inflammatory arthritides, and hematologic disorders.[2] The pathophysiologic mechanism of disease is not completely known but likely related to the cumulative influence of inflammation, immune-mediated neutrophilic dysfunction, and genetic predisposition.[2,4] Women are affected more often than men, and the disease most often occurs between the second to fifth decade of life.[2] Incidence is between 3 and 10 people per million but may be greater due to underrecognition.[2] In this article, we will discuss the diagnostic criteria, disease subtypes, systemic associations, and workup.

DISEASE DIAGNOSTIC CRITERIA

PG is a diagnostic challenge due to its lack of pathognomonic findings. The characteristic lesions were first described by Brocq[5] and later elucidated by Brunsting and colleagues[6] as irregular ulcerations with well-demarcated erythematous-violaceus serpiginous borders and atrophic scarring. Since then, additional clinical characteristics have been described and multiple sets of criteria for the diagnosis of PG have been proposed as described in the next several paragraphs.

Su and colleagues[7] developed a set of criteria from clinical experience using 2 major criteria and 4 minor criteria. The first major criterion is a rapidly progressive (1–2 cm/d or 50% increase in 1 month) painful ulcer with an irregular erythematous-violaceus border and undermined edges. The presence of a papule, pustule, or bulla is common before the development of the ulcer. The second major criterion requires the exclusion of other relevant diseases. The 4 minor criteria include a history of pathergy, presence of an

Department of Dermatology, University of Louisville, 3810 Springhurst Boulevard, Suite 200, Louisville, KY, USA
* Corresponding author.
E-mail address: mlzain01@louisville.edu

Dermatol Clin 42 (2024) 157–170
https://doi.org/10.1016/j.det.2023.08.003

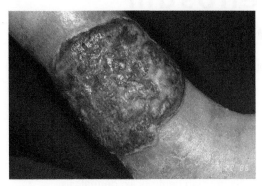

Fig. 1. Purulent necrotic ulcer with reddish-violaceous undermined borders and an inflammatory rim of erythema.

associated systemic disease known to occur in conjunction with PG, neutrophilia on histology, and response to immunosuppressive treatment (eg, prednisone or a traditional immunosuppressive agent). Two major criteria and a minimum of 2 minor criteria are required for diagnosis.

Hadi and colleagues[8] summarized clinical features of PG using 30 case reports in the literature. An ulcerated lesion located on the leg or peristomal skin with undermined borders and history of pathergy were the most common features. Additional findings included concomitant associated disease, purulent discharge, and a preceding pustule. They stated that although no feature is diagnostic in isolation, when used in combination, can aid in clinical diagnosis.

Al Ghazal and colleagues[9] developed a set of primary and secondary criteria following a retrospective chart review of 49 patients with PG, which are similar to those proposed by Su and colleagues. The first of 2 primary criteria is the presence of a sterile ulcer with erythematous-violaceous undermined edges. The second criterion is the exclusion of other related diseases. The 4 secondary criteria include history of pathergy, comorbid associated systemic disease, dermal neutrophilia ± lymphocytic vasculitis on histology, and response to treatment with immunosuppression. These criteria were preceded by a survey study characterizing clinical characteristics of PG from the same group. In this study, the significance of various PG diagnostic criteria was scored as "very important," "important," or "not important." Fifty-seven individuals completed the questionnaire.[10] The most important clinical characteristic was "erythematous-violaceous borders" followed by "rapid progression" and "undermined borders."[10] Sterile ulcerations or "negative swab test" was the lowest scoring criterion.[10]

Since the development of the criteria described above, separate groups of expert physicians have developed their own respective consensus guidelines. The first was the Delphi Consensus of International Experts.[11] Twelve PG expert physicians, including 2 current authors (JPC and CRS) participated in a multiround evaluation of the most important diagnostic criteria of disease, each round revising criteria until a consensus was reached. The result was 1 major criterion and 8 minor criteria consisting of histologic findings, patient history, clinical examination, and response to treatment.

The Delphi Consensus[11] requires 1 major criterion and a minimum of 4 minor criteria. The major criterion is a neutrophilic infiltrate on histology. Once this criterion has been met, additional criteria can be evaluated. Exclusion of infection on histology and tissue culture, history of a preceding papule, pustule, or vesicle, pathergy, and comorbid IBD or arthritis are some of the minor criteria. Additional minor criteria include a painful ulcer with surrounding erythema and undermined borders, multiple ulcerations (one located on the lower leg), cribriform scarring, and reduction in ulcer size in response to immunosuppressive treatment.

The PARACELSUS[12] is the second set of consensus guidelines developed by physician experts comparing 60 patients with PG to 50 patients with venous leg ulcer (controls). The primary purpose of these criteria was to differentiate leg ulcers due to PG from those due to venous insufficiency, and thus these criteria might not be applicable to patients with ulcers in locations other than the legs. The PARACELSUS uses a point system to score the likelihood of disease and consists of 10 diagnostic criteria: *P*rogressive disease, *A*ssessment of relevant differential diagnosis, *R*eddish-violaceous wound border, *A*melioration by immunosuppressive drugs, *C*haracteristically irregular ulcer shape, *E*xtreme pain, *L*ocation of lesion at site of trauma, *S*uppurative inflammation on histopathology, *U*ndermined wound border, and *S*ystemic disease associated. The first 3 criteria are considered major criteria and are each valued at 3 points. The next set of 4 and 3 criteria are the minor and additional criteria, respectively. Minor criteria are each valued at 2 points and additional criteria at 1 point. A score of 10 points or greater represents a high likelihood of disease.

The PARACELSUS, Delphi consensus, and Su and colleagues criteria have all been assessed and compared for PG diagnostic accuracy. The PARACELSUS accurately scored 42 (89%) of 47 patients with PG, followed by the Delphi consensus and Su and colleagues criteria, which each identified 35 (74%) patients with PG.[13] The diagnostic agreement was highest and lowest between the PARACELSUS score and Su and colleagues and the PARACELSUS score and Delphi consensus, respectively.[13]

The use of artificial intelligence (AI)-powered machines to improve PG diagnostic accuracy may also be of use. Convolutional neural networks have been studied in patients with PG to distinguish between PG and venous ulcers.[14] The sensitivity and specificity of these deep learning convolutional neural networks used to compare PG to venous ulcers is 97% and 83.3%, respectively, compared with 72.7% and 88.9% in dermatologists using photographs alone, respectively. Additional algorithms to expand the AI-powered PG differentials are also currently under development.[14]

DISEASE SUBTYPES

PG is multifaceted cutaneous disease of neutrophil dysfunction, aberrant inflammation, and genetic predisposition.[2] The diagnosis is clinical, and the presentation varies. Within the spectrum of disease, 4 subtypes exist (Table 1). These include ulcerative, pustular, bullous, and vegetative PG. Additional variants include postsurgical (also known as postoperative) (Fig. 2) and peristomal PG (Fig. 3), both of which will be addressed in a later article. Patients may present with more than one type, although rare, and a single subtype typically dominates.

Ulcerative PG: Ulcerative PG presents as a progressive purulent necrotic ulcer with reddish-violaceous undermined borders and an inflammatory rim of erythema.[4,15,16] Ulcers can be superficial or deep and may present as a single lesion or as multiple ulcers coalescing into one.[4,15,16] Preceding painful follicular-based papules, pustules, or vesicles are common.[4,15,16] Lesions can seem de novo or secondary to minimal trauma, also known as pathergy.[4,15,16] The clinical course may be rapid and accompanied by pain, fevers, and hemorrhagic or suppurative inflammation or indolent and spreading over the period of months.[4,15,16] Cribriform or "cigarette paper-like" atrophic scarring from secondary intention healing is characteristic.[4,15,16]

Ulcerative PG can occur at any site; however, a predilection for the lower extremities and the trunk does exist.[4,15,16] History of concomitant IBD, inflammatory arthritis, or myeloproliferative disease is common but not required.[4,15,16] Biopsy from the active edge of ulceration shows lymphocytic infiltration and dermal neutrophilia with or without abscess formation.[17] These histopathologic findings are nonspecific but are useful to exclude other ulcerative diseases. Special stains may be used to exclude infection.

Pustular PG: Pustular PG presents as discrete erythematous painful pustules surrounded by a red halo.[4,15,16] Pustules range from 0.5 to 2 cm in size and have a predilection for the trunk or extensor surfaces.[4,15,16] It is frequently associated with IBD, and its clinical course may coincide with IBD acute exacerbations, improving once the flare has resolved.[4,15,16] Pustular PG has been reported in conjunction with chronic gastroduodenal ulcers, cystic fibrosis, and mucosal infections secondary to obstructing neoplasms.[17] Histopathological findings include perifollicular neutrophilic infiltration, dermal neutrophilia, subcorneal neutrophil aggregates, and subepidermal edema.[17]

Within pustular PG, variants exist. Oral pustular PG, likely a variant of pyostomatitis vegetans, has been described in patients with IBD as inflammatory erythematous pustules occurring during active periods of disease.[15,18] Follicular-based necrotic vesiculopustular eruptions with lymphocytic vasculitis and neutrophilic dermolysis on histology have also been described in patients with hepatobiliary disease without IBD.[19]

Bullous PG: Bullous PG, also known as *atypical PG*, presents as a rapidly appearing hemorrhagic painful vesicles or bullae with a blue-gray border (Fig. 4).[4,15,16,20] The bullae typically necrose to a shallow erosion surrounded by a rim of erythema.[4,15,16] Lesions most commonly affect the face, dorsal hands, and extensor surfaces.[4,15,16] It is associated with myeloproliferative disorders and concomitant hematologic malignancy is a poor indicator of disease.[17,20] Bullous PG may remit with treatment of the underlying hematologic disorder.[17] Histology varies according to the stage of disease but may show epidermal necrosis, intraepidermal vesicles, subepidermal bullae, or dense dermal aggregates.[17]

Clinical features of bullous PG may overlap with Sweet syndrome. Sweet syndrome presents with well-demarcated erythematous papules and plaques but bullae and hemorrhagic blisters can occur.[21] Distinction between the 2 may be made by the localization of the neutrophilic infiltrate on biopsy. The infiltrate is often folliculocentric and located in the deep dermis in patients with PG.[22]

Vegetative PG: Vegetative PG, also known as *superficial granulomatous pyoderma*, presents as an indolent solitary nonpurulent superficial ulcer typically accompanied by a verrucous pustular studded plaque.[15,23] It is not painful and reddish-violaceous undermined borders are absent.[4,15,16] The lack of pain and nonpurulent appearance differentiates it from other forms of PG and may lead to delay in diagnosis.[24] It occurs primarily on the trunk, head, and neck.[4,15,16] It is not associated with systemic disease and typically responds

Table 1
Pyoderma gangrenosum subtypes

| Subtypes | Clinical Manifestations | | | | Histologic Findings |
	Clinical Presentation	Localization[a]	Time Course	Associated Disease	Histology
Ulcerative	Purulent necrotic ulcer with reddish-violaceous undermined borders and surrounding erythema	Trunk Lower legs	Rapidly progressive	IBD IRA Myeloproliferative	Lymphocytic infiltration Dermal neutrophilia
Pustular	Discrete erythematous papules (0.5–2 cm) with an inflammatory red halo	Trunk Extensor surfaces	Frequently occurs with acute IBD exacerbation	IBD	Subepidermal edema Perifollicular neutrophil infiltration Subcorneal neutrophil aggregates Dermal neutrophilia
Bullous	Grouped erythematous vesicles or bullae with a gray-blue border necrosing to a shallow erosion	Face Dorsal hands Extensor surfaces	Concomitant hematologic malignancy is a poor prognostic factor	Hematologic malignancy	Intraepidermal vesicles Subepidermal bullae Dermal neutrophilia
Vegetative	Painless, nonpurulent shallow erosion without reddish-violaceus undermined borders	Face Neck Trunk	Slowly progressive	None	Epidermal granuloma Histiocytes Eosinophilia Dermal neutrophilia

Abbreviations: IBD, irritable bowel disease; IRA, inflammatory rheumatoid arthritis.
  [a] Lesions may occur on any part of the body but have a propensity for specific sites.

to topical or intralesional forms of therapy.[4,15,16] Histology shows epidermal granulomatous formation, neutrophilic infiltration with histiocytes, and eosinophilia.[17]

Necrotizing Neutrophilic Dermatosis: Necrotizing neutrophilic dermatosis (NND) describes a set of neutrophilic dermatoses characterized by necrotic reddish-violaceous plaques or ulcers and systemic symptoms, including fever, a leukemoid reaction, and hemodynamic instability.[25] Common sites of involvement are the legs, arms, and trunk.[25] Patients may have PG, necrotizing Sweet syndrome, or overlapping features of both. Distinguishing NND from necrotizing fasciitis (NF) is difficult. In a multicenter retrospective chart review, 51 (94%) of 54 patients with NND were initially misdiagnosed as NF.[25]

NF is a monomicrobial or polymicrobial infection of the skin and soft tissue that presents similarly.[26] Pain out of proportion to examination, positive blood cultures, and subcutaneous gas on radiographic imaging are common but not required.[26] Treatment consists of prompt surgical debridement and antibiotics.[26] In patients with NND, whose presentation is clinically similar, surgical intervention and lack of immunosuppression with systemic corticosteroids risk disease progression and iatrogenic exacerbation.[27] The risk of disease worsening in response to surgical intervention is high given the phenomenon of pathergy in patients

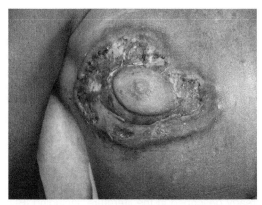

Fig. 2. Necrotic ulcer with ill-defined raised erythematous-violaceous borders.

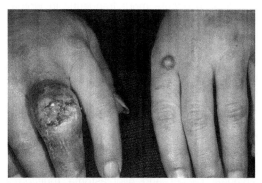

Fig. 4. Erythematous necrotic ulcer with an irregular blue-gray border discharging a hemorrhagic exudate on the proximal interphalangeal joint (left) and a well-circumscribed blue-gray papule with a rim of erythema on the metacarpophalangeal joint (right).

with PG.[15] Approximately one-third of patients with PG experience pathergy, an exaggerated response of injury induced by minimal trauma, which may present as worsening of existing skin lesions or development of new ones.[2,28] If the suspicion is high, concomitant administration of antibiotics and corticosteroids may be considered.

PG in Infants and Children: PG can occur in individuals of all ages, although its presence in infants and children is rare. Less than 5% of all PG cases have been reports in patients aged younger than 18 years.[29,30] PG presents in infants and children similarly to that as adults but are more common on the face and neck of children and perineum and buttocks of infants.[29,31] A preceding pustule is common and pathergy is present in more than half of all cases.[29,30] Associated diseases include IBD, inflammatory arthritis, and hematologic dyscrasias.[31] Osteomyelitis, acquired immune deficiency syndrome, and collagen-vascular disease have also been reported.[31,32]

PG in Pregnancy: PG has been reported in pregnancy, which may be associated with the physiologic increase in inflammation required for labor.[33] Patients have presented from 2 weeks gestation to 4 weeks postpartum.[33] Nine (35%) of 26 pregnant patients with PG reported in the literature had an earlier history of PG and 11 (42%) of the lesions occurring during pregnancy presented at the site of caesarean incision.[33] Additional locations included the arms, legs, and feet.[33] Associated systemic disease mirrored that of the general patient population (IBD, inflammatory arthritis, and hematologic disease), and the response to treatment was similar.[33]

Genital PG: PG has also been reported on the vulva, penis, and scrotum.[4,15] This variant is characterized by its localization for the genitals, although its appearance is like that of ulcerative PG.[4,15] Initial lesions may be misdiagnosed as Behcet disease. However, lack of oral aphthous ulcers, uveitis, and involvement of the cardiovascular, neurologic, or gastrointestinal system favor a diagnosis of PG.[34] Lesions may also be differentiated from Fournier's gangrene by lack of genital edema, fever, and hemodynamic instability.[35]

DISEASE SYSTEMIC ASSOCIATIONS

PG may be idiopathic or associated with systemic disease.[36] Associated diseases are those that occur in patients with PG more than the general population.[20] These include IBD, inflammatory arthritides, and hematologic disorders.[20] The proportion of idiopathic to disease associated PG varies, likely related to the interrater and intrarater reliability that exist when selecting which concomitant disease to report.

PG occurs more often in women than men.[9,20,36,37] Associated inflammatory systemic

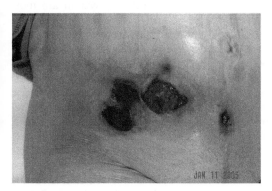

Fig. 3. Multiple well-circumscribed bright red ulcers with dusky borders.

disease also occurs more frequently in women with PG than in men with PG.[36,38] The most common associated disease is IBD and inflammatory rheumatoid and nonrheumatoid arthritis.[20] IBD includes both Crohn disease and ulcerative colitis, the incidence at which each occurs is not consistent. Additional associated diseases include endocrine disorders, solid organ neoplasia, and myeloid or lymphocytic hematopoietic-derived malignancies.[36] In decreasing order of occurrence, solid organ neoplasms included breast, prostate, melanoma, ovary, liver, and colon.[9,36] Laryngeal cancer and glioblastoma multiforme have also been reported.[9,36] Hematologic neoplasms included myelodysplasia and monoclonal gammopathy (immunoglobulin [Ig] A > IgM, IgG) followed by acute myelogenous leukemia (AML), chronic myelogenous leukemia (CML), chronic lymphocytic leukemia, Hodgkin lymphoma, and other non-Hodgkin lymphoma.[9,15,17,36,39] The majority of myelodysplastic cases preceded PG, which was reversed for monoclonal gammopathies of undetermined significance.[39] Of note, myeloproliferative disorders occur more frequently in men with PG than in women and are associated with worse outcomes.[15,40]

In a retrospective review of 103 patients with PG, 86.6% had an associated systemic disease.[38] This included 29.1% with one comorbidity and 35.9% and 13.6% with 2 and 3 or more comorbidities, respectively.[38] Most patients (34%) had concomitant IBD.[38] This was followed by inflammatory arthritis and hematological disorders, respectively.[38] Inflammatory arthritis included rheumatoid arthritis, nonrheumatoid arthritis, and psoriatic arthritis.[38] Associated endocrine disorders included diabetes and Hashimoto thyroiditis.[38] Of those with diabetes mellitus, the majority were type II diabetes.[38]

Diabetes and thyroid disease are the 2 endocrine disorders most associated with PG.[9,36] Cardiovascular, peripheral vascular, metabolic syndrome, and obesity (body mass index >30 kg/m^2) may also be implicated in disease pathogenesis.[9,36] The relationship between obesity and metabolic syndrome as a risk factor for PG is likely related to the influence adipokines have on the inflammatory pathways.[9,36] However, their association may also be confounded by the overall occurrence of systemic disease in individuals of older age, for which PG most often occurs.

Hepatitis has also been reported as an associated comorbid disease.[4,15,17,19,36,41–44] This includes hepatitis C virus infection and autoimmune hepatitis. Although the impact of hepatic disease of PG has not been elucidated, it may be related to altered immune function secondary to hepatic dysfunction. Damage-associated molecular patterns released by hepatocytes leads to an upregulation of proinflammatory chemokines and cytokines. Dysregulated immune signaling may also be affected by reduced renal function. In a retrospective study of 49 patients with PG, 14 (29%) had an elevated creatinine, including 9 (18%) who had stage IIIa chronic kidney disease or worse.[9]

Adults: PG systemic associations may be affected by age. In a retrospective chart review of 267 patients with PG, 238 (66.9%) had an associated comorbid disease.[37] These mirrored those already described in the literature, including IBD, inflammatory arthritides, and hematologic dyscrasias. However, the prevalence of each disease varied by age group. Patients aged younger than 65 years were more likely to have IBD than in older individuals.[37] Patients aged older than or equal to 65 years were more likely to have arthritis, solid organ neoplasia, or hematologic disorder and/or neoplasia than younger individuals.[37] Despite these differences, the prevalence of comorbid disease was the same between groups.[37]

Infants and Children: Associated systemic diseases in infants and children vary. IBD, acquired immune deficiency syndrome, pneumonia, noninfectious necrotizing tracheitis, monoclonal gammopathy (IgM), osteomyelitis, and Takayasu arteritis have been observed in infants.[29,31,32] Comorbid disease in children has been reported as high as 74% in patients with PG and is parallel to those affecting the adult population, particularly IBD, arthritis, and hematologic disorders (AML and CML).[30]

Extracutaneous Manifestations: Extracutaneous manifestation of PG is rare but may occur.[3,4,15] Lesions may develop in isolation or with concomitant eruption on the skin.[3] Patients may be asymptomatic or present with constitutional symptoms and associated organ dysfunction.[3] The diagnosis is clinical and warrants a high index of suspicion. Lesions affecting the pulmonary system are most common.[3,4,15,16]

Pulmonary lesions may present as cavitations, multiple pulmonary nodules, or patchy interstitial infiltrates.[45–60] Patients may be asymptomatic or present with cough, shortness of breath, and chest pain. Respiratory failure and sepsis can occur and is most prevalent in patients with concomitant hematologic malignancy. Cultures from blood, tissue, and sputum are negative and aspirate from bronchoalveolar lavage may show neutrophils.[3] Sterile neutrophilic infiltrates, focal vasculitis, and mixed cellular infiltrates occluding the bronchioles and alveoli may also be observed on biopsy.[3] Pulmonary involvement can coincide with involvement of other tissues and has been observed with simultaneous PG lesions of the genitals and kidney.[52,55] Nonspecific sterile neutrophilic aggregates may also affect the pancreas, spleen, liver, gastrointestinal tract, and lymph nodes.[46,49,60] Patients may or may not have associated symptoms and organ dysfunction and comorbid hematologic disease, primarily monoclonal gammopathies, have been observed.[60]

Additional extracutaneous manifestations of disease include the bone and musculoskeletal system (eg, sterile pyoarthrosis, multifocal sterile osteomyelitis, or neutrophilic myositis).[3,4,15,17] Patients may present with fever, bone pain, joint pain, and muscle aches. Radiographic imaging may show periosteal reaction, osteolysis, or lesions and fibrotic inflammatory change on biopsy.[3] A pituitary pseudotumor negative for sarcoidosis, infection, and malignancy responsive to corticosteroids with mixed inflammatory infiltrates on biopsy has also been suggested as a cerebral manifestation of PG.[61] Ocular involvement of the disease often coincides with the cutaneous manifestation of PG and may present as episcleritis, iritis, and ulcerations.[4,15,17]

Syndromic PG: PG can exist in syndromic forms of autoinflammatory diseases (**Table 2**).[4,62] Autoinflammatory diseases are pleiotropic monogenic or polygenic systemic inflammatory diseases that lack features of autoimmunity.[62] The most common gene involved in PG-associated autoinflammatory diseases is the Proline-Serine-Threonine Phosphatase Interacting Protein 1 (PSTPIP1) gene.[4,62] The PSTPIP1 gene codes for phosphorylating proteins involved in the regulation of pyrin, an inflammatory molecule associated with the inflammasome and capase-1 immune-mediated signaling.[4,62] PSTPIP1 genetic mutations and subsequent altered functions of pyrin leads to proinflammatory signaling and neutrophil-driven inflammation.[4,62] The clinical implication of which is elevated levels of interleukin-1, tumor necrosis factor-alpha, and sterile neutrophilia.[4,62] Additional immune-mediated abnormalities include altered function of matrix metalloproteinases, chemokines, and cytokines.[4,62]

Pyogenic arthritis, PG, and acne (PAPA) syndrome is an autosomal dominant pleomorphic polygenic autoinflammatory disease.[62,63] Patients present with inflammatory joint pain, acne, and PG. History of pathergy is common and appearance of cutaneous lesions may vary. *PG, acne, and suppurative hidradenitis (PASH)* may present similarly.[62,64,65] PAPASH is an acronym coined to describe 2 distinct entities. These include pyogenic arthritis, PG, acne, and suppurative hidradenitis and the other PG, acne, psoriasis, arthritis, and suppurative hidradenitis.[62,66,67] An autoinflammatory disease similar to the latter is PsAPASH, which includes psoriatic arthritis, PG, acne, and suppurative hidradenitis.[68] In all autoinflammatory diseases, PG lesions seem similar to those that develop in isolation, as an erythematous necrotic ulcer with rugged undermined borders.

Medications: PG has been associated with systemic medications. There are reports of patients developing necrotic ulcerative lesions at the site of interferon alpha injections, including PG.[69–71]

Table 2
Autoinflammatory diseases associated with pyoderma gangrenosum

Autoinflammatory Disease	Clinical Manifestation	Genetic Mutation
PAPA	Pyogenic arthritis, PG, and acne	PSTPIP1 gene
PASH	PG, acne, and suppurative hidradenitis	PSTPIP1, MEFV, NOD2, NLRP3, IL1RN, or PSMB8 gene
PAPASH	Pyogenic arthritis, PG, acne, and suppurative hidradenitis	PSTPIP1 gene
PAPASH	PG, acne, psoriasis, arthritis, and suppurative hidradenitis	PSTPIP1 gene
PASS	PG, acne, suppurative hidradenitis, axial spondyloarthritis	n.r.
PsAPASH	Psoriatic arthritis, PG, acne, suppurative hidradenitis	n.r.

Abbreviation: n.r., not reported.

PG lesions have developed in patients who have received granulocyte colony-stimulating factor injections, particularly the bullous subtype.[72-76] PG-like eruptions have also been reported in patients receiving antipsychotic medications, retinoids (isotretinoin and alitretinoin), tyrosine kinase inhibitors (gefitinib, sunitinib, and imatinib), biologics (adalimumab, infliximab, and rituximab), and others (levamisole, azacytidine, and hydroxycarbamide).[77-82] In almost all cases, lesions resolved with cessation of the offending agent and administration of immunosuppression medications.

EVALUATION OF THE PATIENT WITH SUSPECTED PYODERMA GANGRENOSUM

Laboratory and histopathologic findings specific to PG do not exist; however, a medical history, physical examination, and skin biopsy are recommended for every patient suspected of disease.[83] The biopsy should be obtained despite the risk of pathergy, and tissue samples can be sent for routine hematoxylin and eosin processing and microbial stains as well as for culture.[4,15,17,83] The workup is designed to narrow the differential and assess for associated systemic illness. Exclusion of infection and malignancy are also important if treatment with immunosuppressive agents is likely to commence.

The differential diagnosis of PG is broad (**Table 3**), and includes infection, malignancy, and exogenous factors (pustular drug reactions, insect bite, and factitious disorder).[17,83] Infections that may mimic PG include but are not limited to deep fungal (eg, blastomycosis and sporotrichosis), viral (chronic atypical herpes simplex), bacterial (ecthyma gangrenosum and syphilitic ulceration), and protozoal (leishmaniasis).[17,83] Autoimmune diseases may include cryoglobulinemia, antiphospholipid syndrome, systemic lupus erythematosus, and granulomatosis with polyangiitis.[17,83,84] Vasculopathies may include arterial ulcer, venous ulcers, or livedoid vasculopathy.[17,83]

Information pertinent to patient history includes past medical history, previous medications, symptoms of associated disease (IBD, arthritis, and malignancy), and lesions preceding ulceration.[83] The patient should describe the appearance, progression, and associated trauma of the lesion before the development of ulceration.[83] This includes a papular, pustular, or vesicular appearing lesion that rapidly or slowly progressed and may or may not have been in response to trauma with associated pathergy.[83] The clinical examination should consider the location, diameter, border, depth, surrounding erythema, and number of lesions.[83] Patient-reported pain out of proportion to examination is common.[83]

The biopsy should be obtained from the edge of the ulcer via a deep punch or elliptical incision extending into the subcutaneous fat.[85] Acanthosis, polymorphonuclear leukocytes, and a mixed cellular infiltrate of lymphocytes and neutrophils invading the vasculature, dermis, and possibly the panniculus may be observed.[17,83,85] The histopathologic examination will vary by age and location from which the biopsy was performed.[83,85] The erythematous zone surrounding the ulcer will show lymphocytic vasculitis, fibrinoid necrosis, endothelial swelling, extravasation of erythrocytes, and thrombosis.[83,85] Nonspecific findings of necrosis are seen from biopsies taken at the center of the lesion.[83,85] Early lesions may be characterized by mild-to-moderate lymphocytic infiltrates compared with necrosis and dense perivascular lymphocytic infiltrates observed in late-stage lesions.[83,85] Direct immunofluorescence studies may be positive for IgM, complement C3, and fibrin deposition, which are nonspecific but may be performed to rule out autoimmune disease and vasculitis.[83,85]

Histopathologic findings of PG are not diagnostic but characteristic features in combination with clinical presentation may aid in differential diagnosis. The nonnecrotizing mononuclear cell vascular reaction observed in PG may help distinguish the disease from necrotizing mononuclear cell or neutrophil-infiltrated vascular reaction seen in necrotizing pustular follicular reactions with associated vasculitis.[17] These include mixed cryoglobulinemia, rheumatoid vasculitis, and Behcet disease.[17] The folliculocentric features of the vasculitis may also help differentiate the disease from Sweet syndrome.[17] Histologic examination with microbial stains and biopsied tissue cultured for bacteria, viruses, fungi, and atypical mycobacteria may also be used to exclude infection.

Routine laboratory examination is also recommended (**Table 4**).[4,15,83] This includes a complete blood cell count (CBC) with differential and comprehensive metabolic panel (CMP).[4,15,83] The CBC can be used to assess for hematologic disorders and the CMP for electrolytes and hepatorenal function. Elevated liver enzymes may be concerning for associated hepatitis. Leukocytosis and elevated erythrocyte sedimentation rate and C-reactive protein are often present but nonspecific findings of inflammation.

Blood tests to rule out autoimmune skin disease and vasculitis are also advised. These include antinuclear antibodies, antiphospholipid antibodies, circulating antineutrophil cytoplasmic antibodies (ANCA), cryoglobulins, rheumatoid factor, and

Table 3
Pyoderma gangrenosum differential diagnosis

Infectious	
Bacterial	Impetigo
	Ecthyma
	Necrotizing fasciitis
	Anthrax
	Tuberculosis
	Atypical mycobacteria
	Syphilitic gumma
Viral	HSV
Fungal	Blastomycosis
	Histoplasmosis
	Sporotrichosis
	Cryptococcosis
	Aspergillosis
	Penicilliosis
	Zygomycosis
Protozoal	Leishmaniasis
	Schistosomiasis
	Amebiasis cutis
Immune-mediated	
Systemic vasculitis or vasculopathy	Behcet's disease
	ANCA-associated vasculitides
	Mixed cryoglobulinemia
	Rheumatoid vasculitis
	Antiphospholipid antibody syndrome
	Lupus-associated neutrophilic dermatoses
	Polyarteritis nodosa
	Microscopic polyangiitis
Neutrophilic dermatoses	Sweet syndrome
	Subcorneal pustular dermatosis
	Bullous lupus erythematosus
Vascular	Arterial insufficiency
	Venous hypertension
	Hypercoagulopathic thrombosis
	Non-septic emboli
	Livedoid vasculopathy
	Sickle cell disease
Cancer	SCC
	BCC
	Cutaneous T-cell lymphoma
	Cutaneous B-cell lymphoma
	Leukemia cutis
Exogenous	Factitious disorder
	Arthropod bite
	Calciphylaxis
	Halogenodermas
	Drug-induced tissue injury
Other	Necrobiosis lipodoidica with ulceration

anti–cyclic citrullinated peptide antibody.[4,15,83] Perinuclear-ANCA antibodies may occur in patients with IBD, whereas cytoplasmic-ANCA antibodies typically indicate granulomatous polyangiitis.[4,15,83] Antiphospholipid antibodies and cryoglobulins as well as Factor V Leiden mutation, methylene tetrahydrofolate reductase, and a coagulopathy panel can also be used for disorders of hypercoagulability.[4,15,83] Human immunodeficiency virus, hepatitis serologies, and rapid

Table 4
Recommended evaluation for patients with suspected pyoderma gangrenosum

	Patients <65 y of age	Patients ≥65 y of age
History and physical examination	+	+
Skin biopsy with tissue culture (bacterial, viral, fungal, and mycobacterial)	+	+
Complete blood count with differential	+	+
CMP	+	+
Age-appropriate malignancy screening	+/-	+/-
Evaluate for inflammatory arthritis: Anti-CCP and/or RF	+/-	+/-
Evaluate for autoimmune and vasculitis: ANA, ANCA, additional serologic tests, and cryoglobulins	+/-	+/-
Evaluate for signs and symptoms of IBD	+	
Fecal occult blood test and sigmoidoscopy or colonoscopy	+	
Consider referral to gastroenterology	+	
Evaluate for malignant neoplasms		+
Evaluate for signs and symptoms of hematologic disorders		+
SPEP, UPEP, IFE, and peripheral blood smear		+
Consider referral to hematology/oncology		+

Abbreviations: ANCA, antineutrophil cytoplasmic antibody; ANA, antinuclear antibody; anti-CCP, anti–cyclic citrullinated peptide antibody; IBD, inflammatory bowel disease; IFE, immunofixation electrophoresis; RF, rheumatoid factor; SPEP, serum protein electrophoresis; UPEP, urine protein electrophoresis.
For the editor: Table adapted from Ashchyan and colleagues, 2018.

plasma regain may be used to rule out infectious causes of ulceration and serum iodide and bromide levels to assess for halogenodermas.[4,15,83]

Additional tests exist to assess for IBD and hematologic disease.[37,83] Fecal occult blood test, upper gastrointestinal series, barium enema, and flexible sigmoidoscopy and/or colonoscopy may be used to evaluate for IBD.[37,83] Serum protein electrophoresis, urine protein electrophoresis, immunofixation electrophoresis, peripheral blood smear, and bone marrow aspirate and/or biopsy may be used to evaluate for hematologic disorders.[37,83] Referral to gastroenterology and/or

hematology/oncology for patients suspected of associated gastrointestinal or hematologic disease, respectively, may be indicated.[37,83]

Radiographic images may also be considered. Chest radiographs can be used to evaluate for infection, systemic vasculitis, and extracutaneous manifestations of disease.[83] Computed tomography with contrast or MRI may help rule out osteomyelitis.[83] Doppler ultrasonography and/or ankle brachial index to screen for underlying peripheral vascular disease may also be of use.[83]

Despite a thorough examination, diagnosis is a challenge. The threshold for PG diagnosis in patients with associated disease (IBD, inflammatory arthritis, and hematologic disorder) should be low and lack of response to antibiotics or worsening with surgery should prompt an evaluation for PG diagnosis. In patients diagnosed with PG without associated disease, workup for comorbid systemic illness is advised, and age-appropriate malignancy assessments may be considered but is controversial.[37,83]

CLINICS CARE POINTS

- Pyoderma gangrenosum (PG) is an inflammatory neutrophilic dermatosis that classically presents as an ulceration with an erythematous to violaceous undermined border.

- PG may be idiopathic or associated with systemic disease and the most common associated diseases include inflammatory bowel disease, inflammatory arthritides, and hematologic disorders.

- PG diagnosis is a challenge due to its lack of pathognomonic findings and multiple sets of criteria for the diagnosis of PG have been proposed.

- A medical history, physical examination, complete blood cell count, comprehensive metabolic panel, and skin biopsy are recommended for every patient suspected of having PG.

DISCLOSURE

Zaino and Schadt have no interests to disclose. Callen receives honorarium for the following work: Serono - adjudication for entry into a study of Cutaneous Lupus Erythematosus; Biogen - adjudication for entry into a study of Cutaneous Lupus Erythematosus; Riovant - Adjudication for entry into a study of Dermatomyositis.

REFERENCES

1. Callen JP. Pyoderma gangrenosum. Lancet 1998; 351(9102):581–5.
2. Braswell SF, Kostopoulos TC, Ortega-Loayza AG. Pathophysiology of pyoderma gangrenosum (PG): an updated review. J Am Acad Dermatol 2015;73(4): 691–8.
3. Borda LJ, Wong LL, Marzano AV, et al. Extracutaneous involvement of pyoderma gangrenosum. Arch Dermatol Res 2019;311(6):425–34.
4. Alavi A, French LE, Davis MD, et al. Pyoderma Gangrenosum: An Update on Pathophysiology, Diagnosis and Treatment. Am J Clin Dermatol 2017;18(3):355–72.
5. Brocq L. Nouvelle contribution a l'etude du phagedenisme geo- metrique. Paris: Ann Dermatol Syphiligr; 1916. p. 1–39.
6. BRUNSTING L, GOECKERMAN W, O'LEARY P. Pyoderma (echthyma) gangrenosum : clinical and experimental observations in five cases occurring in adults. Arch Dermatol Syphilol 1930;655–80.
7. Su WP, Davis MD, Weenig RH, et al. Pyoderma gangrenosum: clinicopathologic correlation and proposed diagnostic criteria. Int J Dermatol 2004;43(11):790–800.
8. Hadi A, Lebwohl M. Clinical features of pyoderma gangrenosum and current diagnostic trends. J Am Acad Dermatol 2011;64(5):950–4.
9. Al Ghazal P, Körber A, Klode J, et al. Investigation of new co-factors in 49 patients with pyoderma gangrenosum. J Dtsch Dermatol Ges 2012;10(4):251–7.
10. Al Ghazal P, Klode J, Dissemond J. Diagnostic criteria for pyoderma gangrenosum: results of a survey among dermatologic wound experts in Germany. J Dtsch Dermatol Ges 2014;12(12):1129–31.
11. Maverakis E, Ma C, Shinkai K, et al. Diagnostic Criteria of Ulcerative Pyoderma Gangrenosum: A Delphi Consensus of International Experts. JAMA Dermatol 2018;154(4):461–6.
12. Jockenhöfer F, Wollina U, Salva KA, et al. The PARACELSUS score: a novel diagnostic tool for pyoderma gangrenosum. Br J Dermatolr 2019;180(3):615–20.
13. Haag C, Hansen T, Hajar T, et al. Comparison of Three Diagnostic Frameworks for Pyoderma Gangrenosum. J Invest Dermatol 2021;141(1):59–63.
14. Birkner M, Schalk J, von den Driesch P, et al. Computer-Assisted Differential Diagnosis of Pyoderma Gangrenosum and Venous Ulcers with Deep Neural Networks. J Clin Med 2022;(23):11.
15. Ruocco E, Sangiuliano S, Gravina AG, et al. Pyoderma gangrenosum: an updated review. J Eur Acad Dermatol Venereol 2009;23(9):1008–17.
16. Conrad C, Trüeb RM. Pyoderma gangrenosum. J Dtsch Dermatol Ges 2005;3(5):334–42.
17. Crowson AN, Mihm MC, Magro C. Pyoderma gangrenosum: a review. J Cutan Pathol 2003;30(2): 97–107.
18. Clark LG, Tolkachjov SN, Bridges AG, et al. Pyostomatitis vegetans (PSV)-pyodermatitis vegetans (PDV): A clinicopathologic study of 7 cases at a tertiary referral center. J Am Acad Dermatol 2016; 75(3):578–84.
19. Magro CM, Crowson AN. A distinctive vesiculopustular eruption associated with hepatobiliary disease. Int J Dermatol 1997;36(11):837–44.
20. Bennett ML, Jackson JM, Jorizzo JL, et al. Pyoderma gangrenosum. A comparison of typical and atypical forms with an emphasis on time to remission. Case review of 86 patients from 2 institutions. Medicine (Baltim) 2000;79(1):37–46.

21. Heath MS, Ortega-Loayza AG. Insights Into the Pathogenesis of Sweet's Syndrome. Front Immunol 2019;10:414.

22. Wallach D, Vignon-Pennamen MD. Pyoderma gangrenosum and Sweet syndrome: the prototypic neutrophilic dermatoses. Br J Dermatol 2018; 178(3):595–602.

23. Wilson-Jones E, Winkelmann RK. Superficial granulomatous pyoderma: a localized vegetative form of pyoderma gangrenosum. J Am Acad Dermatol 1988;18(3):511–21.

24. Gibson LE. Superficial granulomatous pyoderma: who are you? J Eur Acad Dermatol Venereol 2002; 16(2):97.

25. Sanchez IM, Lowenstein S, Johnson KA, et al. Clinical Features of Neutrophilic Dermatosis Variants Resembling Necrotizing Fasciitis. JAMA Dermatol 2019;155(1):79–84.

26. Stevens DL, Bryant AE. Necrotizing Soft-Tissue Infections. N Engl J Med 2017;377(23):2253–65.

27. Callen JP. Necrotizing Neutrophilic Dermatitis, an Often-Misdiagnosed Entity With Potentially Severe Consequences. JAMA Dermatol 2019;155(1):17–8.

28. Rahman S, Daveluy S. Pathergy Test. (Updated 2023 May 1(. In: StatPearls (Internet). Treasure Island (FL): StatPearls Publishing; 2023 Jan-. Available from: https://www.ncbi.nlm.nih.gov/books/NBK558909/.

29. Schoch JJ, Tolkachjov SN, Cappel JA, et al. Pediatric Pyoderma Gangrenosum: A Retrospective Review of Clinical Features, Etiologic Associations, and Treatment. Pediatr Dermatol 2017;34(1):39–45.

30. Graham JA, Hansen KK, Rabinowitz LG, et al. Pyoderma gangrenosum in infants and children. Pediatr Dermatol 1994;11(1):10–7.

31. Crouse L, McShane D, Morrell DS, et al. Pyoderma gangrenosum in an infant: A case report and review of the literature. Pediatr Dermatol 2018;35(5): e257–61.

32. McAleer MA, Powell FC, Devaney D, et al. Infantile pyoderma gangrenosum. J Am Acad Dermatol 2008;58(2 Suppl):S23–8.

33. Steele RB, Nugent WH, Braswell SF, et al. Pyoderma gangrenosum and pregnancy: an example of abnormal inflammation and challenging treatment. Br J Dermatol 2016;174(1):77–87.

34. Greco A, De Virgilio A, Ralli M, et al. Behçet's disease: New insights into pathophysiology, clinical features and treatment options. Autoimmun Rev 2018;17(6):567–75.

35. Hagedorn JC, Wessells H. A contemporary update on Fournier's gangrene. Nat Rev Urol 2017;14(4): 205–14.

36. Al Ghazal P, Herberger K, Schaller J, et al. Associated factors and comorbidities in patients with pyoderma gangrenosum in Germany: a retrospective multicentric analysis in 259 patients. Orphanet J Rare Dis 2013;8:136.

37. Ashchyan HJ, Butler DC, Nelson CA, et al. The Association of Age With Clinical Presentation and Comorbidities of Pyoderma Gangrenosum. JAMA Dermatol 2018;154(4):409–13.

38. Binus AM, Qureshi AA, Li VW, et al. Pyoderma gangrenosum: a retrospective review of patient characteristics, comorbidities and therapy in 103 patients. Br J Dermatol 2011;165(6):1244–50.

39. Montagnon CM, Fracica EA, Patel AA, et al. Pyoderma gangrenosum in hematologic malignancies: A systematic review. J Am Acad Dermatol 2020; 82(6):1346–59.

40. von den Driesch P. Pyoderma gangrenosum: a report of 44 cases with follow-up. Br J Dermatol 1997;137(6):1000–5.

41. Burns DA, Sarkany I. Active chronic hepatitis and pyoderma gangrenosum: report of a case. Clin Exp Dermatol 1979;4(4):465–9.

42. Byrne JP, Hewitt M, Summerly R. Pyoderma gangrenosum associated with active chronic hepatitis: report of two cases. Arch Dermatol 1976;112(9):1297–301.

43. Keane FM, MacFarlane CS, Munn SE, et al. Pyoderma gangrenosum and hepatitis C virus infection. Br J Dermatol 1998;139(5):924–5.

44. Marshall AW, Slonim JM, Smallwood RA, et al. The association of chronic active hepatitis with pyoderma gangrenosum. Aust N Z J Med 1978;8(6): 656–8.

45. Akyol Ş, Ö Tüfekçi, Baysal B, et al. Abscess-like skin and lung lesions in a patient with acute lymphoblastic leukemia: Pyoderma gangrenosum. Pediatr Blood Cancer 2022;69(10):e29655.

46. Allen CP, Hull J, Wilkison N, et al. Pediatric pyoderma gangrenosum with splenic and pulmonary involvement. Pediatr Dermatol 2013;30(4):497–9.

47. Arai S, Furukawa N, Takahama M, et al. Extracutaneous neutrophilic infiltration of the spleen and lung associated with pyoderma gangrenosum of the skin. Clin Exp Dermatol 2022;47(4):775–8.

48. Brown TS, Marshall GS, Callen JP. Cavitating pulmonary infiltrate in an adolescent with pyoderma gangrenosum: a rarely recognized extracutaneous manifestation of a neutrophilic dermatosis. J Am Acad Dermatol 2000;43(1 Pt 1):108–12.

49. Contreras-Verduzco FA, Espinosa-Padilla SE, Orozco-Covarrubias L, et al. Pulmonary nodules and nodular scleritis in a teenager with superficial granulomatous pyoderma gangrenosum. Pediatr Dermatol 2018;35(1):e35–8.

50. Field S, Powell FC, Young V, et al. Pyoderma gangrenosum manifesting as a cavitating lung lesion. Clin Exp Dermatol 2008;33(4):418–21.

51. Kasuga I, Yanagisawa N, Takeo C, et al. Multiple pulmonary nodules in association with pyoderma gangrenosum. Respir Med 1997;91(8):493–5.

52. Lebbé C, Moulonguet-Michau I, Perrin P, et al. Steroid-responsive pyoderma gangrenosum with vulvar

and pulmonary involvement. J Am Acad Dermatol 1992;27(4):623–5.

53. Maritsi DN, Tavernaraki K, Vartzelis G. Pyoderma gangrenosum with systemic and pulmonary involvement in a toddler. Pediatr Int 2015;57(3):505–6.

54. McCulloch AJ, McEvoy A, Jackson JD, et al. Severe steroid responsive pneumonitis associated with pyoderma gangrenosum and ulcerative colitis. Thorax 1985;40(4):314–5.

55. Mercer JM, Kuzel P, Mahmood MN, et al. Fatal case of vulvar pyoderma gangrenosum with pulmonary involvement: case presentation and literature review. J Cutan Med Surg 2014;18(6):424–9.

56. Sakata KK, Penupolu S, Colby TV, et al. Pulmonary pyoderma gangrenosum without cutaneous manifestations. Clin Respir J 2016;10(4):508–11.

57. Scherlinger M, Guillet S, Doutre MS, et al. Pyoderma gangrenosum with extensive pulmonary involvement. J Eur Acad Dermatol Venereol 2017;31(4):e214–6.

58. Shands JW, Flowers FP, Hill HM, et al. Pyoderma gangrenosum in a kindred. Precipitation by surgery or mild physical trauma. J Am Acad Dermatol 1987; 16(5 Pt 1):931–4.

59. Vignon-Pennamen MD, Zelinsky-Gurung A, Janssen F, et al. Pyoderma gangrenosum with pulmonary involvement. Arch Dermatol 1989;125(9):1239–42.

60. Xing F, Chiu KH, Yang J, et al. Pyoderma gangrenosum with pulmonary involvement: a pulmonary special report and literature review. Expet Rev Respir Med 2022;16(2):149–59.

61. Chanson P, Timsit J, Kujas M, et al. Pituitary granuloma and pyoderma gangrenosum. J Endocrinol Invest 1990;13(8):677–81.

62. Cugno M, Borghi A, Marzano AV. PAPA, PASH and PAPASH Syndromes: Pathophysiology, Presentation and Treatment. Am J Clin Dermatol 2017;18(4): 555–62.

63. Lindor NM, Arsenault TM, Solomon I I, et al. A new autosomal dominant disorder of pyogenic sterile arthritis, pyoderma gangrenosum, and acne: PAPA syndrome. Mayo Clin Proc 1997;72(7):611–5.

64. Braun-Falco M, Kovnerystyy O, Lohse P, et al. Pyoderma gangrenosum, acne, and suppurative hidradenitis (PASH)–a new autoinflammatory syndrome distinct from PAPA syndrome. J Am Acad Dermatol 2012;66(3):409–15.

65. Marzano AV, Ceccherini I, Gattorno M, et al. Association of pyoderma gangrenosum, acne, and suppurative hidradenitis (PASH) shares genetic and cytokine profiles with other autoinflammatory diseases. Medicine (Baltim) 2014;93(27):e187.

66. Garzorz N, Papanagiotou V, Atenhan A, et al. Pyoderma gangrenosum, acne, psoriasis, arthritis and suppurative hidradenitis (PAPASH)-syndrome: a new entity within the spectrum of autoinflammatory syndromes? J Eur Acad Dermatol Venereol 2016; 30(1):141–3.

67. Marzano AV, Trevisan V, Gattorno M, et al. Pyogenic arthritis, pyoderma gangrenosum, acne, and hidradenitis suppurativa (PAPASH): a new autoinflammatory syndrome associated with a novel mutation of the PSTPIP1 gene. JAMA Dermatol 2013;149(6): 762–4.

68. Saraceno R, Babino G, Chiricozzi A, et al. PsAPASH: a new syndrome associated with hidradenitis suppurativa with response to tumor necrosis factor inhibition. J Am Acad Dermatol 2015;72(1):e42–4.

69. Montoto S, Bosch F, Estrach T, et al. Pyoderma gangrenosum triggered by alpha2b-interferon in a patient with chronic granulocytic leukemia. Leuk Lymphoma 1998;30(1–2):199–202.

70. Sanders S, Busam K, Tahan SR, et al. Granulomatous and suppurative dermatitis at interferon alfa injection sites: report of 2 cases. J Am Acad Dermatol 2002;46(4):611–6.

71. Yurci A, Guven K, Torun E, et al. Pyoderma gangrenosum and exacerbation of psoriasis resulting from pegylated interferon alpha and ribavirin treatment of chronic hepatitis C. Eur J Gastroenterol Hepatol 2007;19(9):811–5.

72. Lewerin C, Mobacken H, Nilsson-Ehle H, et al. Bullous pyoderma gangrenosum in a patient with myelodysplastic syndrome during granulocyte colony-stimulating factor therapy. Leuk Lymphoma 1997;26(5–6):629–32.

73. Mizushima M, Miyoshi H, Yonemori K. Pyoderma Gangrenosum After Total Hip Arthroplasty Associated with Administration of Granulocyte Colony-Stimulating Factor: A Case Report. JBJS Case Connect 2021;(2):11.

74. Ross HJ, Moy LA, Kaplan R, et al. Bullous pyoderma gangrenosum after granulocyte colony-stimulating factor treatment. Cancer 1991;68(2):441–3.

75. Takagi S, Ohsaka A, Taguchi H, et al. Pyoderma gangrenosum following cytosine arabinoside, aclarubicin and granulocyte colony-stimulating factor combination therapy in myelodysplastic syndrome. Intern Med 1998;37(3):316–9.

76. White LE, Villa MT, Petronic-Rosic V, et al. Pyoderma gangrenosum related to a new granulocyte colony-stimulating factor. Skinmed 2006;5(2):96–8.

77. Dean SM, Zirwas M. A Second Case of Sunitinib-associated Pyoderma Gangrenosum. J Clin Aesthet Dermatol 2010;3(8):34–5.

78. Freiman A, Brassard A. Pyoderma gangrenosum associated with isotretinoin therapy. J Am Acad Dermatol 2006;55(5 Suppl):S107–8.

79. Jeong HS, Layher H, Cao L, et al. Pyoderma gangrenosum (PG) associated with levamisole-adulterated cocaine: Clinical, serologic, and histopathologic findings in a cohort of patients. J Am Acad Dermatol 2016;74(5):892–8.

80. Srebrnik A, Shachar E, Brenner S. Suspected induction of a pyoderma gangrenosum-like

eruption due to sulpiride treatment. Cutis 2001; 67(3):253–6.

81. ten Freyhaus K, Homey B, Bieber T, et al. Pyoderma gangrenosum: another cutaneous side-effect of sunitinib? Br J Dermatol 2008;159(1):242–3.

82. Tinoco MP, Tamler C, Maciel G, et al. Pyoderma gangrenosum following isotretinoin therapy for acne nodulocystic. Int J Dermatol 2008;47(9):953–6.

83. Ahronowitz I, Harp J, Shinkai K. Etiology and management of pyoderma gangrenosum: a comprehensive review. Am J Clin Dermatol 2012; 13(3):191–211.

84. Genovese G, Tavecchio S, Berti E, et al. Pyoderma gangrenosum-like ulcerations in granulomatosis with polyangiitis: two cases and literature review. Rheumatol Int 2018;38(6):1139–51.

85. Su WP, Schroeter AL, Perry HO, et al. Histopathologic and immunopathologic study of pyoderma gangrenosum. J Cutan Pathol 1986;13(5):323–30.

Postoperative and Peristomal Pyoderma Gangrenosum
Subtypes of Pyoderma Gangrenosum

Théodora Kipers, JD, MS[a], Stanislav N. Tolkachjov, MD[b],*

KEYWORDS

- Pyoderma gangrenosum • Postoperative pyoderma gangrenosum
- Peristomal pyoderma gangrenosum • Neutrophilic dermatoses • Ulcer • Neutrophil • Postsurgical
- Surgical wounds

KEY POINTS

- Both postoperative and peristomal pyoderma gangrenosum are diagnoses of exclusion, and they present as rapidly progressing ulcers with violaceous, irregular, and undermined borders.
- Postoperative pyoderma gangrenosum may occur after surgery or trauma.
- A majority of peristomal pyoderma gangrenosum cases occur in patients with inflammatory bowel disease.
- Effective management requires local or systemic immunomodulation and wound care.
- Surgical management for peristomal pyoderma gangrenosum may include stoma closure or relocation/revision but must be done with caution and while controlling inflammation with immunomodulation.

INTRODUCTION/BACKGROUND

Pyoderma gangrenosum (PG) is a type of dermatosis characterized by inflammation, ulcers, and an abundance of neutrophils. It can emerge following trauma at any site on the skin. Louis-Anne-Jean Brocq first described this skin disorder in 1916 followed by Brunsting and colleagues in 1930.[1] Patients with PG often have an underlying systemic illness, with the most common associated being inflammatory bowel disease (IBD). Other associated diseases include inflammatory arthritis, myeloproliferative disorders, solid organ malignancies, and hepatitis, particularly hepatitis C.[2,3] There are 4 clinical subtypes of PG: classic ulcerative, pustular, bullous (or atypical), and vegetative (superficial granulomatous) PG.[4] The classic ulcerative subtype typically starts as a pustule on an erythematous or violaceous base that then rapidly transforms into an ulcer with a necrotic undermined border.[4] Pustular PG, frequently linked to IBD, manifests as a generalized pustular eruption without eventual ulceration.[4] The bullous (atypical) form presents as painful superficial blisters to bullae with associated necrosis and erosion and is seen in the setting of myeloproliferative disease.[4] Vegetative PG is commonly found on the trunk, appearing as less painful, superficially ulcerative, and verrucous lesions.[4]

The clinical differential diagnosis associated with PG encompasses various conditions such as infections (commonly deep fungal infection), vasculitis, vasculopathies, neoplasms (eg, leukemia and

a School of Medicine, Texas A&M University School of Medicine, 5536 Tremont Street, Dallas, TX 75214, USA;
b Mohs Micrographic & Reconstructive Surgery, Epiphany Dermatology; Department of Dermatology, Baylor University Medical Center; University of Texas at Southwestern; Texas A&M University School of Medicine, 1640 FM 544, Suite 100, TX 75056, USA
* Corresponding author.
E-mail address: stan.tolkachjov@gmail.com

Dermatol Clin 42 (2024) 171–181
https://doi.org/10.1016/j.det.2023.12.001
0733-8635/24/© 2023 Elsevier Inc. All rights reserved.

lymphoma cutis, squamous or basal cell carcinoma, and other malignancies), drug reactions, and factitious ulcerations.[4,5] The histopathologic hallmark of PG involves the formation of dermal neutrophilic abscesses.[4] Pustular PG is characterized by the presence intraepidermal neutrophilic abscesses and perifollicular neutrophilic inflammation on histologic examination.[4] Bullous PG exhibits intraepidermal blister formation and intraepidermal neutrophilic abscesses, while vegetative PG is distinguished by epidermal hyperplasia and dermal granulomas.[4] The histopathologic differential diagnosis of PG includes infections and other neutrophilic dermatoses which may be on a clinical continuum (eg, Sweet syndrome, neutrophilic dermatosis of the dorsal hand, and bowel bypass syndrome).[4] Clinicopathologic correlations, tissue cultures, and special microorganism stains on skin biopsy sections including stains for bacteria, mycobacteria, and fungi are ways to distinguish the diagnosis.[4]

Pathergy is a phenomenon observed in PG, where pustular and subsequent ulcerative PG lesions develop at sites of trauma.[2,6] Unlike the Koebner phenomenon, which involves the appearance of disease-specific lesions in areas of trauma, pathergy refers to the formation of nonspecific lesions unrelated to the underlying disease and not necessarily limited to the skin.[4] Pathergy can be observed in various conditions such as Behcet's disease, PG, Sweet syndrome, and IBD.[4]

Postoperative Pyoderma Gangrenosum

Postoperative PG, also referred to as postsurgical or pathergic PG or postoperative progressive gangrene of Cullen, was described by Cullen in 1924[7] and is documented in various surgical disciplines such as orthopedic, cardiothoracic, general, plastic, and gynecologic fields.[4,8–13] The diagnosis is often delayed and initial treatment may be inappropriate due to its lack of recognition and resemblance of wound infection and necrotizing fasciitis (NF).[4,8] Debridement is often performed as a standard treatment for wound infection; however, this can be detrimental to postoperative PG due to pathergy.[4]

Postoperative PG is characterized by the development of PG-like lesions within surgical sites.[14,15] Postoperative PG can lead to slow wound healing and dehiscence.[4] A retrospective chart review by Tolkachjov and colleagues found it is more common at surgical sites of the breast (eg, breast reconstruction, reduction, or revision), with the nipple-areolar complex spared, and the abdomen in women.[1,8] This association of postoperative PG with breast surgery may be secondary to the

enhancement of the inflammatory and immunologic neutrophilic response to the skin of microbiologic agents in the mammary ducts.[16,17]

In postoperative PG, most patients do not have an underlying disorder, a direct contrast to PG. Tolkachjov and colleagues conducted a study revealing that 22% of patients with postoperative PG had associated systemic diseases.[8] An additional review of literature by Tolkachjov and colleagues found that 64% of postoperative PG patients had no underlying disease,[1] suggesting that surgical trauma alone might trigger this phenomenon. This observation is similar to that of superficial granulomatous pyoderma (SGP).[14] While postoperative PG often has the clinical appearance of SGP, it is typically very painful and rapidly ulcerates, as seen in classic PG.

Postoperative PG typically presents with initial erythema at the surgical site with extreme pain out of proportion to the clinical examination.[18] The onset of pain and symptoms usually occurs between 7 and 11 days after surgery or wound dehiscence.[8,19] The wound may develop small punctate ulcerations with discharge, eventually merging and dehiscing.[16] Patients report pain at the site usually without fever and it may be misdiagnosed as a wound infection, as disproportionate pain and rapid wound breakdown are hallmarks of NF.[4,8] NF may present with patchy discoloration of skin and poorly-defined erythema. This can be followed by tight edema, along with vesicles, bullae, or necrosis. Similar to postoperative PG, pain can be excessive compared to the clinical examination, but the critical distinction is that patients with NF can quickly become septic and systemically unwell.[20–22]

Ehrl and colleagues[23] established a set of diagnostic criteria in 2018 to aid in the diagnosis of postoperative PG based on a systematic review of PG after breast surgery. Major criteria included (1) rapid progression (1–2 cm/day or 50% increase in size of the ulcer within 1 month) of a necrolytic ulcer with a violaceous, irregular, and undermined border associated with pain out of proportion and (2) exclusion of other causes of cutaneous ulceration.[23,24] Minor criteria included (1) cribriform scarring or history or pathergy; (2) history of systemic disease such as IBD, immunoglobulin A gammopathy, rheumatoid arthritis (RA), or underlying malignancy; (3) sterile dermal neutrophilia with or without lymphocytic vasculitis with or without mixed inflammation on biopsy; and (4) rapid response to systemic corticosteroid treatment (1–2 mg/kg per day and a 50% decrease in size within 1 month).[23,24]

Due to the potential misdiagnosis of wound infection or NF, surgeons may initiate antibiotic therapy and wound debridement.[4] However, prolonged use of potent antibiotics may increase the risk of drug-resistant bacteria and lead to adverse drug reactions.[24] While the initiation of antibiotics can have anti-inflammatory effects and help with any superinfection, debridement can lead to further progression of the PG or due to pathergy and wound breakdown.[4] Being aware of pathergy and early recognition of postoperative PG, as well as consultation with a dermatologist, can facilitate accurate diagnosis and the timely initiation of appropriate treatment. A review of published cases on postoperative PG indicated a latency period ranging from symptom onset to diagnosis of 14 to 15 days.[1]

Postoperative PG continues to be a diagnosis of exclusion and needs to be correlated to clinical presentation, negative culture results, histologic characteristics, pathergy, and response to immunologic agents/systemic corticosteroids.[25] To rule out lesions caused by autoimmune diseases, blood work testing for antinuclear antibodies, rheumatoid factor, anticyclic citrullinated peptide antibodies, antineutrophilic cytoplasmic antibodies (ANCAs), antiphospholipid antibody assays, and possibly other markers should be obtained.[2] It is prudent for the patient to undergo testing for active bowel disease, infections, vasculitis, and malignancy.[26]

Time to resolution is variable and is dependent on the involved area, time to diagnosis, and therapy.[1] Yet due to how uncommon postoperative PG is as compared to wound infection, empirical antibiotic therapy should be initiated until infection and other causes can be effectively ruled out, being sure to not utilize antibiotics longer than necessary.[5] Prior to starting antibiotics, photographs and pan cultures are encouraged.[1] Ideally, debridement is avoided. If debridement takes place prior to the recognition of postoperative PG, a skin biopsy of the ulcer edge may be obtained and sent for routine histopathologic evaluation and tissue culture (ie, bacteria, fungi, mycobacteria). The risk of pathergy should not deter a diagnostic biopsy if PG is suspected. A full-thickness biopsy at the periphery of the ulcer will often show a neutrophilic ulcer with possible vasculitis, undermined edges, and confinement to the epidermis and dermis.[27] Systemic corticosteroids may be tried if the patient is not responding to topical corticosteroids or the postoperative PG is rapidly progressing.[28] If postoperative PG is recognized early, however, systemic corticosteroids are the first line. Signs of positive response are a rapid decrease in pain and the slowing of wound breakdown[1] **(Figs. 1–3) (Table 1).**

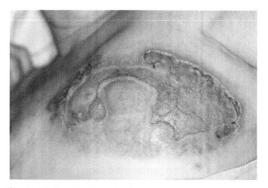

Fig. 1. Postoperative pyoderma gangrenosum encompassing the majority of the left periareolar breast with characteristic sparing of the nipple-areolar complex after a breast reduction. Painful, necrotic ulceration with slightly violaceous, undermined edges.[8]

Peristomal Pyoderma Gangrenosum

Peristomal PG (PPG) is a relatively uncommon condition, accounting for approximately 15% of all PG cases.[19] Its first report dates back to 1984 when 3 patients with Crohn's disease (CD) were identified with this condition.[19] PPG develops around a stoma site following surgical placement of an ileostomy or colostomy, often associated with underlying IBD.[29] IBD was seen in 80% of cases of PPG, while 30% to 65% of patients with PG had IBD.[29–36] A literature review conducted by Afifi and colleagues[37] on PPG cases revealed that most patients with PPG were female and had a diagnosis of IBD. The average age of patients was 48 years old, with those having CD or ulcerative colitis being younger than those patients without IBD.[37] Additionally, most patients reported a concurrent flare of the underlying systemic

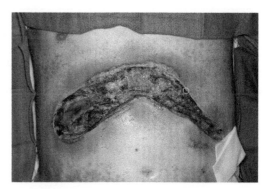

Fig. 2. Postoperative pyoderma gangrenosum of the abdomen after insulinoma resection. The green circle corresponds to the suggested skin biopsy site for peristomal pyoderma gangrenosum. (Tolkachjov SN, Fahy AS, Cerci FB, Wetter DA, Cha SS, Camilleri MJ. Postoperative Pyoderma Gangrenosum: A Clinical Review of Published Cases. Mayo Clin Proc. 2016;91(9):1267-1279.)

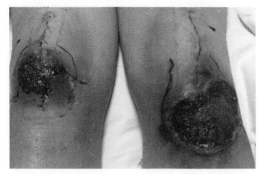

Fig. 3. Postoperative pyoderma gangrenosum of bilateral knees. (Used with permission of Mayo Foundation for Medical Education and Research, all rights reserved.)

disease at the time of PPG onset.[37] Clinically, PPG is characterized by a painful, erythematous, rapidly progressing ulcer with undermined, irregular, and violaceous borders.[37]

The occurrence of PPG after stoma creation may be variable, ranging from 1.5 months to greater than 23 months.[37] PPG may be misdiagnosed as a suture abscess, contact dermatitis, irritation from stoma leakage, infection, or extension of underlying CD.[19] Skin biopsies and cultures play a crucial role in diagnosing PPG. Cultures are particularly helping in ruling out infection since PPG ulcers are either sterile or grow commensal skin and gut flora.[38] In conditions that do not typically present with ulcerations such as contact dermatitis, ulcers may appear in the peristomal region due to exposure to enzyme-rich ileal output, leading to erosions.[39]

Various conditions can present with similar symptoms to PPG, making the differential diagnosis essential. These include trauma, infection, ischemia, drug-induced lupus, brown recluse spider bite, folliculitis, and malignancy.[40,41] PPG is a diagnosis of exclusion; however, misdiagnosis and resultant inappropriate treatment can lead to adverse outcomes such as decreased quality of life and potential life-threatening sequelae

Table 1
Considerations when approaching postoperative pyoderma gangrenosum[1]

Postoperative Approach	Consideration
Consider demographic characteristics of the patient	Female sex Age: 45–50y Previous pyoderma gangrenosum Systemic disease Breast or abdomen involvement
Consider presentation	Severe pain Nonhealing wound Wound dehiscence Time: about 7d postoperatively Violaceous undermined border Rapid evolution Refractory to antibiotic drug therapy Refractory to or worsening with debridement Negative wound cultures
Perform evaluation and management	Obtain photographs of affected tissue area Obtain pan cultures (ie, bacteria, fungi, and mycobacteria) Initiate broad spectrum or site-specific antibiotic drug therapy Consider skin biopsy alone or during debridement of ulcer edge and send for routine histopathologic evaluation and tissue culture (ie, bacteria, fungi, and mycobacteria) Consider dermatologic evaluation or dermatologic teleconsultation
Consider trial of systemic corticosteroids if not responding to topical corticosteroids or postoperative PG is rapidly progressing	If ulceration is unresponsive to standard treatment, has the clinical characteristics of postoperative PG, and exhibits rapid progression despite debridement and negative wound cultures Corticosteroid-sparing agents may be added, with a slow taper in corticosteroid administration

Abbreviation: PG, pyoderma gangrenosum.

like bowel evisceration through the abdominal wall.[37]

Risk factors contributing to pathergy development include peristomal hernias, repetitive peristomal stress, irritation from ostomy leakage or appliance change, and tension or ischemia due to the ostomy appliance.[42–47] PPG ulcers disrupt the adhesion of ostomy appliances, leading to leakage that then further aggravates PPG and delays wound healing.[48] Clinicians should consider the possibility of PPG in a patients exhibiting painful, rapidly expanding peristomal ulcers that do not respond to treatment, along with characteristic features of pathergy and concurrent IBD[37] (Fig 4) (Table 2).

PATHOPHYSIOLOGY

The etiology of PG remains uncertain, but research indicates that an overexpression of proinflammatory cytokines, including tumor necrosis factor-α and interleukin (IL)−1α, 1β, IL-8, IL-12, IL-15, IL-17, IL-23, IL-26, is involved in the pathogenesis.[49] As a consequence, autoinflammation occurs, leading to an imbalanced regulatory T-cell and T-helper 17 cell response, alongside abnormal neutrophil chemotaxis.[50–58] Variants of genes involved in inflammasome formation, such as PSTPIP1, MEFV, NLRP3, NLRP12, and NOD2, which lead to an excessive release of IL-1β, have been documented in PG cases.[49] Recent findings suggest that PG is a T-cell mediated disease, specifically targeting follicular adnexal structures.[59] Additional culprits of PG include the complement system, neutrophil-attractant anaphylatoxin C5a, NETosis, regulatory T-cell unbalance, B cells, fibroblasts, and monocytes/macrophages.[49] Research initiated due to the response of PG to ustekinumab, an IL-12/23 antagonist, demonstrated an overexpression

of IL-23 and a diminished ratio of regulator T-cell to T-helper 17 cells in the skin lesions of patients with PG.[51,60,61] A majority of cases do not report a personal or familial history of PG, but familial PG and PG in the setting of autoinflammatory syndromes have been described.[32]

Postoperative Pyoderma Gangrenosum

Pathergy in PG is most likely initiated by surgical trauma, leading to cytokine release and polymorphonuclear neutrophil (PMN) chemotaxis.[52,62] Predisposed individuals may experience an exaggerated response by PMNs to the surgery itself resulting in postoperative PG, rather than the systemic inflammation typically associated with co-morbid conditions related to nonsurgical PG.[53,63–65] This can be seen in major surgery or even minor procedures like skin excisions and phlebotomy.

Predisposing factors for postoperative PG may include genetic mutations in the coding of methylenetetrahydrofolate reductase and Janus kinase 2. However, these associations have only been reported in small case reports and have not been confirmed in all cases of PG.[32] Postoperative PG is likely a multifactorial response in a predisposed individual.

Peristomal Pyoderma Gangrenosum

The mechanism linking IBD and PG remains unknown, but it is believed to involve cross-reacting antigens in bowel and skin or shared pathways of autoinflammation.[66] In the context of IBD, the underlying pathogenesis of PPG involves proinflammatory immune complexes and cytokines from active bowel disease.[67,68] While the majority of PPG cases occur in patients with IBD, some patients may have stomas outside of IBD. Therefore, patients presenting without IBD should not be disregarded.[37]

TREATMENT

Treatment of PG depends on factors such as the underlying associated disease, the setting of the PG, and the extent of involvement. Typically, corticosteroids and corticosteroid-sparing agents are used as primary therapies. Corticosteroid-sparing agents include tetracyclines, dapsone, mycophenolate mofetil, intravenous immunoglobin, tumor necrosis factor-α inhibitors, and other immunomodulatory or immunosuppressive agents.[4] A new target for PG therapy is the Janus kinase/signal transducer and activator of transcription (JAK/STAT) signaling proinflammatory pathway.[69] Tofacitinib, a JAK-1 and JAK-3 inhibitor, has been

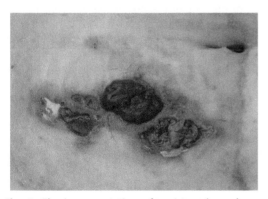

Fig. 4. Classic presentation of peristomal pyoderma gangrenosum, showing superficial ulcers with well-defined, undermined violaceous border and craterlike holes.[19]

Table 2
Considerations when approaching peristomal pyoderma gangrenosum

Postoperative Approach	Consideration
Consider demographic characteristics of the patient	Female sex Age: 45–50y History of IBD with possible current flare
Consider presentation	Pain Rapidly progressing ulcer Time: about 1.5–23 m after ostomy placement Violaceous undermined border Refractory to antibiotic drug therapy Negative wound cultures
Perform evaluation and management	Obtain photographs of affected tissue area Obtain pan cultures (ie, bacteria, fungi, and mycobacteria) Consider skin biopsy of ulcer edge and send for routine histopathologic evaluation and tissue culture (ie, bacteria, fungi, and mycobacteria) Consider dermatologic evaluation or dermatologic teleconsultation
Topical agents vs systemic therapy	Mild cases with no active IBD can be managed with topical corticosteroids and calcineurin and wound care Severe/rapidly progressing cases require systemic therapy (corticosteroids, cyclosporine, dapsone) Biologics and alternative treatments available Surgical management, if necessary

Abbreviation: IBD, inflammatory bowel disease.

successful in the treatment of refractory PG.[69] In cases where PG is associated with systemic disease, disease-specific therapy may be added to corticosteroids.[4] Surgical intervention such as split-thickness skin grafting (STSG), along with associated immunosuppressive therapy, can be considered to expedite wound healing, though this approach remains somewhat controversial.[4] Commonly used dressings for PG ulcers are antimicrobial dressings and hyperabsorbent dressings.[70] These dressings require less frequent changes and manipulation.[70]

Postoperative Pyoderma Gangrenosum

The treatment of postoperative PG closely resembles that of typical PG. The primary therapies, as supported by the literature, include systemic corticosteroids and cyclosporine, either as standalone treatments or in combination.[18] The positive response to treatment is characterized by rapid improvement in erythema and edema, accompanied by pain relief.[9] The duration of immunotherapy treatment may vary, ranging from single dose to up to 2 years.[23] Although corticosteroids are the gold standard, the Study of Treatments for PG (STOP GAP) randomized controlled trial reported a failed response to corticosteroid therapy.[28,71] In this trial, only 47% of patients achieved complete ulcer

recovery at 6 months with the use of either oral prednisolone or oral cyclosporine.[28,71] Less frequently used treatments are corticosteroid-sparing agents (either with or without systemic corticosteroids), anti-inflammatory antibiotics, topical therapy, and hyperbaric oxygen.[18] While most investigators recommend against surgery due to the potential for pathergy, some reported surgical interventions such as full-thickness, split-thickness, pinch grafts, and radical debridement as potential therapeutic options.[16,72–74] In cases where surgery is pursued, perioperative immunomodulators or corticosteroids should be administered in conjunction to surgical intervention.[18,72,73,75–80] A partial response is more likely to be seen in male patients and those with comorbid conditions.[8] Recurrence or no response is more likely in patients with prior PG.[8]

Patients with a history of PG (up to 21% of postoperative PG cases occur in patients with prior disease[18]) or a history of prolonged wound healing may be at an increased risk for postoperative PG.[1] Additionally individuals undergoing surgeries involving the breast or abdomen or those with hematologic dyscrasias, IBD, RA, and genetic syndromes commonly associated with PG may be at an increased risk of developing postoperative PG.[81,82] Perioperative corticosteroid coverage should be considered in patients at increased risk when surgery is unavoidable.[1] A systematic review by Tuffaha and colleagues[83] demonstrated success in 9 out of 12 cases when patients received corticosteroid therapy prior to undergoing STSG reconstruction of PG breast wounds.[24] However, for patients with a history of postoperative PG, perioperative immunosuppressive treatment may not always be necessary. A case report described a patient with a history of postoperative PG who declined perioperative corticosteroids during a series of surgeries over a 10 year period without recurrence.[84] Patients with a history of PG, RA, IBD, or hematologic malignancy who underwent breast, cardiothoracic, or abdominal surgeries and were administered perioperative corticosteroids had favorable outcomes as shown in a systematic review by Zuo and colleagues.[18] To prevent postoperative PG, it has been suggested by Long and colleagues[76] to close surgical wound edges only by subcuticular synthetic sutures and to avoid skin surface puncture and the presence of potentially proinflammatory materials but the literature on these techniques is limited.

Peristomal Pyoderma Gangrenosum

In contrast to other peristomal ulcers that often show improvement with conservative management and local wound care, the treatment of PPG requires long-term and multimodal approaches.[19,41–43]

Topical and systemic medications, such as corticosteroids, immunosuppressive agents, and biologic therapies, have been utilized with PPG, often in conjunction with surgical intervention, with no single treatment showing consistent efficacy.[19] Mild cases of PPG, not associated with active systemic disease, can often be effectively managed with topical agents.[37] Commonly, topical corticosteroids, calcineurin inhibitors, and wound care are used in these cases.[19]

For severe or rapidly progressing PPG, systemic therapies are employed.[37] These treatments include systemic corticosteroids, with similar effectiveness observed for cyclosporine and dapsone.[37] Less commonly used therapies but still effective alternatives are systemic metronidazole, azathioprine, sulfasalazine, and tacrolimus.[37] In cases of refractory PPG, intravenous immunoglobulin may be considered.[37] Tumor necrosis factor–α inhibitors, such as infliximab and adalimumab, may provide concomitant control of any active IBD.[37] Etanercept and ustekinumab have also demonstrated effectiveness in the treatment of PPG.[37] Newer therapies have shown promising results for those patients with IBD and include topical crushed prednisone,[45] topical sucralfate,[85] cultured keratinocyte autografts,[86] mycophenolate mofetil,[87–89]

and other biologic agents, such as the JAK/STAT inhibitors used for PG.[61,90–92]

Surgical management of PPG is indicated in cases of intractability, severe colitis, or the presence of complications such as perforation, stenosis, bowel obstruction, herniation, perianal disease, and dysplasia.[37] A retrospective chart review conducted by Barbosa and colleagues found that stoma closure or relocation/revision resulted in a complete response in all studied patients.[19] Complete closure had a zero recurrence rate; however, recurrence was very high in patients who underwent relocation/revision.[19] Stoma-related complications including ischemia, prolapse, stenosis, bowel obstruction, parastomal hernia, recalcitrant peristomal skin irritation, or ulceration may provide reason for relocation or revision.[19] It is essential to avoid aggressive debridement during inflammation to minimize pathergy, but gentle debridement can be beneficial in removing nonviable tissue.[41,43]

Wound care is important for PPG management with the goals being to provide a clean wound environment, absorb exudate, maintain moisture, and prevent additional skin irritation or maceration.[93] Occlusive dressings should be employed to create a protective barrier against infection while promoting reepithelialization, angiogenesis, and collagen synthesis.[29] Using nonadherent dressings can reduce the risk of minor skin trauma.[41] To minimize pathergy risk, it is essential to limit adhesion and pressure, prevent wound disruption during appliance changes, and avoiding leakage through proper fit.[37]

Overall it was found that providing adequate immunomodulator coverage during surgery could potentially reduce the recurrence of PPG.[19] Despite availability of treatment options, the recurrence rate of PPG remains high at 61%, confirming the challenging nature of this condition.[40] Consequently, effective PPG management requires a multidisciplinary approach involving wound care nurses, gastroenterologists, surgeons, and dermatologists working collaboratively.[37] (Table 3).

PG is a rare cutaneous inflammatory condition that, if left untreated, can result in significant morbidity and deformity, especially following surgery or stomal placement. Postoperative PG and PPG are uncommon subtypes of PG. Keys to successful management include early suspicion for any nonhealing wound at or near the incision line that does not respond to therapy. First-line therapy involves the use of topical and systemic corticosteroids, with alternative treatments available for cases that are unresponsive to initial therapy. Surgical stoma closure and relocation have shown promise in cases of PPG, but this should be done with caution and with immunomodulation,

Table 3
Treatment options for postoperative pyoderma gangrenosum and peristomal pyoderma gangrenosum

	Postoperative Pyoderma Gangrenosum	Peristomal Pyoderma Gangrenosum
Systemic therapy	Corticosteroids or cyclosporine Corticosteroids-sparing agents may be used alone or in conjunction with corticosteroids	Used for severe or rapidly progressing peristomal pyoderma gangrenosum Includes corticosteroid, cyclosporine, dapsone Alternatives include metronidazole, azathioprine, sulfasalazine, tacrolimus
Biologic agents and other therapies	Anti-inflammatory antibiotics Topical corticosteroids Hyperbaric oxygen	Infliximab, adalimumab Etanercept, ustekinumab Tofacitinib
Surgical management	Usually discouraged Potential therapeutic options include full-thickness, split-thickness, pinch grafts, radical debridement Consider perioperative corticosteroid coverage when surgery unavoidable	Stoma closure or relocation/revision Gentle debridement for removal of nonviable tissue which must be done while the patient is on immunomodulatory therapy to avoid further pathergy
Wound care	Subcuticular synthetic sutures to close wound edges Avoid skin surface puncture and the presence of proinflammatory materials	Occlusive, nonadherent dressings

as pathergy can lead to additional ulceration at surgical sites.

CLINICS CARE POINTS

- Early recognition of postoperative and peristomal pyoderma gangrenosum may help prevent improper therapy like debridement.
- After a proper diagnosis is made, immunomodulating therapy should be initiated to treat active inflammatory pyoderma gangrenosum.
- Gentle wound care in conjunction with immunomodulation must be done during active therapy until wound healing occurs or a chronic non-inflammatory wound remains, which can be treated with wound care alone.
- The patients and their treating providers should be aware of the chance for recurrence with future trauma or surgery.

DISCLOSURE

T. Kipers: No disclosures or conflicts of interest; S.N. Tolkachjov: Speaker: Bioventus/LifeNet; CASTLE Biosciences; Investigator: Bioventus; CASTLE Biosciences.

REFERENCES

1. Tolkachjov SN, Fahy AS, Cerci FB, et al. Postoperative Pyoderma Gangrenosum: A Clinical Review of Published Cases. Mayo Clin Proc 2016;91(9):1267–79.
2. Callen JP, Jackson JM. Pyoderma gangrenosum: an update. Rheum Dis Clin N Am 2007;33(4):787–802, vi.
3. Ashchyan HJ, Butler DC, Nelson CA, et al. The Association of Age With Clinical Presentation and Comorbidities of Pyoderma Gangrenosum. JAMA Dermatol 2018;154(4):409–13.
4. Tolkachjov SN, Wetter DA, Fahy AS, et al. Necrotic ulcerations after splenectomy. Int J Dermatol 2015;54(3):251–4.
5. Weenig RH, Davis MD, Dahl PR, et al. Skin ulcers misdiagnosed as pyoderma gangrenosum. N Engl J Med 2002;347(18):1412–8.
6. Boyd AS, Neldner KH. The isomorphic response of Koebner. Int J Dermatol 1990;29(6):401–10.
7. Grillo MA, Cavalheiro TT, da Silva Mulazani M, et al. Postsurgical pyoderma gangrenosum complicating reduction mammaplasty. Aesthetic Plast Surg 2012;36(6):1347–52.

8. Tolkachjov SN, Fahy AS, Wetter DA, et al. Postoperative pyoderma gangrenosum (PG): the Mayo Clinic experience of 20 years from 1994 through 2014. J Am Acad Dermatol 2015;73(4):615–22.

9. Davis MD, Alexander JL, Prawer SE. Pyoderma gangrenosum of the breasts precipitated by breast surgery. J Am Acad Dermatol 2006;55(2):317–20.

10. de Thomasson E, Caux I. Pyoderma gangrenosum following an orthopedic surgical procedure. Orthop Traumatol Surg Res 2010;96(5):600–2.

11. Bryan CS. Fatal pyoderma gangrenosum with pathergy after coronary artery bypass grafting. Tex Heart Inst J 2012;39(6):894–7.

12. Guth U, Wagner S, Huang DJ, et al. Pyoderma gangrenosum of the vaginal vault after vaginal hysterectomy: only the correct diagnosis of a rare entity can prevent long-term morbidity. Arch Gynecol Obstet 2013;288(1):79–82.

13. Liaqat M, Elsensohn AN, Hansen CD, et al. Acute postoperative pyoderma gangrenosum case and review of literature identifying chest wall predominance and no recurrence following skin grafts. J Am Acad Dermatol 2014;71(4):e145–6.

14. Quimby SR, Gibson LE, Winkelmann RK. Superficial granulomatous pyoderma: clinicopathologic spectrum. Mayo Clin Proc 1989;64(1):37–43.

15. Wilson-Jones E, Winkelmann RK. Superficial granulomatous pyoderma: a localized vegetative form of pyoderma gangrenosum. J Am Acad Dermatol 1988;18(3):511–21.

16. Ouazzani A, Berthe JV, de Fontaine S. Post-surgical pyoderma gangrenosum: a clinical entity. Acta Chir Belg 2007;107(4):424–8.

17. Collis N, Mirza S, Stanley PR, et al. Reduction of potential contamination of breast implants by the use of 'nipple shields'. Br J Plast Surg 1999;52(6):445–7.

18. Zuo KJ, Fung E, Tredget EE, et al. A systematic review of post-surgical pyoderma gangrenosum: identification of risk factors and proposed management strategy. J Plast Reconstr Aesthetic Surg 2015;68(3):295–303.

19. Barbosa NS, Tolkachjov SN, El-Azhary RA, et al. Clinical features, causes, treatments, and outcomes of peristomal pyoderma gangrenosum (PPG) in 44 patients: The Mayo Clinic experience, 1996 through 2013. J Am Acad Dermatol 2016;75(5):931–9.

20. Bisarya K, Azzopardi S, Lye G, et al. Necrotizing fasciitis versus pyoderma gangrenosum: securing the correct diagnosis! A case report and literature review. Eplasty 2011;11:e24.

21. Green RJ, Dafoe DC, Raffin TA. Necrotizing fasciitis. Chest 1996;110(1):219–29.

22. Wilkerson R, Paull W, Coville FV. Necrotizing fasciitis. Review of the literature and case report. Clin Orthop Relat Res 1987;216:187–92.

23. Ehrl DC, Heidekrueger PI, Broer PN. Pyoderma gangrenosum after breast surgery: A systematic review. J Plast Reconstr Aesthetic Surg 2018;71(7):1023–32.

24. Hammond D, Chaudhry A, Anderson D, et al. Postsurgical Pyoderma Gangrenosum After Breast Surgery: A Plea for Early Suspicion, Diagnosis, and Treatment. Aesthetic Plast Surg 2020;44(6):2032–40.

25. Su WP, Davis MD, Weenig RH, et al. Pyoderma gangrenosum: clinicopathologic correlation and proposed diagnostic criteria. Int J Dermatol 2004;43(11):790–800.

26. Edinger KM, Rao VK. The Management of Postsurgical Pyoderma Gangrenosum following Breast Surgery. Plast Reconstr Surg Glob Open 2022;10(4):e4282.

27. Touil LL, Gurusinghe DA, Sadri A, et al. Postsurgical Pyoderma Gangrenosum Versus Necrotizing Fasciitis: Can We Spot the Difference? Ann Plast Surg 2017;78(5):582–6.

28. Ormerod AD, Thomas KS, Craig FE, et al. Comparison of the two most commonly used treatments for pyoderma gangrenosum: results of the STOP GAP randomised controlled trial. BMJ 2015;350:h2958.

29. Ahronowitz I, Harp J, Shinkai K. Etiology and management of pyoderma gangrenosum: a comprehensive review. Am J Clin Dermatol 2012;13(3):191–211.

30. Brooklyn T, Dunnill G, Probert C. Diagnosis and treatment of pyoderma gangrenosum. BMJ 2006;333(7560):181–4.

31. Callen JP. Pyoderma gangrenosum. Lancet 1998;351(9102):581–5.

32. DeFilippis EM, Feldman SR, Huang WW. The genetics of pyoderma gangrenosum and implications for treatment: a systematic review. Br J Dermatol 2015;172(6):1487–97.

33. Mir-Madjlessi SH, Taylor JS, Farmer RG. Clinical course and evolution of erythema nodosum and pyoderma gangrenosum in chronic ulcerative colitis: a study of 42 patients. Am J Gastroenterol 1985;80(8):615–20.

34. Powell FC, Su WP, Perry HO. Pyoderma gangrenosum: classification and management. J Am Acad Dermatol 1996;34(3):395–409 [quiz 410-392].

35. Weizman A, Huang B, Berel D, et al. Clinical, serologic, and genetic factors associated with pyoderma gangrenosum and erythema nodosum in inflammatory bowel disease patients. Inflamm Bowel Dis 2014;20(3):525–33.

36. Wu XR, Shen B. Diagnosis and management of parastomal pyoderma gangrenosum. Gastroenterol Rep (Oxf) 2013;1(1):1–8.

37. Afifi L, Sanchez IM, Wallace MM, et al. Diagnosis and management of peristomal pyoderma gangrenosum: A systematic review. J Am Acad Dermatol 2018;78(6):1195–1204 e1191.

38. Ye MJ, Ye JM. Pyoderma gangrenosum: a review of clinical features and outcomes of 23 cases requiring inpatient management. Dermatol Res Pract 2014; 2014:461467.

39. Ng CS, Wolfsen HC, Kozarek RA, et al. Chronic parastomal ulcers: spectrum of dermatoses. J Nurs 1992;19(3):85–90.

40. Hughes AP, Jackson JM, Callen JP. Clinical features and treatment of peristomal pyoderma gangrenosum. JAMA 2000;284(12):1546–8.

41. Kiran RP, O'Brien-Ermlich B, Achkar JP, et al. Management of peristomal pyoderma gangrenosum. Dis Colon Rectum 2005;48(7):1397–403.

42. McGarity WC, Robertson DB, McKeown PP, et al. Pyoderma gangrenosum at the parastomal site in patients with Crohn's disease. Arch Surg 1984; 119(10):1186–8.

43. Lyon CC, Smith AJ, Beck MH, et al. Parastomal pyoderma gangrenosum: clinical features and management. J Am Acad Dermatol 2000;42(6): 992–1002.

44. Ahmadi S, Powell FC. Pyoderma gangrenosum: uncommon presentations. Clin Dermatol 2005;23(6): 612–20.

45. DeMartyn LE, Faller NA, Miller L. Treating peristomal pyoderma gangrenosum with topical crushed prednisone: a report of three cases. Ostomy/Wound Manag 2014;60(6):50–4.

46. Ohashi T, Yasunobu K, Yamamoto T. Peristomal pyoderma gangrenosum: A report of three cases. J Dermatol 2015;42(8):837–8.

47. Vornehm ND, Kelley SR, Ellis BJ. Parastomal small bowel evisceration as a result of parastomal pyoderma gangrenosum in a patient with Crohn's disease. Am Surg 2011;77(7):E150–1.

48. Lyon CC, Smith AJ, Griffiths CE, et al. The spectrum of skin disorders in abdominal stoma patients. Br J Dermatol 2000;143(6):1248–60.

49. Maronese CA, Pimentel MA, Li MM, et al. Pyoderma Gangrenosum: An Updated Literature Review on Established and Emerging Pharmacological Treatments. Am J Clin Dermatol 2022;23(5):615–34.

50. Oka M, Berking C, Nesbit M, et al. Interleukin-8 overexpression is present in pyoderma gangrenosum ulcers and leads to ulcer formation in human skin xenografts. Lab Invest 2000;80(4):595–604.

51. Caproni M, Antiga E, Volpi W, et al. The Treg/Th17 cell ratio is reduced in the skin lesions of patients with pyoderma gangrenosum. Br J Dermatol 2015; 173(1):275–8.

52. Malech HL, Gallin JI. Current concepts: immunology. Neutrophils in human diseases. N Engl J Med 1987;317(11):687–94.

53. Adachi Y, Kindzelskii AL, Cookingham G, et al. Aberrant neutrophil trafficking and metabolic oscillations in severe pyoderma gangrenosum. J Invest Dermatol 1998;111(2):259–68.

54. Johnson ML, Grimwood RE. Leukocyte colony-stimulating factors. A review of associated neutrophilic dermatoses and vasculitides. Arch Dermatol 1994;130(1):77–81.

55. Su WP, Schroeter AL, Perry HO, et al. Histopathologic and immunopathologic study of pyoderma gangrenosum. J Cutan Pathol 1986;13(5):323–30.

56. Wollina U, Haroske G. Pyoderma gangraenosum. Curr Opin Rheumatol 2011;23(1):50–6.

57. Braswell SF, Kostopoulos TC, Ortega-Loayza AG. Pathophysiology of pyoderma gangrenosum (PG): an updated review. J Am Acad Dermatol 2015;73(4):691–8.

58. Marzano AV, Borghi A, Meroni PL, et al. Pyoderma gangrenosum and its syndromic forms: evidence for a link with autoinflammation. Br J Dermatol 2016;175(5):882–91.

59. Wang EA, Steel A, Luxardi G, et al. Classic Ulcerative Pyoderma Gangrenosum Is a T Cell-Mediated Disease Targeting Follicular Adnexal Structures: A Hypothesis Based on Molecular and Clinicopathologic Studies. Front Immunol 2017;8:1980.

60. Marzano AV, Fanoni D, Antiga E, et al. Expression of cytokines, chemokines and other effector molecules in two prototypic autoinflammatory skin diseases, pyoderma gangrenosum and Sweet's syndrome. Clin Exp Immunol 2014;178(1):48–56.

61. Guenova E, Teske A, Fehrenbacher B, et al. Interleukin 23 expression in pyoderma gangrenosum and targeted therapy with ustekinumab. Arch Dermatol 2011;147(10):1203–5.

62. Miller ME. Pathology of chemotaxis and random mobility. Semin Hematol 1975;12(1):59–82.

63. Prat L, Bouaziz JD, Wallach D, et al. Neutrophilic dermatoses as systemic diseases. Clin Dermatol 2014;32(3):376–88.

64. Vignon-Pennamen MD, Wallach D. Cutaneous manifestations of neutrophilic disease. A study of seven cases. Dermatol 1991;183(4):255–64.

65. Wallach D, Vignon-Pennamen MD. From acute febrile neutrophilic dermatosis to neutrophilic disease: forty years of clinical research. J Am Acad Dermatol 2006;55(6):1066–71.

66. Boh EE, al-Smadi RM. Cutaneous manifestations of gastrointestinal diseases. Dermatol Clin 2002; 20(3):533–46.

67. Tjandra JJ, Hughes LE. Parastomal pyoderma gangrenosum in inflammatory bowel disease. Dis Colon Rectum 1994;37(9):938–42.

68. Cairns BA, Herbst CA, Sartor BR, et al. Peristomal pyoderma gangrenosum and inflammatory bowel disease. Arch Surg 1994;129(7):769–72.

69. Orfaly VE, Kovalenko I, Tolkachjov SN, et al. Tofacitinib for the treatment of refractory pyoderma gangrenosum. Clin Exp Dermatol 2021;46(6):1082–5.

70. Strunck JL, Cutler B, Latour E, et al. Wound care dressings for pyoderma gangrenosum. J Am Acad Dermatol 2022;86(2):458–60.

71. Soto Vilches F, Vera-Kellet C. Pyoderma gangreno-sum: Classic and emerging therapies. Med Clin 2017;149(6):256–60.

72. Cabalag MS, Wasiak J, Lim SW, et al. Inpatient man-agement of pyoderma gangrenosum: treatments, outcomes, and clinical implications. Ann Plast Surg 2015;74(3):354–60.

73. Shands JW Jr, Flowers FP, Hill HM, et al. Pyoderma gangrenosum in a kindred. Precipitation by surgery or mild physical trauma. J Am Acad Dermatol 1987; 16(5 Pt 1):931–4.

74. Saracino A, Kelly R, Liew D, et al. Pyoderma gangre-nosum requiring inpatient management: a report of 26 cases with follow up. Australas J Dermatol 2011;52(3):218–21.

75. Seok HH, Kang MS, Jin US. Treatment of atypical pyoderma gangrenosum on the face. Arch Plast Surg 2013;40(4):463–5.

76. Long CC, Jessop J, Young M, et al. Minimizing the risk of post-operative pyoderma gangrenosum. Br J Dermatol 1992;127(1):45–8.

77. Cliff S, Holden CA, Thomas PR, et al. Split skin grafts in the treatment of pyoderma gangrenosum. A report of four cases. Dermatol Surg 1999;25(4): 299–302.

78. Havlik RJ, Giles PD, Havlik NL. Pyoderma gangreno-sum of the breast: sequential grafting. Plast Re-constr Surg 1998;101(7):1909–14.

79. Rozen SM, Nahabedian MY, Manson PN. Manage-ment strategies for pyoderma gangrenosum: case studies and review of literature. Ann Plast Surg 2001;47(3):310–5.

80. Kaddoura IL, Amm C. A rationale for adjuvant surgi-cal intervention in pyoderma gangrenosum. Ann Plast Surg 2001;46(1):23–8.

81. Marzano AV, Trevisan V, Gattorno M, et al. Pyogenic arthritis, pyoderma gangrenosum, acne, and hidra-denitis suppurativa (PAPASI I): a new autoinflamma-tory syndrome associated with a novel mutation of the PSTPIP1 gene. JAMA Dermatol 2013;149(6): 762–4.

82. Smith EJ, Allantaz F, Bennett L, et al. Clinical, Molec-ular, and Genetic Characteristics of PAPA Syn-drome: A Review. Curr Genom 2010;11(7):519–27.

83. Tuffaha SH, Sarhane KA, Mundinger GS, et al. Pyo-derma Gangrenosum After Breast Surgery: Diag-nostic Pearls and Treatment Recommendations Based on a Systematic Literature Review. Ann Plast Surg 2016;77(2):e39–44.

84. Canzoneri CN, Taylor DL, Freet DJ. Is Prophylactic Immunosuppressive Therapy for Patients with a His-tory of Postsurgical Pyoderma Gangrenosum Necessary? J Cutan Aesthetic Surg 2018;11(4): 234–6.

85. Lyon CC, Stapleton M, Smith AJ, et al. Topical su-cralfate in the management of peristomal skin dis-ease: an open study. Clin Exp Dermatol 2000; 25(8):584–8.

86. Limova M, Mauro T. Treatment of pyoderma gangre-nosum with cultured keratinocyte autografts. J Dermatol Surg Oncol 1994;20(12):833–6.

87. Daniels NH, Callen JP. Mycophenolate mofetil is an effective treatment for peristomal pyoderma gangre-nosum. Arch Dermatol 2004;140(12):1427–9.

88. Eaton PA, Callen JP. Mycophenolate mofetil as ther-apy for pyoderma gangrenosum. Arch Dermatol 2009;145(7):781–5.

89. Wollina U, Karamfilov T. Treatment of recalcitrant ul-cers in pyoderma gangrenosum with mycopheno-late mofetil and autologous keratinocyte transplantation on a hyaluronic acid matrix. J Eur Acad Dermatol Venereol 2000;14(3):187–90.

90. Alkhouri N, Hupertz V, Mahajan L. Adalimumab treatment for peristomal pyoderma gangrenosum associated with Crohn's disease. Inflamm Bowel Dis 2009;15(6):803–6.

91. Goldminz AM, Botto NC, Gottlieb AB. Severely recalcitrant pyoderma gangrenosum successfully treated with ustekinumab. J Am Acad Dermatol 2012;67(5):e237–8.

92. Kloinponning MM, Langcwoutors AM, Van Do Kerkhof PC, et al. Severe pyoderma gangrenosum unresponsive to etanercept and adalimumab. J Dermatol Treat 2011;22(5):261–5.

93. Stamm L, Swatske ME, Hickey S, et al. Caring for the patient with peristomal pyoderma gangrenosum. J Wound, Ostomy Cont Nurs 1995;22(5):237–41.

Treatment of Pyoderma Gangrenosum

Marcus G. Tan, MD, FAAD, FRCPC[a,1,*], Stanislav N. Tolkachjov, MD, FAAD, FACMS[b]

KEYWORDS

- Pyoderma gangrenosum • Ulcer • Therapy • Treatment • Review • Neutrophil

KEY POINTS

- Pyoderma gangrenosum (PG) is a rare neutrophilic dermatosis that results in painful cutaneous ulcers and is frequently associated with underlying hematologic disorders, inflammatory bowel disease, or other autoimmune conditions.
- The pathogenesis involves dysregulation of both innate and adaptive immunity, with imbalance between proinflammatory and anti-inflammatory mediators, leading to neutrophilic inflammation and tissue damage.
- First-line treatment options with the best evidence are systemic corticosteroids, cyclosporine, and tumor necrosis factor alpha inhibitors. Topical corticosteroids, intralesional corticosteroids, and calcineurin inhibitors are often used as adjuncts and are well tolerated.
- Other steroid-sparing therapies include dapsone, mycophenolate mofetil, intravenous immunoglobulin, and targeted biologic or small molecule inhibitors.
- Patients without associated comorbidities respond better to treatment and suffered fewer adverse events. Wound care and management of underlying disorders are also critical parts of care.

INTRODUCTION

Pyoderma gangrenosum (PG) is a rare neutrophilic dermatosis that results in painful cutaneous ulcers. The classic lesion of PG begins as a tender pustule that rapidly enlarges into a painful, irregularly shaped ulcer with purulent base and gunmetal gray-violaceous undermined borders, and perilesional erythema. The ulcers typically heal with atrophic cribriform scars and dyspigmentation. Besides the ulcerative form of PG, other possible variants include bullous, pustular, vegetative, and peristomal presentation. PG most commonly affects the lower extremities but can occur anywhere including the genitalia.

The cause of PG remains unclear but approximately half of all patients presenting with PG have a concomitant underlying hematologic disorder, inflammatory bowel disease or other autoimmune disorders, or malignancy (**Box 1**). Certain medications have also been implicated in PG, including isotretinoin, propylthiouracil, and sunitinib. The diagnosis of PG requires clinicopathologic correlation and the exclusion of other potential causes of cutaneous ulceration. The diagnostic criteria of PG have been listed in **Table 1**.[1–7]

The pathogenesis of PG is complex and thought to be due to immune dysregulation in both the innate and adaptive immune pathways. PG lesions or serums of patients with PG have shown to contain elevated levels of proinflammatory molecules and cytokines C5a, interleukin (IL)-1, IL-4, IL-5 IL-8, IL-12, IL-15, IL-17, IL-23, IL-36, tumor necrosis factor alpha (TNF-α), Janus Kinase (JAK)-1,

Funding sources, IRB approval status, and patient consent: Not applicable.
[a] Division of Dermatology, University of Ottawa, 737 Parkdale Avenue, 4th Floor Dermatology, Ottawa, ON K1Y1J8, Canada; [b] Mohs Micrographic & Reconstructive Surgery, Epiphany Dermatology, Department of Dermatology, Baylor University Medical Center, University of Texas at Southwestern, Texas A&M University School of Medicine, 1640 FM 544, Suite 100, Lewisville, TX 75056, USA
[1] Present address: 1920 N Collins Boulevard, Richardson, TX 75080, USA
* Corresponding author.
E-mail address: marcusg.tan@gmail.com

Dermatol Clin 42 (2024) 183–192
https://doi.org/10.1016/j.det.2023.12.002

Hematologic disorders

- Monoclonal gammopathy (especially immunoglobulin A)
- Polycythemia vera
- Acute myelogenous leukemia
- Chronic myelogenous leukemia
- Hairy cell leukemia
- Lymphoma
- Myelodysplasia

Autoimmune disorders

- Inflammatory bowel disease
- Rheumatoid arthritis
- Sjogren syndrome
- Systemic lupus erythematosus
- Granulomatosis with polyangiitis

Medications

- Cocaine laced with levamisole
- Isotretinoin
- Propylthiouracil
- Sunitinib

Others

- Neutrophilic disorder
  - Behçet disease
  - Subcorneal pustular dermatosis
  - Sweet syndrome
  - Bowel-associated dermatosis arthritis syndrome
- Autoinflammatory disorders
  - PAPA syndrome (pyogenic arthritis, pyoderma gangrenosum, acne)
  - PASH syndrome (pyogenic arthritis, hidradenitis suppurativa)
  - PAPASH syndrome (Pyogenic arthritis, pyoderma gangrenosum, acne, hidradenitis suppurativa)
- Solid tumor malignancies

JAK-2, JAK-3, interferon (IFN)-γ, chemokine receptors, and reduced levels of anti-inflammatory cytokines IL-10, transforming growth factor beta (TGF-β), Foxhead box P3 (FOXP3), and regulatory T-cells (T-reg).[8] This imbalance leads to a predominant neutrophilic inflammation, tissue necrosis, and ulceration. Skin trauma results in the release of IL-8 and IL-36 inflammatory cytokines by keratinocytes. Hence, PG may be triggered or aggravated by minor trauma (ie, pathergy).

Since the discovery of novel therapies, the treatment of PG has evolved from a blanket immunosuppression to a more targeted immunomodulation. The goals of therapy should be to reduce inflammation to allow healing to place, pain control, and management of underlying comorbidities. Multidisciplinary management involving dermatology, wound care, pain, plastic surgery, rheumatology, gastroenterology, hematology, and oncology are often required to achieve disease control and prevent recurrence. Herein, we discuss various treatment options stratified by level of evidence (**Box 2**) and propose an algorithm to approach PG (**Fig. 1**).

DISCUSSION
Level 1 Evidence (Randomized Controlled Trials)

Systematic corticosteroids
Corticosteroids (CS) asserts its immunosuppressive effects by binding to glucocorticoid receptors and affecting transcription factors, leading to a reduction in proinflammatory cytokines such as IL-1 and TNF-α, while increasing anti-inflammatory mediators such as T-reg and IL-10. CS has a rapid onset of action, making it an excellent first-line treatment option for PG.

Prednisolone 0.75 mg/kg/d resulted in resolution in 47% of PG by 6 months.[9] Patients with milder disease and without underlying PG-associated disorders had better response to CS. Steroid-sparing agents should be initiated concurrently with CS to allow tapering once disease remission is achieved. Serious adverse events (AEs) associated with CS included hyperglycemia, diabetes mellitus, serious infections, and bowel perforation. Patient characteristics discouraging the use of prednisone include obesity, impaired fasting glucose, osteoporosis, gastrointestinal ulcers, and mental illness.

Calcineurin inhibitors (cyclosporine and tacrolimus)
Cyclosporine and tacrolimus are calcineurin inhibitors that predominantly reduce IL-2, IFN-γ, and T-cells proliferation.

Cyclosporine 4 mg/kg/d resulted in complete resolution in 47% of PG lesions by 6 months.[9] Serious AEs associated with cyclosporine included abdominal aortic aneurysm rupture and renal dysfunction. Patient characteristics discouraging the use of cyclosporine include hypertension, renal insufficiency, and malignancy. Compared with prednisolone, cyclosporine showed similar treatment

Table 1
Diagnostic criteria for pyoderma gangrenosum[1-4]

Criteria by Su et al (2004)	Delphi Consensus Criteria (2018)	Paracelsus Score (2019)
Diagnosis requires 2 major and ≥2 minor criteria	Diagnosis requires 1 major and ≥4 minor criteria	Diagnosis (highly likely) requires a score of ≥10 points
Major Criteria	Major Criterion	3 points each
• Rapidly developing painful, necrolytic ulcer with an irregular, violaceous, and undermined border • Ruled out other causes of ulcers	• Biopsy of ulcer edge demonstrates neutrophilic infiltrate	• Progressive disease • Excluded other potential causes • Red-violet wound border
Minor Criteria	Minor Criteria	2 points each
• History suggestive of pathergy or cribriform scarring on examination • Underlying systemic disease with known association to PG • Histopathology consistent with PG (sterile neutrophilic dermal infiltrate, ± mixed infiltrates, ± lymphocytic vasculitis) • Rapid response to systemic CS	• Infection excluded on histology (with appropriate stains and tissue culture) • Pathergy • Underlying inflammatory bowel disease or inflammatory arthritis • Papule, pustule, or vesicle that rapidly evolves into an ulcer within 4 d • Ulcer with undermined borders and peripheral erythema • Multiple ulcers including ≥1 on anterior lower leg • Cribriform atrophic scarring after ulcer heals • Ulcer decreases in size within 1 mo of starting immunosuppressive medication	• Ameliorates with immunosuppressive medications • Irregularly shaped (bizarre) ulcer • Pathergy • Significant pain (>4/10 on the visual analog scale)
		1 point each
		• Suppurative inflammation on histopathology • Undermined wound edge • Associated systemic disease

efficacy while having fewer serious AEs.[9] Cyclosporine was also found to be a more cost-effective treatment option, especially for larger lesions (20 cm^2 or greater).[10]

Oral tacrolimus is more potent than cyclosporine. Oral tacrolimus has been used in the management of PG.[11-13] Four patients with PG refractory to conventional immunosuppressive medications developed significant clinical improvements within 1 week of initiating oral tacrolimus, and 3 of them had complete resolution by 8 weeks.[11] Potential AEs were similar to that of cyclosporine.

Tumor necrosis factor alpha inhibitors

TNF-α is a proinflammatory cytokine that leads to the downstream production of IL-17, IL-23, and further TNF-α cytokines, which propagates the proinflammatory state. TNF-α inhibitors used in the treatment of PG have included adalimumab, certolizumab pegol, etanercept, infliximab, and golimumab.

Clinical improvement and complete resolution of PG was seen in 87% and 67% of lesions treated with TNF-α inhibitors.[14,15] Complete resolution was seen in 87% of PG with disease duration less than 12 weeks, compared with 69% of PG with disease duration greater than 12 weeks.[14] Infliximab had the greatest evidence supporting its use in PG, followed by adalimumab and then by etanercept. Infliximab and adalimumab trended toward greater clinical improvements compared with etanercept but this difference was not statistically significant.[14] Certolizumab pegol and golimumab had the fewest evidence in PG.

<table>
<tr><td>

Box 2
Systemic treatment options stratified by available level of evidence

Level 1 (Randomized controlled trials)
- Systemic corticosteroids[9]
- Calcineurin inhibitors (cyclosporine and tacrolimus)[9]
- TNF-α inhibitors[15]

Level 2 (cohort studies)
- Topical corticosteroids[16]
- Topical calcineurin inhibitors[18]
- Dapsone[23]
- Mycophenolate mofetil
- IL-1 inhibitors[26]
- IL-17 inhibitors[28]

Level 3 (case-control studies)
- Intravenous immunoglobulin (IVIG)[36]
- IL-12/23[14]

Level 4 (case series or case reports)
- Azathioprine[38]
- Colchicine[41]
- Methotrexate[62]
- Thalidomide[50]
- IL-23 inhibitors[57]
- IL-36R inhibitor[62]
- JAK inhibitors[64]
- PDE-4 inhibitors[68]

Highest (Level 1) to lowest.

</td></tr>
</table>

Level 2 Evidence (Cohort Studies)

Topical corticosteroids and intralesional corticosteroids

High-potency topical corticosteroids (TCSs) have been evaluated in the treatment of PG.[16] Clobetasol propionate 0.05% resulted in complete resolution in 43% of PG lesions within 6 months.[16] Intralesional CS have also been successfully used for the treatment of PG lesions.[17] Lesion size at time of presentation was an important prognostic factor because smaller lesions resolved more quickly.[16]

Topical calcineurin inhibitors

Topical calcineurin inhibitors (TCIs) work via a similar mechanism to cyclosporine and reduce IL-2, IFN-γ, and T-cells proliferation. Topical tacrolimus 0.1% ointment resulted in complete resolution in 50% to 100% of PG lesions within 2 to 6 months.[16,18] Caution should be paid when using TCI in extensive PG because one patient experienced acute renal dysfunction with elevated serum levels of tacrolimus after applying topical tacrolimus repeatedly to PG.[19] Topical pimecrolimus has less systemic absorption compared with topical tacrolimus and may be a safer choice in extensive PG.[20–22]

Dapsone

Dapsone is an antineutrophilic medication that works by inhibiting myeloperoxidase in neutrophils and preventing cellular damage from reactive oxygen species. Dapsone has been evaluated as an adjunct to other first-line immunosuppressive therapies.[23] When used as an adjuvant to systemic CS, antibiotics, intralesional CS, or TNF-α inhibitors, dapsone at 50 to 100 mg/d resulted in clinical improvements in 96.9% patients with PG, of which 81.3% had partial response and 15.6% had complete resolution of PG after a mean therapy duration of 14.3 months.[23] AEs included hemolytic anemia and methemoglobinemia in 9.4% and 3.7% of patients, respectively.

Mycophenolate mofetil

Mycophenolate mofetil (MMF) is an immunosuppressive agent that inhibits inosine monophosphate dehydrogenase, a key enzyme preferentially expressed in activated lymphocytes but not in nonactivated lymphocytes or other inflammatory cells. MMF also inhibits antibody production by B cells, tissue fibrosis by fibroblast, and recruitment of inflammatory cells. MMF was evaluated as a steroid-sparing agent and used concomitantly with systemic CS to reduce the overall dose of CS necessary to achieve clinical improvement.[24,25] When used alongside systemic CS, MMF at starting doses of 1 to 2 g/d and increasing to maintenance doses of 2 to 3 g/d resulted in clinical improvements in 85% to 93% of patients with PG, with 36% to 50% having complete resolution of PG lesions within 12 months.[24,25] Adding MMF to the treatment regimen allowed patients to reduce their mean doses of systemic CS from 35 to 40 mg/d to 9 to 18 mg/d.[24] MMF was overall tolerable, with minor GI discomfort being the most commonly reported SE.

Interleukin-1 inhibitors

IL-1 is an inflammatory cytokine that recruits and activates neutrophils, in addition to its involvement in inflammasome formation. Anakinra, an IL-1 receptor antagonist, and canakinumab, IL-1β inhibitor, have been successfully used for the treatment of PG. Among 12 patients treated with anakinra, clinical improvements or complete resolution was

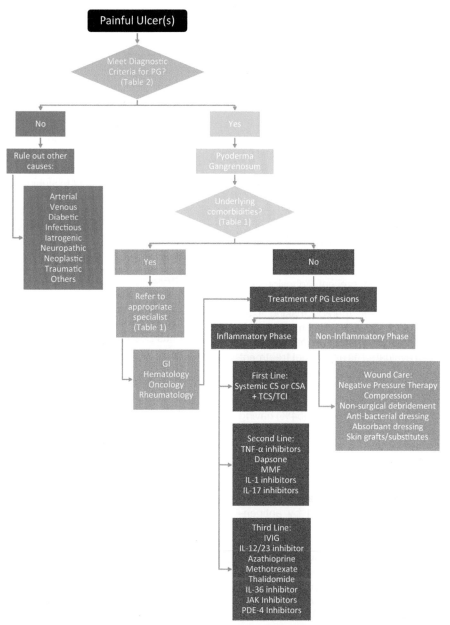

Fig. 1. Management algorithm for PG. CS, corticosteroids; CSA, cyclosporine; GI, gastroenterology; IL, interleukin; IVIG, intravenous immunoglobulin; MMF, mycophenolate mofetil; PDE-4, phosphodiesterase-4; TCI, topical calcineurin inhibitors; TCSs, topical corticosteroids.

observed in 10 patients (83.3%).[26] Among 10 patients with PG, treatment with canakinumab resulted in complete resolution of PG in 6 patients and clinical improvements in 1 patient.[26] In a separate case series of 5 patients with steroid-resistant PG, canakinumab resulted in clinical improvements in 4 patients (80%) after 16 weeks.[27]

Interleukin-17 inhibitors

IL-17 inhibitors secukinumab, brodalumab, and ixekizumab have all been successfully used for the treatment of PG. A small phase I-II investigator-initiated trial found that secukinumab reduced pain significantly in all 7 patients, and resulted in significant clinical improvements in 2 patients after 32 weeks (28%).[28] Secukinumab resulted in complete resolution of PG in 1 patient within 3 months.[29] Brodalumab resulted in complete resolution of PG in 3 patients within 12 weeks, including one that had been previously refractory to secukinumab.[30,31] It was postulated that brodalumab but not secukinumab inhibited IL-17E, which is responsible for the recruitment of neutrophils by activated macrophages.[31] Ixekizumab resulted in complete resolution of PG in 4 patients within 3 months.[32] Interestingly, IL-17 inhibitors have also been implicated in triggering PG.[33] It is postulated that the inhibition of IL-17 leads to a paradoxic increase in IL-23, thereby inducing PG. Hence, clinicians need to be cautious when choosing IL-17 inhibitors for PG.

Level 3 Evidence (Case-Control Studies)

Intravenous immunoglobulin
Intravenous immunoglobulin (IVIG) is derived from purified plasma pooled from more than 1000 healthy donors and contains supraphysiologic amounts of immunoglobulin G primarily. IVIG has been shown to neutralize pathogenic antibodies in circulation, inhibit antibody production, inhibit complement activation, induce selective apoptosis of autoreactive T cells, and prevent adhesion and migration of inflammatory cells. IVIG is not an immunosuppressive agent, thereby making it an excellent choice in those with concomitant infections or sepsis or steroid-sparing agent.

IVIG has been evaluated as an adjunct treatment of refractory PG.[34–36] Among 50 patients with refractory PG, IVIG as an adjunct to systemic CS or cyclosporine resulted in clinical improvements in 44 patients (88%), with 27 patients (54%) having complete resolution of PG by 6 months.[34,35] No major AEs occurred.

Interleukin-12/23 inhibitors
Ustekinumab targets the common p40 subunit of IL-12 and IL-23 cytokines. IL-12 and IL-23 are proinflammatory cytokines released by antigen-presenting cells that result in the activation of T-helper 1 (Th1) and T-helper 17 (Th17) cellular pathway respectively that lead to downstream inflammatory cytokines that were found to be elevated in PG lesions. Th1 cells produce proinflammatory cytokines IL-2, TNF-α, and IFN-γ, whereas Th17 cells produce proinflammatory cytokines IL-17, IL-22, and TNF-α.

Ustekinumab has been used for the treatment of PG.[14,37] Among 34 patients with PG who received ustekinumab, clinical improvement and complete resolution were seen in 79% and 71% of patients, respectively.[14] Ustekinumab was effective in all types of PG but patients without associated comorbidities had better response to ustekinumab.[37] No major AEs were reported.

Level 4 Evidence (Case Series or Case Reports)

Azathioprine
Azathioprine works by inhibiting purine metabolism and cell division, thereby selectively affecting lymphocyte activation and antibody production. Azathioprine has been used as a steroid-sparing agent in combination with prednisolone, infliximab, and topical tacrolimus for the successful treatment of PG.[38,39]

Colchicine
Colchicine has antimitotic and anti-inflammatory properties. It prevents the proliferation of lymphocytes, reduces recruitment and activation of inflammatory cells including neutrophils, and inhibits inflammasome-mediated IL-1β.[40]

Colchicine has been successful in the management of PG.[41,42] Low-dose colchicine monotherapy was used as a maintenance therapy in 3 patients and allowed for the tapering of traditional immunosuppressive medications without disease recurrence.[41,42]

Methotrexate
Methotrexate is an immunosuppressant that inhibits cellular division through the inhibition of nucleotides necessary for DNA synthesis. Methotrexate has been reported to be successful in the management of PG primarily as a steroid-sparing agent and in combination with adalimumab, infliximab, cyclosporine, dapsone, and systemic CS.[43–47]

Intralesional methotrexate was used as an adjuvant to oral CS.[48] The patient had a lack of response to oral methotrexate, so intralesional methotrexate was instead administered to the borders of PG lesions weekly and the patient had almost complete resolution after 7 weeks.[48] Low-dose methotrexate was also used as an adjuvant to reduce neutralizing antidrug antibodies to infliximab (ADA-I).[46] Among 6 patients with PG who initially responded well to infliximab but subsequently developed ADA-I and lost clinical response, adding low-dose methotrexate resulted in restoration of infliximab's efficacy and complete resolution of PG in 4 patients.[46]

Thalidomide
Thalidomide inhibits neutrophil chemotaxis and phagocytosis and inhibits the production of proinflammatory mediators IL-12, TNF-α, and IFN-γ, whereas it upregulates anti-inflammatory mediators IL-4 and IL-5. Major AEs associated with thalidomide include irreversible peripheral neuropathy and teratogenicity. Thalidomide should be strictly avoided in women of childbearing potential due to the almost 100% incidence of birth defects.[49]

Thalidomide has been successful in the management of numerous neutrophilic disorders including PG. Thalidomide was added as one of the last resorts after patients had failed numerous conventional immunosuppressants and antibiotics.[50–55] A 49-year-old patient with 27-year history of recalcitrant PG developed significant improvement after 6 months of thalidomide.[50] Thalidomide resulted in complete resolution of lesions in 2 patients with PG involving their penis.[52,56] Thalidomide has also been successful for PG in the pediatric population.[55,56]

Interleukin-23 inhibitors

In contrast to ustekinumab, the IL-23 inhibitors guselkumab, risankizumab, and tildrakizumab target the p19 subunit of IL-23 only and have no effect on IL-12. All 3 IL-23 inhibitors have been used in the treatment of PG. Significant clinical improvements or complete resolution of PG lesions were observed within 3 to 4 months of initiating guselkumab, risankizumab, or tildrakizumab.[57–61]

Interleukin-36R inhibitor

IL-36 is a proinflammatory cytokine released by keratinocytes in response to cutaneous injury that plays a key role in the unrelenting inflammation in PG. Activated IL-36 causes downstream release of neutrophil-recruiting cytokines IL-6, IL-8, IL-17A, and TNF-α, to drive the innate immune response. IL-36 also upregulates the adaptive immunity by skewing Th1 differentiation and reducing T-reg differentiation.

Spesolimab, an IL-36 receptor inhibitor approved for the treatment of generalized pustular psoriasis, has been used in 2 patients with severe, recalcitrant PG.[62] In the first patient, repeated attempts at tapering prednisone and cyclosporine led to disease flare up. Adding spesolimab to his treatment regimen resulted in significant clinical improvements and allowed the tapering of systemic CS and cyclosporine within 5 weeks.[62] Of note, the first patient developed epididymitis on spesolimab requiring treatment with doxycycline. In the second patient, spesolimab added to a regimen consisting of prednisone, cyclosporine, hydroxychloroquine, and IVIG. The patient experienced dramatic improvement in pain and reduced purulent discharge within 48 hours of spesolimab infusion and complete resolution of PG lesions after several weeks.

Janus kinase inhibitors

JAK is a family of tyrosine kinases that respond to proinflammatory cytokines such as IFN-γ and further propagate the proinflammatory response. JAK inhibitors are a newer class of medications that have been approved for other inflammatory or autoimmune disorders including atopic dermatitis and psoriatic arthritis.

JAK inhibitors, baricitinib, ruxolitinib, tofacitinib, and upadacitinib, have been successful in the treatment of 15 cases of PG.[63–67] Patients without underlying comorbidities responded to JAK inhibitors more quickly and without AEs, as compared with patients with underlying associated inflammatory disorders.[63] Potential AEs of JAK inhibitors include reactivation of latent infections including herpes zoster or tuberculosis, liver or lipid abnormalities, or other infections. There are no reports of topical JAK inhibitor use in PG. Of note, in our opinion, JAK inhibitors will be increasingly used for PG and the level of evidence should improve over time because it has been used effectively in recalcitrant PG.

Phosphodiesterase-4 inhibitors

Phosphodiesterase-4 (PDE-4) is an enzyme present mainly in immune cells and is responsible for the downstream expression of proinflammatory cytokines IL-17, TNF-α, and IFN-γ and downregulation of anti-inflammatory cytokines IL-10. PDE-4 inhibitor apremilast has been approved for the treatment of psoriasis, and oral ulcers in Behçet disease recently.

Apremilast has been used either as a monotherapy or adjuvant steroid-sparing agent in the management of PG.[68–70] Apremilast monotherapy was initiated in a patient with 5-year history of PG without underlying associated disorders and resulted in significant clinical improvements within 4 months, and complete resolution after 3 years.[68] Apremilast was used as a steroid-sparing agent in 2 cases of PG and allowed the tapering of systemic CS.[69,70] Side effects reported include diarrhea, nausea, and weight loss. There are no reports of topical PDE-4 inhibitors crisaborole and roflumilast for PG.

SUMMARY

PG remains an orphan disease that neither has any approved treatments nor has active clinical trials evaluating potential treatments.[71] Management of PG requires a multidisciplinary approach, involving but not limited to dermatology, pain, wound care, plastic surgery, and management of underlying associated disorders.

Systemic CS, cyclosporine, and TNF-α inhibitors have the strongest evidence supporting their efficacy and safety in PG. Although systemic CS is the most popular first-line option, it has been associated with higher incidence of serious AEs compared with cyclosporine and TNF-α inhibitors.[9,72] The choice between systemic CS and cyclosporine should be based on the patient's pre-existing comorbidities and lesion size.[9] Ultrapotent TCSs, intralesional CS, or TCI should be used in conjunction with systemic therapies to minimize overall dose required to achieve disease remission.

Once inflammation of PG is in remission, then the focus should be redirected to other factors that may affect wound healing. A useful mnemonic, TIME, has been proposed: tissue, infection, moisture, and epithelization.[73] Although surgical debridement is contraindicated due to the risk of pathergy, the use of nonsurgical debridement, negative pressure wound therapy, and compression, have shown to be safe and effective for PG.[73,74] Patients without underlying associated comorbidities tended to have better response to treatment and suffered fewer treatment-related AEs.

CLINICS CARE POINTS

- PG remains an orphan disease with no approved treatment
- Multidisciplinary approach to PG is necessary for optimal management, especially for wound care and underlying comorbidities
- Systemic CS, cyclosporine, and TNF-α inhibitors have the greatest body of evidence supporting their use in PG
- Patients receiving systemic CS suffered more serious AEs than patients receiving cyclosporine. The choice of medication should be based on the patient's preexisting comorbidities and size of PG lesions. Patient characteristics discouraging the use of prednisone include obesity, impaired fasting glucose, osteoporosis, gastrointestinal ulcers, mental illness, and large lesion size ($\geq$20 cm). Patient characteristics discouraging the use of cyclosporine include hypertension, renal insufficiency, and malignancy
- Topical CS, intralesional CS and/or TCI should be incorporated into most treatment regimen due to low risk of AEs
- Spesolimab, a new IL-36 receptor antagonist, has demonstrated preliminary evidence for treating neutrophilic disorders including PG
- Patients without underlying associated disorders tended to have better response to treatment and suffered fewer incidences of treatment-related AEs

DISCLOSURE

The authors have nothing to disclose.

REFERENCES

1. Haag C, Hansen T, Hajar T, et al. Comparison of Three Diagnostic Frameworks for Pyoderma Gangrenosum. J Invest Dermatol 2021;141(1):59–63.

2. Su WPD, Davis MDP, Weenig RH, et al. Pyoderma gangrenosum: clinicopathologic correlation and proposed diagnostic criteria. Int J Dermatol 2004; 43(11):790–800.

3. Maverakis E, Ma C, Shinkai K, et al. Diagnostic Criteria of Ulcerative Pyoderma Gangrenosum: A Delphi Consensus of International Experts. JAMA Dermatol 2018;154(4):461–6.

4. Jockenhöfer F, Wollina U, Salva KA, et al. The PARACELSUS score: a novel diagnostic tool for pyoderma gangrenosum. Br J Dermatol 2019;180(3): 615–20.

5. Kamal K, Xia E, Li SJ, et al. Eligibility Criteria for Active Ulcerative Pyoderma Gangrenosum (PG) in Clinical Trials: A Delphi Consensus on Behalf of the Understanding PG: Review and Assessment of Disease Effects (UPGRADE) Group. J Invest Dermatol. 2023:S0022-202X(23)03193-7.

6. Nusbaum KB, Boettler M, Korman AM, et al. Subjective assessments in pyoderma gangrenosum diagnostic frameworks undermine framework agreement. Int J Dermatol 2023. https://doi.org/10.1111/ijd.16952.

7. Jacobson ME, Rick JW, Gerbens LAA, et al. A core domain set for pyoderma gangrenosum trial outcomes - an international e-Delphi and consensus study from the UPGRADE initiative. Br J Dermatol 2023;ljad420.

8. Flora A, Kozera E, Frew JW. Pyoderma gangrenosum: A systematic review of the molecular characteristics of disease. Exp Dermatol 2022;31(4):498–515.

9. Ormerod AD, Thomas KS, Craig FE, et al. Comparison of the two most commonly used treatments for pyoderma gangrenosum: results of the STOP GAP randomised controlled trial. BMJ 2015;350:h2958.

10. Mason JM, Thomas KS, Ormerod AD, et al. Ciclosporin compared with prednisolone therapy for patients with pyoderma gangrenosum: cost-effectiveness analysis of the STOP GAP trial. Br J Dermatol 2017;177(6):1527–36.

11. Abu-Elmagd K, Jegasothy BV, Ackerman CD, et al. Efficacy of FK 506 in the treatment of recalcitrant pyoderma gangrenosum. Transplant Proc 1991; 23(6):3328–9.

12. Baumgart DC, Wiedenmann B, Dignass AU. Successful therapy of refractory pyoderma gangrenosum and periorbital phlegmona with tacrolimus (FK506) in ulcerative colitis. Inflamm Bowel Dis 2004;10(4):421–4.

13. Deckers-Kocken J, Pasmans S. Successful tacrolimus (FK506) therapy in a child with pyoderma gangrenosum. Arch Dis Child 2005;90(5):531.

14. Ben Abdallah H, Fogh K, Bech R. Pyoderma gangrenosum and tumour necrosis factor alpha inhibitors: A semi-systematic review. Int Wound J 2019; 16(2):511–21.

15. Brooklyn TN, Dunnill MGS, Shetty A, et al. Infliximab for the treatment of pyoderma gangrenosum: a

randomised, double-blind, placebo-controlled trial. Gut 2006;55(4):505–9.

16. Thomas KS, Ormerod AD, Craig FE, et al. Clinical outcomes and response of patients applying topical therapy for pyoderma gangrenosum: A prospective cohort study. J Am Acad Dermatol 2016;75(5): 940–9.

17. Keltz M, Lebwohl M, Bishop S. Peristomal pyoderma gangrenosum. J Am Acad Dermatol 1992;27(Part 2):360–4.

18. Marzano AV, Trevisan V, Lazzari R, et al. Topical tacrolimus for the treatment of localized, idiopathic, newly diagnosed pyoderma gangrenosum. J Dermatol Treat 2010;21(3):140–3.

19. Wollina U. Letter to the editor: Temporary renal insufficiency associated with topical tacrolimus treatment of multilocal pyoderma gangrenosum. J Dermatol Case Rep 2013;7(3):106–7.

20. Yan AC, Honig PJ, Ming ME, et al. The Safety and Efficacy of Pimecrolimus, 1%, Cream for the Treatment of Netherton Syndrome: Results From an Exploratory Study. Arch Dermatol 2010;146(1):57–62.

21. Cecchi R, Pavesi M, Bartoli L, Brunetti L. Successful Treatment of Localized Pyoderma Gangrenosum with Topical Pimecrolimus. https://journals-sagepub-com.proxy.bib.uottawa.ca/doi/10.1177/120347541201 600503. Accessed September 8, 2023.

22. Bellini V, Simonetti S, Lisi P. Successful treatment of severe pyoderma gangrenosum with pimecrolimus cream 1. J Eur Acad Dermatol Venereol 2008; 22(1):113–5.

23. Din RS, Tsiaras WG, Li DG, et al. Efficacy of Systemic Dapsone Treatment for Pyoderma Gangrenosum: A Retrospective Review. J Drugs Dermatol JDD 2018;17(10):1058–60.

24. Li J, Kelly R. Treatment of pyoderma gangrenosum with mycophenolate mofetil as a steroid-sparing agent. J Am Acad Dermatol 2013;69(4):565–9.

25. Hrin ML, Bashyam AM, Huang WW, et al. Mycophenolate mofetil as adjunctive therapy to corticosteroids for the treatment of pyoderma gangrenosum: a case series and literature review. Int J Dermatol 2021;60(12):e486–92.

26. McKenzie F, Cash D, Gupta A, et al. Biologic and small-molecule medications in the management of pyoderma gangrenosum. J Dermatol Treat 2019; 30(3):264–76.

27. Kolios AGA, Maul JT, Meier B, et al. Canakinumab in adults with steroid-refractory pyoderma gangrenosum. Br J Dermatol 2015;173(5):1216–23.

28. Lauffer F, Seiringer P, Böhmer D, et al. 044 Safety and efficacy of anti-IL-17 (Secukinumab) for the treatment of pyoderma gangrenosum. J Invest Dermatol 2021;141(10 Supplement):S156.

29. McPhie ML, Kirchhof MG. Pyoderma gangrenosum treated with secukinumab: A case report. SAGE Open Med Case Rep 2020;8. 2050313X20940430.

30. Tee MW, Avarbock AB, Ungar J, et al. Rapid resolution of pyoderma gangrenosum with brodalumab therapy. JAAD Case Rep 2020;6(11):1167–9.

31. Huang CM, Tsai TF. Use of brodalumab for the treatment of pyoderma gangrenosum: A case report. Dermatol Sin 2021;39(1):57.

32. Kao AS, King AD, Bardhi R, et al. Targeted therapy with ixekizumab in pyoderma gangrenosum: A case series and a literature overview. JAAD Case Rep 2023;37:49–53.

33. Petty AJ, Whitley MJ, Balaban A, et al. Pyoderma gangrenosum induced by secukinumab in a patient with psoriasis successfully treated with ustekinumab. JAAD Case Rep 2020;6(8):731–3.

34. Song H, Lahood N, Mostaghimi A. Intravenous immunoglobulin as adjunct therapy for refractory pyoderma gangrenosum: systematic review of cases and case series. Br J Dermatol 2018;178(2): 363–8.

35. De Zwaan SE, Iland HJ, Damian DL. Treatment of refractory pyoderma gangrenosum with intravenous immunoglobulin. Australas J Dermatol 2009;50(1): 56–9.

36. Haag CK, Ortega-Loayza AG, Latour E, et al. Clinical factors influencing the response to intravenous immunoglobulin treatment in cases of treatment-resistant pyoderma gangrenosum. J Dermatol Treat 2020;31(7):723–6.

37. Westerdahl JS, Nusbaum KB, Chung CG, et al. Ustekinumab as adjuvant treatment for all pyoderma gangrenosum subtypes. J Dermatol Treat 2022; 33(4):2386–90.

38. Nazir A, Zafar A. Management of idiopathic pyoderma gangrenosum with azathioprine as the primary adjunct in an asian man: a case report. Cureus 2022;14(5):e25177. https://doi.org/10.7759/cureus.25177.

39. Chatzinasiou F, Polymeros D, Panagiotou M, et al. Generalized Pyoderma Gangrenosum Associated with Ulcerative Colitis: Successful Treatment with Infliximab and Azathioprine. Acta Dermatovenerol Croat ADC 2016;24(1):83–5.

40. Wolverton SE, Wu JJ. Comprehensive dermatologic drug therapy. 4th edition. Philadelphia, PA: Elsevier; 2020.

41. Paolini O, Hébuterne X, Flory P, et al. Treatment of pyoderma gangrenosum with colchicine. Lancet Lond Engl 1995;345(8956):1057–8.

42. Kontochristopoulos GJ, Stavropoulos PG, Gregoriou S, et al. Treatment of Pyoderma gangrenosum with Low-Dose Colchicine. Dermatology 2004;209(3):233–6.

43. Spangler JG. Pyoderma gangrenosum in a patient with psoriatic arthritis. J Am Board Fam Pract 2001;14(6):466–9.

44. Loloi J, MacDonald SM. Pyoderma gangrenosum of the penis. Can J Urol 2021;28(1):10560–4.

45. Vekic DA, Woods J, Lin P, et al. SAPHO syndrome associated with hidradenitis suppurativa and pyoderma gangrenosum successfully treated with adalimumab and methotrexate: a case report and review of the literature. Int J Dermatol 2018;57(1):10–8.

46. Wang LL, Micheletti RG. Low-dose methotrexate as rescue therapy in patients with hidradenitis suppurativa and pyoderma gangrenosum developing human antichimeric antibodies to infliximab: A retrospective chart review. J Am Acad Dermatol 2020;82(2):507–10.

47. Sardana K, Bajaj S, Bose SK. Successful treatment of PAPA syndrome with minocycline, dapsone, deflazacort and methotrexate: a cost-effective therapy with a 2-year follow-up. Clin Exp Dermatol 2019;44(5):577–9.

48. Del Puerto C, Navarrete-Dechent CP, Carrasco-Zuber JE, et al. Intralesional methotrexate as an adjuvant treatment for pyoderma gangrenosum: A case report. Indian J Dermatol Venereol Leprol 2017;83(2):277.

49. Tseng S, Pak G, Washenik K, et al. Rediscovering thalidomide: a review of its mechanism of action, side effects, and potential uses. J Am Acad Dermatol 1996;35(6):969–79.

50. Hecker MS, Lebwohl MG. Recalcitrant pyoderma gangrenosum: Treatment with thalidomide. J Am Acad Dermatol 1998;38(3):490–1.

51. Federman GL, Federman DG. Recalcitrant Pyoderma Gangrenosum Treated With Thalidomide. Mayo Clin Proc 2000;75(8):842–4.

52. Farrell AM, Black MM, Bracka A, et al. Pyoderma gangrenosum of the penis. Br J Dermatol 1998;138(2):337–40.

53. Rustin MHA, Gilkes JJH, Robinson TWE. Pyoderma gangrenosum associated with Behçet's disease: Treatment with thalidomide. J Am Acad Dermatol 1990;23(5, Part 1):941–4.

54. Malkan UY, Gunes G, Eliacik E, et al. Treatment of pyoderma gangrenosum with thalidomide in a myelodysplastic syndrome case. Int Med Case Rep J 2016;9:61–4.

55. Venencie PY, Saurat JH. Pyoderma gangrenosum in a child. Treatment with thalidomide. Ann Pediatr (Paris) 1982;29(1):67–9.

56. Hu YQ, Yao XX, Zhang JZ, et al. Penile pyoderma gangrenosum: Successful treatment with thalidomide. Dermatol Ther 2019;32(4):e12952.

57. Baier C, Barak O. Guselkumab as a treatment option for recalcitrant pyoderma gangrenosum. JAAD Case Rep 2021;8:43–6.

58. Reese AM, Erickson K, Reed KB, et al. Modified dose of guselkumab for treatment of pyoderma gangrenosum. JAAD Case Rep 2022;21:38–42.

59. Burgdorf B, Schlott S, Ivanov IH, et al. Successful treatment of a refractory pyoderma gangrenosum with risankizumab. Int Wound J 2020;17(4):1086–8.

60. Leow LJ, Zubrzycki N. Recalcitrant Ulcerative Pyoderma Gangrenosum of the Leg Responsive to Tildrakizumab: A Case Report. Clin Cosmet Investig Dermatol 2022;15:1729–36.

61. John JM, Sinclair RD. Tildrakizumab for treatment of refractory pyoderma gangrenosum of the penis and polymyalgia rheumatica: Killing two birds with one stone. Australas J Dermatol 2020;61(2):170–1.

62. Guénin SH, Khattri S, Lebwohl MG. Spesolimab use in treatment of pyoderma gangrenosum. JAAD Case Rep 2023;34:18–22.

63. Castro LGM. JAK inhibitors: a novel, safe, and efficacious therapy for pyoderma gangrenosum. Int J Dermatol 2023;62(8):1088–93.

64. Scheinberg M, Machado LA, Castro LG, et al. Successful treatment of ulcerated pyoderma gangrenosum with baricitinib, a novel JAK inhibitor. J Transl Autoimmun 2021;4:100099.

65. Sitaru S, Biedermann T, Lauffer F. Successful treatment of pyoderma gangrenosum with Janus kinase 1/2 inhibition. JEADV Clin Pract 2022;1(4):420–3.

66. Orfaly VE, Kovalenko I, Tolkachjov SN, et al. Tofacitinib for the treatment of refractory pyoderma gangrenosum. Clin Exp Dermatol 2021;46(6):1082–5.

67. Van Eycken L, Dens AC, de Vlam K, et al. Resolution of therapy-resistant pyoderma gangrenosum with upadacitinib. JAAD Case Rep 2023;37:89–91.

68. Bordeaux ZA, Kwatra SG, West CE. Treatment of pyoderma gangrenosum with apremilast monotherapy. JAAD Case Rep 2022;30:8–10.

69. Vernero M, Ribaldone DG, Cariti C, et al. Dual-targeted therapy with apremilast and vedolizumab in pyoderma gangrenosum associated with Crohn's disease. J Dermatol 2020;47(6):e216–7.

70. Laird ME, Tong LX, Lo Sicco KI, et al. Novel use of apremilast for adjunctive treatment of recalcitrant pyoderma gangrenosum. JAAD Case Rep 2017;3(3):228–9.

71. Alston D, Eggiman E, Forsyth RA, et al. Pyoderma gangrenosum and dehydrated human amnion/chorion membrane: a potential tool for an orphan disease. J Wound Care 2022;31(10):808–14.

72. Kolios AGA, Gübeli A, Meier B, et al. Clinical Disease Patterns in a Regional Swiss Cohort of 34 Pyoderma Gangrenosum Patients. Dermatology 2017;233(4):268–76.

73. Janowska A, Oranges T, Fissi A, et al. A practical approach to the clinical management of pyoderma gangrenosum. Dermatol Ther 2020;33(3):e13412.

74. Bazaliński D, Krawiec A, Kucharzewski M, et al. Negative Pressure Wound Therapy in Pyoderma Gangrenosum Treatment. Am J Case Rep 2020;21:e922581.

75. Schmieder SJ, Krishnamurthy K. Pyoderma Gangrenosum. In: StatPearls. StatPearls Publishing; 2023. Available at: http://www.ncbi.nlm.nih.gov/books/NBK482223/. Accessed September 11, 2023.

Sweet Syndrome and Neutrophilic Dermatosis of the Dorsal Hands

Matthew L. Hrin, MD[a],*, William W. Huang, MD, MPH[b]

KEYWORDS

- Acute febrile neutrophilic dermatosis • Dorsal hands • Sweet syndrome

KEY POINTS

- Sweet syndrome is generally categorized into 1 of 3 forms: classic, malignancy-associated, and drug-induced.
- Onset of malignancy-associated Sweet syndrome can be a sign of cancer recurrence and/or development of a new cancer.
- Extracutaneous involvements are uncommon and can be life-threatening.
- Systemic corticosteroids can provide rapid improvements; several nonsteroidal agents seem to be effective with growing evidence.
- There are a multitude of possible triggers, and Sweet syndrome's pathogenesis is incompletely characterized.

INTRODUCTION
History

Sweet syndrome (acute febrile neutrophilic dermatosis) is a rare cutaneous condition originally described by Dr Robert Douglas Sweet in 1964.[1] While Dr Sweet's case series included several patients with preceding mucosal tract infections, Sweet syndrome is also associated with several autoimmune diseases, pregnancy, malignancies (hematologic and solid tumors), and medication exposures.[2] Although the pathogenesis of Sweet syndrome is not well characterized, it can be classified into 3 main categories based on the clinical context in which it presents: classic (idiopathic), malignancy-associated, and drug-induced. In this article, the authors summarize and discuss the up-to-date medical literature on Sweet syndrome and neutrophilic dermatosis of the dorsal hands—a condition that is frequently recognized as a clinical variant of Sweet syndrome.

DEFINITIONS
Background

Epidemiology

Sweet syndrome is a rare entity, and its incidence is difficult to precisely estimate. Classic Sweet syndrome comprises roughly 28% to 61% of cases, malignancy-associated Sweet syndrome has been reported in frequencies between 3% and 67%, and drug-induced Sweet syndrome has been reported at rates between 1% and 27%.[3] Typically, disease onset occurs in middle-aged individuals, and malignancy-associated cases seem to tend to occur in slightly older patients (average age 68 years) than classic cases (average age 51 years).[4] Although Sweet syndrome can also affect children (average age 5 years), pediatric patients comprise less than 10% of cases.[5] Women generally seem to be affected more commonly than men in the classic variant (roughly 4:1 ratio); however, malignancy-associated (1:1), solid-tumor associated (1.4:1),

[a] Department of Dermatology, Wake Forest School of Medicine, Medical Center Boulevard, 4618 Country Club Road, Winston-Salem, NC 27157-1071, USA; [b] Department of Dermatology, Wake Forest School of Medicine, 4618 Country Club Road, Winston-Salem, NC 27104, USA
* Corresponding author.
E-mail address: matthewhrin@virginia.edu

Dermatol Clin 42 (2024) 193–207
https://doi.org/10.1016/j.det.2023.08.007
0733-8635/24/© 2023 Elsevier Inc. All rights reserved.

and drug-induced (2.4:1) cases tend to be slightly less female predominant, and there is growing evidence that suggests there may not be a significant sex predilection.[6–8]

Evaluation

Observation/assessment

Clinical hallmarks of Sweet syndrome include an acute onset of tender, nonpruritic, erythematous or violaceous papules/plaques with or without central yellow discoloration and/or mammillated surfaces; lesions can also present as vesicles, pustules, and bullae (Fig. 1).[9]

Cutaneous findings characteristically asymmetrically involve the head, neck, and upper extremities (such as the dorsal hands) and can onset either concurrently with constitutional signs and symptoms (fever, malaise, arthralgia, myalgia, headache, and so forth) or manifest days to weeks after. An estimated 28% to 85% of patients experience fevers.[3]

Extracutaneous manifestations

Although uncommon, multiorgan involvement in Sweet syndrome can be serious and potentially life-threatening.[8] A wide variety of systemic manifestations have been reported involving the cardiovascular (myocarditis, aortitis, coronary artery occlusion, neutrophilic infiltration of myocardium), nervous (meningitis, encephalitis), gastrointestinal (hepatomegaly, splenomegaly, intestinal neutrophilic inflammation), musculoskeletal (osteomyelitis), pulmonary (pleurisy, alveolitis, radiologic findings of infiltrations, pleural effusions), and renal (glomerulonephritis, hematuria, proteinuria) systems.[10,11]

Hisanaga and colleagues coined the term "neuro-Sweet disease" in 1999 after managing a patient with recurrent encephalitis found to have associated biopsy-proven Sweet syndrome.[12]

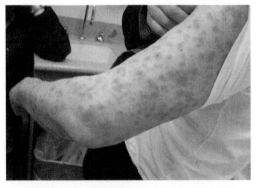

Fig. 1. Clinical findings of Sweet syndrome: erythematous edematous papules and plaques involving the upper extremity. (Image courtesy of PathPresenter.)

The most common neurologic manifestations are aseptic meningitis and encephalitis; other complications include epilepsy, paresis, dyskinesia, and psychiatric disorders.[13]

Mucous membrane involvement is relatively rare and tends to occur more often in malignancy-associated cases compared with classic.[10,14–16] Ocular Sweet syndrome typically presents as a mild-moderate conjunctivitis with characteristic rapid responsiveness to corticosteroids; however, several ophthalmologic pathologies have been reported (retinal vasculitis, choroiditis, scleritis, episcleritis, iritis, central retinal artery occlusion), some of which can lead to blindness.[8,15,17,18] The oral cavity may also be affected and present with ulcers.

Pulmonary manifestations can be resistant to treatment and fatal.[19] Symptoms can range from mild dyspnea to acute respiratory distress syndrome. Diagnostic bronchoalveolar lavages and/or pleural fluid analyses are often obtained to assess for malignancy/infection and typically exhibit characteristic neutrophilic predominance and negative microbial cultures. Bronchoscopy may reveal erythematous pustules with ulcerations.[20]

Systemic inflammatory response syndrome may also occur in the setting of Sweet syndrome.[21–25]

Approach

Diagnosis

Establishing a diagnosis of classic or malignancy-induced Sweet syndrome relies on meeting both 2 major ([1] abrupt onset of painful erythematous plaques or nodules occasionally with vesicles, pustules, or bullae; [2] histopathology consistent with Sweet syndrome) and 2 of 4 minor clinical criteria ([1] preceded by one of the following: an associated infection, vaccination, malignancy, inflammatory disorder, drug exposure, or pregnancy; [2] presence of fever > 38°C [100.4°F], general malaise, constitutional signs and symptoms; [3] three of the following 4 laboratory values: erythrocyte sedimentation rate (ESR) > 20 mm, c-reactive protein (CRP) positive, segmented nuclear neutrophils, and stabs > 70% in peripheral blood smear, leukocytosis > 8000; [4] excellent response to systemic corticosteroids or potassium iodide) developed by Su and colleagues in 1986 and revised by von den Driesch in 1994.[26,27] Drug-induced cases are diagnosed using similar and distinct criteria: (1) abrupt onset of painful erythematous plaques or nodules, (2) histopathologic evidence of a dense neutrophilic infiltrate without evidence of leukocytoclastic vasculitis, (3) pyrexia greater than 38°C (100.4°F), (4) temporal relationship between drug ingestion and clinical presentation or temporally related recurrence after oral challenge, (5) temporally related resolution of lesions after drug withdrawal or treatment with systemic corticosteroids.[10]

Classic (idiopathic) Sweet syndrome

Classic Sweet syndrome is the most common form and typically presents 1 to 3 weeks following an upper respiratory tract and/or gastrointestinal infection. The most highly associated infectious causes include various viruses (cytomegalovirus, hepatitis B and C, human immunodeficiency virus, coronavirus-19), bacteria (yersinia, streptococcus, chlamydia, treponema palladium, helicobacter pylori, typical and atypical mycobacteria [*Mycobacterium tuberculosis* and *Mycobacterium leprae*]), and fungi (sporotrichosis, coccidiomycosis).[9,28–31] Other associated conditions include inflammatory bowel disease (ulcerative colitis and Crohn disease), Behcet disease, relapsing polychondritis, erythema nodosum, rheumatoid arthritis, dermatomyositis, relapsing polychondritis, Sjogren syndrome, sarcoidosis, and autoimmune thyroid disease (Hashimoto and Graves).[11,32–37] There are many other disorders with growing evidence for potential associations, including autoimmune diseases, vasculitides, immunodeficiencies, hereditary syndromes, and a wide variety of infections.[10,11] A more detailed list of disorders potentially associated with Sweet syndrome can be found in **Table 1**.

Similar to pyoderma gangrenosum, pathergy is a feature that may occur in Sweet syndrome as a hypersensitivity reaction to skin trauma such as biopsies, injections, and line placements.[5] Sweet syndrome has developed after relatively minor traumas such as hair plucking and tattoos.[38,39]

Pregnancy-associated Sweet syndrome (classic)

Pregnancy-associated disease rarely occurs (1%–4% of cases) and typically presents in either the first or the second trimester.[3] Prognosis is favorable with spontaneous resolution after delivery and is not associated with a significantly increased risk for infant or maternal morbidity or mortality. However, extra-cutaneous manifestations may cause complications, and spontaneous abortions have been reported.[40–42] Recurrence can occur before, during, and after pregnancy and may present in sequential pregnancies.[40]

Atypical clinical and histologic variants

Less common presentations of Sweet syndrome include bullous Sweet syndrome, pustular Sweet syndrome, subcutaneous panniculitis Sweet syndrome, cryptococcoid Sweet syndrome, histiocytoid Sweet syndrome, giant cellulitis-like Sweet syndrome, and necrotizing Sweet syndrome. Although bullous Sweet syndrome is rare, it is most commonly malignancy-associated and can clinically resemble pyoderma gangrenosum.[9,20,43] Subcutaneous Sweet syndrome presents with nodules that may clinically mimic erythema nodosum and have biopsies demonstrating neutrophilic infiltration of the subcutaneous fat instead of the dermis (correlating clinically with nodules with minimal superficial changes).[44] Cryptococcoid Sweet syndrome was initially described by Ko and colleagues in 2013 and assigned its "cryptococcoid" nomenclature by Wilson and colleagues in 2017 due to its characteristic microscopic findings of vacuolated mononuclear cells with basophilic yeast bodies.[45,46] It can be distinguished from cryptococcosis through negative periodic acid Schiff staining, lack of fungal elements on biopsy, and nonresponsiveness to antifungal therapy.[8] Histiocytoid Sweet syndrome was initially reported by Requena and colleagues in 2005.[47] It can be particularly difficult to distinguish both clinically and histologically from leukemia cutis, and leukemia cutis lesions may occur within the same lesion as Sweet syndrome; the main distinguishing factor is the presence of polymorphonuclear neutrophils of myeloid lineage in Sweet syndrome versus malignant immature leukocytes in leukemia cutis.[48,49] Both the histiocytoid and subcutaneous histologic variants of Sweet syndrome may be associated with increased risk for malignancy, although reporting bias of malignancy-induced cases may exist.[50,51] Giant cellulitis-like Sweet syndrome is another rare presentation characterized by large infiltrated inflammatory plaques and bullae that can clinically resemble bacterial cellulitis and be differentiated through negative bacterial cultures and nonresponsiveness to antibiotics.[8,52] Necrotizing Sweet syndrome resembles necrotizing fasciitis and presents as rapidly progressive lesions with underlying soft tissue necrosis; it is crucial to swiftly and accurately distinguish it from necrotizing fasciitis, as surgical debridement can cause lesion expansion and disease exacerbation.[8] It may have underlying risk factors such as granulocyte colony-stimulating factor and malignancy.[53,54] In 2021, a new variant of Sweet syndrome associated with myelodysplastic syndrome was described: normolipemic xanthomatized Sweet syndrome, characterized histologically by infiltration of CD163 (+) xanthomatous cells and neutrophils with leukocytoclasia.[55] Because the aforementioned patterns include both clinical and histologic findings that can represent atypical presentations of Sweet syndrome, there may be overlap, and variants can evolve over time.[56,57]

Malignancy-associated Sweet syndrome

Roughly 21% of Sweet syndrome cases are associated with malignancies, and cutaneous findings

Table 1
Conditions possibly associated with Sweet syndrome

Disease Process	Conditions
Autoimmune rheumatologic disorders	Ankylosing spondylitis [18204874, 25201185, 10544847], lupus erythematous (systemic and subacute) [23682962, 15934441, 1568805, 22937442, 19276309, 21550284], pemphigus vulgaris [22513066, 15482319], mixed connective tissue disease [33040354], polymyalgia rheumatica [31921506], Still disease [15097938]
Cardiovascular	Dressler syndrome [2411241]
Dermatologic	Acquired cutis lava (Marshall syndrome) [31437319], chronic urticaria, eosinophilic granuloma, granuloma annulare [11722452], Grover disease (transient acantholytic dermatosis) [10877140], hidradenitis suppurativa [32274056, 27002570, 32567672], middermal elastolysis [14675289], psoriasis vulgaris, urticaria pigmentosa
Environmental exposure	Chemical fertilizer [15482306], thermal injury [14641120]
Gastrointestinal	Autoimmune hepatitis [10599643], celiac [19658449], cirrhosis (cryptogenic) [22735879, 29054908, 1794170], common bile duct and intrahepatic duct stones, malabsorption
Hematologic derangements	Aplastic anemia [11902745, 8689342, 7519039], congenital dyserythropoietic anemia [17671383, 2809904], congenital neutropenia (Kostmann syndrome) [15858487, 24387761, 8859296], Fanconi anemia [34403507, 18300309, 21501135, 11196274], hemophagocytic syndrome [18289342, 23955621]
Hereditary syndromes and inherited disorders	Alpha-1-antitrypsin deficiency [7574835], antifactor 8 inhibitor [10759106], antiphospholipid syndrome, glycogen storage disease (type Ib) [8604280], POEMS syndrome (polyneuropathy, organomegaly, endocrinopathy, M protein, and skin changes) [8479179], VEXAS syndrome (vacuoles, E1 enzyme, X-linked, autoinflammatory, somatic) [17655751, 22508923]
Infectious	Anaplasma phagocytophilum (human granulocytic anaplasmosis) [16027306], aseptic meningitis [1488383], bacterial endocarditis [15097971, 17292496, 22605716], campylobacter [22723255], *Capnocytophaga canimorsus* [11411932], *Chlamydia pneumoniae* [11312438], cholangitis [18360136], cholecystitis [27060356], coccidioidomycosis [16027305, 10923132], cytomegalovirus [14693024], dermatophyte [17076728], *Entamoeba histolytica* [16179788], Epstein-Barr virus, *Francisella tularensis* [11903682, 21699525], *Helicobacter pylori* [9216537], hepatitis B [22735879, 11069494], hepatitis C [25348767, 25348767, 12823297, 19052408], herpes simplex [12854387, 29054908, 12100632], herpes zoster [22220147, 10354095], histoplasmosis [32035234], human immunodeficiency virus [10397569, 26396453, 21679803, 18206098, 10545563, 33052291], leprosy, leptospirosis [21771425], lymphadenitis [1504437, 7653187], *Mycobacterium avium* [29171446, 18485019], *Mycobacterium chelonae* [12854387], nontuberculous mycobacteria [9764159, 15222531], otitis media, pancreatitis, parvovirus B19 [23113722, 20534986], *Pasteurella multocida* [10871983], penicillium spp., *Pneumocystis carinii* [10914942, 6816688], sialadenitis

(continued on next page)

Table 1
(continued)

Disease Process	Conditions
	[18420076], sporotrichosis [33025874, 21711340], *Staphylococcus aureus* [15569025], *Staphylococcus epidermidis* [17352724], tonsillitis [34054456], toxoplasmosis [4043468, 30918190], tuberculosis [29332658, 30238576, 23669432, 26891891, 21717890, 11229305]
Immunodeficiencies	Adult-onset immunodeficiency precipitated by antiinterferon gamma antibodies [34676591], chronic granulomatous disease [22246153], common variable immunodeficiency [31089823, 18782323], complement deficiency [2803964], human immunodeficiency virus [10397569, 26396453, 21679803, 18206098, 10545563, 33052291], primary T-cell immunodeficiency disease [10321630], T-cell lymphopenia [10321630]
Musculoskeletal	Chronic recurrent multifocal osteomyelitis [3591758, 19840301, 10383779, 2809904]
Pulmonary	Bronchiolitis obliterans [11460854, 1951419, 17071150], lung transplant [34366039], organizing pneumonia [11460854, 25196175, 1951419, 25163580, 17071150], postoperative pneumonectomy [15223465], rhinosinusitis [16527036]
Renal/genitourinary	Amyloid nephropathy [32681397], end-stage renal disease [22605810], IgA nephropathy (Berger disease), ureter obstruction [2618175], urinary stone disease [1628515]
Vasculitides	ANCA vasculitis [35495970], eosinophilic granulomatosis with polyangiitis [32611774, 33060325], granulomatosis with polyangiitis [22605810], microscopic polyangiitis [22513149], Takayasu arteritis [15608327, 19569285, 35925217, 22011145]
Miscellaneous, autoinflammatory, and complex multisystem disorders	Chronic fatigue syndrome, differentiation syndrome [34026142, 34970368, 25685768], familial Mediterranean fever [19586502], 34159892, 18824843], Kikuchi disease [23955621]

Pubmed Identifiers for associated references are enclosed in brackets.
Abbreviations: ANCA, antineutrophilic cytoplasmic antibody; IgA, immunoglobulin A.
Adapted from Cohen, P.R. and Kurzrock, R. (2003), Sweet's syndrome revisited: a review of disease concepts. International Journal of Dermatology, 42: 761-778. https://doi.org/10.1046/j.1365-4362.2003.01891.x.

can precede, follow, or onset concurrently with a hematologic or solid tumor malignancy.[58] The first reported malignancy-induced case was in 1955 by Costello and colleagues (acute myelogenous leukemia); the first solid-tumor associated case (testicular carcinoma) was reported by Shapiro and colleagues in 1971.[59,60]

Most of the malignancy-associated cases are linked to hematologic disorders (82%), most commonly acute myelogenous leukemia.[50] Other relatively common hematogenous disorders that might be correlated with Sweet syndrome include myelodysplasia, chronic myelogenous leukemia, multiple myeloma, and monoclonal gammopathy. Differences in clinical course between acute myelogenous leukemia (commonly a single episode) and myelodysplasia-associated (usually chronic relapsing) Sweet syndrome seem to exist.[61]

Solid tumors comprise a smaller proportion (18%) of malignancy-associated cases and typically include carcinomas of the breast, genitourinary, and gastrointestinal systems.[50,58,62] The rash can precede the associated hematologic malignancy by up to 11 years and/or can occur as a paraneoplastic syndrome.[58]

Development of Sweet syndrome can be an initial sign of cancer recurrence in patients with histories of malignancy and/or a sign that a new cancer has emerged.[10] Although it can sometimes be difficult to gauge whether suspicion for an underlying neoplasm is warranted, leukopenia, anemia, thrombocytopenia, and absence of arthralgia may be associated with malignancy-associated disease.[50]

There are other neutrophilic dermatoses associated with hematologic malignancies (eg, atypical bullous pyoderma gangrenosum, neutrophilic eccrine hidradenitis) that may present similarly to Sweet syndrome; however, Sweet syndrome can be differentiated from these conditions through its histopathology and systemic manifestations (neutrophilia vs neutropenia in neutrophilic eccrine hidradenitis; lack of systemic features in atypical bullous pyoderma gangrenosum).[9]

Drug-induced Sweet syndrome
Drug-induced cases are a relatively uncommonly observed disease form and typically develop a couple of weeks after an inciting drug exposure. The first report of drug-induced Sweet syndrome involved trimethoprim-sulfamethoxazole and was published by Su and Liu in 1986.[26] Since then, there have been reports involving a broad spectrum of medications from a wide variety of drug classes, including antibiotics, antihypertensive medications, nonsteroidal antiinflammatory drugs, immunosuppressive and immunomodulating therapies, immunostimulants, antiepileptic drugs, antineoplastic agents, antipsychotics, immune checkpoint inhibitors, antithyroid medications, and antidepressants, among others. The most common iatrogenic trigger is granulocyte colony-stimulating factor.[11] A more detailed list of reported contributors can be found in **Table 2**. Disease oftentimes resolves on discontinuation of the provoking medication.

Other potential triggers
In addition to the iatrogenic triggers listed in **Table 2**, there are reports of Sweet syndrome developing following exposures to ultraviolet light, areas of long-standing lymphedema, radioiodine contrast, and vaccines.[63–74] Several coronavirus-19 vaccine–induced Sweet syndrome cases have been reported as well as a few cases involving measles-mumps-rubella-varicella, pneumococcal, influenza, and Bacillus Calmette–Guérin vaccines.[75–92] It is unclear what role, if any, pathergy and/or immune dysregulation played in the development of Sweet syndrome following vaccination. Sweet syndrome has also developed in other altered states of immunity such as renal transplants and autologous stem cell transplants.[93,94]

Neutrophilic dermatosis of the dorsal hands
Neutrophilic dermatosis of the dorsal hands is a condition that clinically and histologically resembles Sweet syndrome and is sometimes considered a subset of Sweet syndrome; however, larger ulcerated plaques and nodules may resemble and be on a spectrum with bullous pyoderma gangrenosum.[95] It was initially described by Strutton and colleagues in 1995 as a pustular vasculitis, although assigned its current name by Galaria and colleagues in 2000.[96,97] Although it is sometimes classified as a cutaneous vasculitis due to a few reported cases demonstrating leukocytoclastic vasculitis, a relatively small proportion of cases display this secondary effect, and the primary pathogenic mechanism is dermal infiltration.[96,98–100] Clinically, it is a localized cutaneous condition characterized by tender erythematous nodules and plaques that can form pustules, bullae, and ulcers. Lesions tend to affect the dorsal aspect of the hand between thumb and index finger bilaterally, although it may involve other areas of the body (eg, mucous membranes, arms, legs, trunk, and face).[95,101] Its morphology, treatment regimens, and response to treatment closely follow Sweet syndrome, predominantly corticosteroids, with alternative options including dapsone, colchicine, and potassium iodide.[102] There may also be an overlap in human leukocyte antigen markers.[103] Nonspecific systemic inflammatory markers, such as ESR and CRP, may be less frequently elevated compared with Sweet syndrome because it is a localized variant; however, they are still elevated most of the time (as are leukocytosis and neutrophilia).[104] Triggers generally closely mirror inciting factors for Sweet syndrome; patients may have coexistent comorbidities that can occur before, during, or after diagnosis, such as hematologic disorders, solid tumors, inflammatory bowel disease, and mucosal tract infections—most commonly respiratory tract infections.[104] It may also be triggered by trauma (eg, gardening injuries, thermal injuries, intravenous line insertion), exposures to chemicals such as fertilizer, and cocaine use.[98,105–108] Thus timely and accurate diagnosis is crucial, as procedural interventions, such as surgical debridement, can exacerbate the condition.[98] Medications may also be related to disease onset such as thalidomide, lenalidomide, and indomethacin.[109–111] Other possible factors, similar to Sweet syndrome, include vaccines.[112]

Although its rarity has generally precluded extensive study, a 123-patient case series reported a slight female predominance 58%, mean age 62 years (range 3–89 years).[104] Other case series have reported incidences in older individuals with a lower female predominance.[98,113] Concomitant pulmonary disease (eg, chronic obstructive pulmonary disease, asthma, secondhand smoke

Table 2
Drugs associated with development of Sweet syndrome

Drug Class	Medication Name
Analgesics	Aceclofenac [21506881], acetaminophen codeine [29121137], aspirin [28300447], celecoxib [11464196, 27060586], diclofenac [26288456], ibuprofen [28300447], metamizole [19702979], phenylbutazone [18420076]
Antibiotics	Amoxicillin-clavulanate [35170473], azithromycin [28300447], cephalexin [28300447], ciprofloxacin [21893237], clindamycin [20398826, 17723089], doxycycline [18779110], levofloxacin [35170473], minocycline [23158645, 1469130, 1826487], nitrofurantoin [10190073], norfloxacin [14702513], ofloxacin [16213026], piperacillin-tazobactam [18360136], quinupristin-dalfopristin [14619389], tetracyclines [12207601], trimethoprim-sulfamethoxazole [8621829, 35866718, 29538086, 20199454, 19221284, 19002360, 18576306]
Anticoagulants	Dabigatran [36041703], low-molecular-weight heparin [30907689]
Antidepressants	Amoxapine [14690466], citalopram [14690466]
Antiepileptic drugs	Carbamazepine [21152216], diazepam [11095204], gabapentin [28958741], lamotrigine [32995432]
Antifungals	Fluconazole [28891066], ketoconazole [25590289]
Antigout	Allopurinol [26684631]
Anti-HIV drugs	Abacavir [15337997]
Antihypertensives	Captopril [28300447], enalapril [28300447], hydralazine [8547013, 1895286, 2193156, 31720352, 22530328, 2944382]
Antimalarial	Chloroquine [19171233], hydroxychloroquine [31540835]
Antineoplastics	Azacitidine [33406304, 31820051, 29044459, 26327709, 24341928, 22555082, 21496689], bortezomib [25784226, 24338786, 23905772, 19442799, 19231647, 16464758, 16197442], capecitabine [28011887], carboplatin [35725278], cytosine arabinoside [10914942], dabrafenib [30724336, 29683894], dasatinib [30932238, 26825166], decitabine [23178879], docetaxel [35725278], enasidenib [34026142], erlotinib [35841359], gemcitabine [22082849], gilteritinib [26886840], ibrutinib [33112465], imatinib [15781678], ipilimumab [32089071, 29396853, 25437997, 24629370, 24113862], ixazomib [34114780, 31828594, 31455150], lenalidomide [19577327], letrozole [32206641], midostaurin [35495179, 34417240], mitoxantrone [21148263], nilotinib [18347292], palbociclib [32598526], pemetrexed [33028131], quizartinib [26886840], ruxolitinib [33112465, 34529266, 28824063, 25707420], sorafenib [23687091], topotecan [24371676], trametinib [30724336, 29683894], vedolizumab [29900741], vemurafenib [24617955, 24372055], vorinostat [21870904]
Antiplatelets	Clopidogrel [32888004], ticagrelor [27146134]
Antipsychotics	Clozapine [12411238], perphenazine [14690466]

(continued on next page)

Table 2
(continued)

Drug Class	Medication Name
Antiviral	Acyclovir [28300447], interferon beta [23786157, 25756490], pegylated interferon alpha [18937663], ribavirin [18937663]
Biological immunomodulators	Abatacept [25117161], adalimumab [22670004, 32567672], infliximab [21798483], risankizumab [35135798], toclizumab [31921506]
Diabetes/heart failure medications	Dapagliflozin [31603973]
Diuretics	Furosemide [15954518]
Erythropoiesis-stimulating agents	Erythropoietin [18457725]
Hormonal agents	Benzylthiouracil [19442798], levonorgestrel-releasing intrauterine device [15086998], oral contraceptives [25772734, 11834860, 1834046], propylthiouracil [10583195], triphasil [1834046]
Immunostimulants	Granulocyte colony-stimulating factor (pegfilgrastim [35389579, 15858487, 1375012]), granulocyte-monocyte colony-stimulating factor (sargramostim [15224368]), IL-2 [20486462]
Other small molecule antiinflammatory agents	Mesalamine [29574433], sulfasalazine [27235662, 23879316]
Proton pump inhibitors	Esomeprazole, omeprazole [26114067]
Retinoids	13-cis retinoid acid [12461805], acitretin, all-trans retinoid acid [9922053], isotretinoin [25324016, 12461805]
Small molecule immunosuppressives	Azathioprine [35983669, 30074533, 28203157, 27090551, 26299606, 26219289, 25791317, 26120462, 23955987, 23294021, 22448458, 18775203, 18623176, 23677084]

Pubmed Identifiers for associated references are enclosed in brackets.

Abbreviation: IL-2, interleukin-2.

Adapted from Cohen, P.R. Sweet's syndrome - a comprehensive review of an acute febrile neutrophilic dermatosis. Orphanet J Rare Dis 2, 34 (2007). https://doi.org/10.1186/1750-1172-2-34.

exposures, oxygen dependence) was reported in 66% of patients in a 2019 retrospective case series; it is possible that disease onset may be related to vascular disruption and/or acral cyanosis.[113]

Histopathology

The clinical differential for Sweet syndrome is broad, and thus, histologic correlation can facilitate an accurate diagnosis. Lesional punch biopsies extending into the subcutis of active papules/plaques are standard. In some cases, a second biopsy specimen may be useful for bacterial, fungal, and mycobacterial cultures. Swab specimens can be obtained from pustules to be sent for culture, and the authors recommend microbial pathology, as Sweet syndrome can present similarly, both clinically and histologically, to skin infections such as cellulitis and/or abscesses.

Typical histologic features include prominent superficial edema, dense neutrophilic infiltrate in the upper and middermis, leukocytoclasia, endothelial swelling, possible eosinophils, and/or lymphocytes/macrophages in older lesions. However, several atypical histologic variants exist as mentioned earlier (**Fig. 2**).

Imaging

Laboratory testing

Leukocytosis with neutrophilia is common in all forms, and ESR and CRP elevations are also common. Extracutaneous involvement may drive abnormalities on a complete metabolic panel and/or urinalysis. Thus, obtaining a complete blood count with differential, complete metabolic panel, ESR, CRP, urinalysis, and pregnancy test (in childbearing aged women) is recommended. Additional tests may be appropriate depending on the clinical context, such as chest radiographs for patients with suspected pulmonary involvement. Computerized tomography scans to assess for underlying malignancy may be warranted, although further

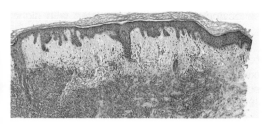

Fig. 2. Typical histopathologic findings of Sweet syndrome: prominent superficial edema with a dense neutrophilic infiltrate primarily in the dermis. (Image courtesy of PathPresenter.)

workup with laboratory tests and/or imaging is generally appropriate only when suspicion is relatively high (ie, weight loss and so on). Age-appropriate cancer screening and a comprehensive review of medications are advised in all patients with Sweet syndrome.

DISCUSSION
Guidelines/Therapeutic Options

Current evidence
Therapeutic ladder Evidence to guide management for Sweet syndrome is primarily limited to small nonexperimental descriptive studies. Although classic Sweet syndrome may resolve spontaneously, its disease course can be unpredictable, and treatment may accelerate resolution.[1] In addition, reports of spontaneous resolution seem to be relatively sparse; in a retrospective study of 80 patients, resolution without treatment occurred in 20% of patients.[114] Another retrospective case series of 48 patients reported resolution without therapy in only 6% of patients.[115] Malignancy-associated cases tend to be recalcitrant and warrant treatment.

Systemic corticosteroids (oral prednisone, 0.5–1 mg/kg/d) are first-line therapy for Sweet syndrome and typically result in rapid improvement (within 48 hours), which can aid in establishing a diagnosis.[4,116] After achieving disease control, corticosteroids can be tapered over 4 to 6 weeks.[116] However, they are associated with potential side effects, and several common comorbidities can make systemic corticosteroids unfavorable such as hypertension, hypercholesterolemia, diabetes, and osteoporosis. Patients with extensive disease severity typically require oral systemic treatment, and severe refractory disease may warrant pulse-dosed intravenous corticosteroids (methylprednisolone 500–1000 mg daily for 3–5 days).[11] Because Sweet syndrome can exhibit pathergy, it may be appropriate to attempt oral pharmacologic management before intravenous medications, injectables, and/or procedural intervention.[5] High-potency topical (clobetasol 0.05% ointment) and/or

intralesional corticosteroids (triamcinolone 3–10 mg/mL) may be appropriate for localized involvement and/or as adjunctive therapies to systemic treatment.[116]

The most commonly used nonsteroidal systemic therapies are dapsone, colchicine, and potassium iodide.

Dapsone (25–200 mg daily) can be a favorable treatment option for Sweet syndrome.[116,117] Improvements are generally observed within 1 to 3 weeks.[117] Because dapsone is associated with agranulocytosis and drug-induced hemolytic anemia in patients with glucose-6-phosphate dehydrogenase (G6PD) deficiency, it is important to test G6PD enzyme levels before initiation of therapy and routinely monitor blood counts.

Colchicine (0.6 mg 2 to 3 times daily) is used for several neutrophilic dermatoses, including Sweet syndrome. Similar to dapsone, small uncontrolled studies have reported high response rates and improvements within 1 to 3 weeks.[118–120] Colchicine is associated with several side effects such as myelosuppression, neuropathy, and myopathy; however, the most common treatment-limiting side effect is gastrointestinal upset.[121]

Potassium iodide (20–30 drops [1000–1500 mg] saturated solution daily or 300 mg pills 3 times daily) has shown comparable response times as corticosteroids (within 48 hours) and may be a particularly effective option for cases associated with underlying vasculitis and thyroid disease.[20] Potential side effects include gastrointestinal upset, reversible hypothyroidism, acneiform skin eruptions, and headache.[122]

Other small molecule immunosuppressants and nonsteroidal antiinflammatory drugs can be effective. Cyclosporine (2–4 mg/kg/d) is a fast-acting steroid-sparing option (initial responses within 1 week) although its side effects (hypertension and nephrotoxicity) can preclude prolonged use.[20] Methotrexate (5–20 mg weekly) can address inflammatory conditions associated with Sweet syndrome and, in our experience, may be favored by oncologists for malignancy-associated cases. Initial responses (median 1.5 months) may occur slightly slower than both systemic corticosteroids (0.25–0.5 months) and dapsone (1 month).[27,117,123] Indomethacin (150 mg daily for 1 week then 100 mg daily for 2 weeks) has been studied prospectively (n = 18) with a high (94%) response rate.[124]

Other systemic therapies with growing evidence can be found in **Table 3**.

Pediatric Sweet syndrome lacks extensive study, and approach to treatment follows the management ladder for adults.

Treatment of neutrophilic dermatosis of the dorsal hands also closely follows Sweet syndrome; oral glucocorticoids and dapsone have been effective in small case series.[97,98,125] It is unclear whether minocycline can yield sustained responses.[125]

CLINICAL OUTCOMES

Prognosis and risk of recurrence vary based on the underlying cause. Classic Sweet syndrome can spontaneously resolve within 5 to 12 weeks or within a few weeks in patients who receive systemic treatment.[9] In contrast, malignancy-associated disease is typically more resistant to treatment and may take longer to resolve. Relapses may occur on tapering or discontinuation of therapy and seem to be more likely in patients with malignancy-associated disease; recurrence rates are roughly 69% in patients with underlying hematologic malignancy compared with 30% in patients with classic Sweet syndrome.[10,126,127]

Leukocytoclasia may be associated with higher recurrence rates.[128]

On healing, milia and scarring may occur, and postinflammatory hyperpigmentation typically takes several months to resolve.[6,40] However, cutaneous lesions of Sweet syndrome usually heal without scarring if ulceration does not occur.[10]

CONTROVERSIES AND CONSIDERATIONS

There are several limitations that preclude definitive conclusions.

Regarding interpretation of treatment data, the characteristic relapsing-remitting course of Sweet syndrome can make outcomes difficult to interpret. Furthermore, studies to support these medications are limited by their sample size and, in some cases, by the concomitant use of corticosteroids. Numerous studies had heterogeneous

---

Table 3
Medications with growing evidence for the treatment of Sweet syndrome

Drug Class	Medication Name
Antibiotics	
Antimycobacterial	Clofazimine [8089280, 11893223]
Nitroimidazoles	Metronidazole [7799365]
Tetracyclines	Doxycycline [8504055, 11893223, 28108184], minocycline [2099706]
Antineoplastics	Azacitidine, chlorambucil [2758862], cyclophosphamide [22115387, 12072085, 1466198]
Biologics	
Anti-CD20	Rituximab [26998300, 35333375]
IL-1 antagonists	Anakinra [18192308, 21464561, 31263644], rilonacept [21464561]
IL-12, IL-23 antagonists	Ustekinumab [36447766, 30003991]
JAK inhibitors	Baricitinib [27051705, 26998300, 27028556, 35157247, 33914946], tocilizumab [32681397, 31089823]
TNF-alpha inhibitors	Adalimumab [27028556, 32833303, 34897822], etanercept [19509095, 17043542], infliximab [30376667, 30074533, 32901971, 29474532]
Immune globulins	Intravenous immunoglobulin [24395855, 20369066, 16354255]
Immunosuppressive small molecules	Azathioprine [11893223, 8089280, 17655751, 9091476], cyclosporine [8033398, 1637692, 24750407, 1467297, 11893223], lenalidomide [24850455], tacrolimus [11253280], thalidomide [16021163]
Other immunomodulator	Interferon alpha [11893223, 7727840]
Other small molecule antiinflammatory agents	Sulfasalazine [21062595]
Retinoids	Acitretin [32207168, 34676629], etretinate [8900854, 11893223]

Pubmed Identifiers for associated references are enclosed in brackets.
Abbreviations: IL, interleukin; JAK, Janus kinase; TNF, tumor necrosis factor.

samples with a combination of classic, malignancy-associated, and drug-induced cases that may have variable responses to therapy. Recurrence rates and time to relapse are also not well characterized.

Determining precise triggers and underlying causes can be difficult. Several medications effective at treating Sweet syndrome have paradoxically been associated with induction of disease such as azathioprine, ipilimumab, adalimumab, nivolumab, abatacept, tocilizumab, and vedolizumab, among others.[129–131] Because several reports of drug-induced disease have involved therapies that can be used to treat Sweet syndrome and/or underlying conditions associated with Sweet syndrome, it is unclear whether the conditions contributed to the onset of disease versus solely the drug. Some drug reactions can also present as neutrophilic dermatoses and closely resemble Sweet syndrome such as azathioprine hypersensitivity syndrome.[132] Nevertheless, there is an increasing incidence of reports of drug-induced disease that has occurred in conjunction with more widespread use of cancer therapies.[20] It has also been hypothesized that malignancy-associated disease and anticancer therapy–induced disease may exhibit distinguishable behavior; however, further study is needed to more clearly define these differences.[20]

SUMMARY
Recommendations

Conclusions and future directions
In summary, the precise cause of Sweet syndrome remains unclear. It seems to be multifactorial and related to immune stimulation/alteration/dysregulation (infection, autoimmune disease/malignancy, transplant, immunodeficient states), chemical and physical insults, and various medication exposures. It may share features with other neutrophil-rich cutaneous disorders such as pyoderma gangrenosum. Although systemic corticosteroids provide rapid improvements and are first-line therapy for Sweet syndrome, there are a multitude of steroid-sparing small molecule and biological therapies that seem effective with variable response times. However, most of the evidence is limited to retrospective nonexperimental descriptive studies such as case series and case reports. Although more robust investigations with larger sample sizes are needed, future studies might consider separating malignancy-induced cases from classic and drug-induced for analyzing disease courses and responses to therapy.

CLINICS CARE POINTS

- Lesional biopsies of active lesions and tissue cultures should be obtained to evaluate for alternative diagnoses.
- Basic laboratory workup is indicated in all patients with Sweet syndrome, and in some cases, additional imaging/specimen sampling is warranted based on suspected underlying cause and/or extracutaneous involvements.
- There are several nonsteroidal small molecule and biological therapies with growing evidence for their effectiveness that can be used for patients who cannot tolerate corticosteroids and/or require prolonged therapy.

DISCLOSURES

The authors have no relevant conflicts to disclose.

REFERENCES

1. Sweet RD. An acute febrile neutrophilic dermatosis. Br J Dermatol 1964;76:349–56.
2. Heath MS, Ortega-Loayza AG. Insights Into the Pathogenesis of Sweet's Syndrome. Front Immunol 2019;10:414.
3. Nelson CA, Stephen S, Ashchyan HJ, et al. Neutrophilic dermatoses: Pathogenesis, Sweet syndrome, neutrophilic eccrine hidradenitis, and Behçet disease. J Am Acad Dermatol 2018;79(6):987–1006.
4. Rochet NM, Chavan RN, Cappel MA, et al. Sweet syndrome: clinical presentation, associations, and response to treatment in 77 patients. J Am Acad Dermatol 2013;69(4):557–64.
5. Halpern J, Salim A. Pediatric Sweet syndrome: case report and literature review. Pediatr Dermatol 2009;26(4):452–7.
6. Kemmett D, Hunter JA. Sweet's syndrome: a clinicopathologic review of twenty-nine cases. J Am Acad Dermatol 1990;23(3 Pt 1):503–7.
7. Amouri M, Masmoudi A, Ammar M, et al. Sweet's syndrome: a retrospective study of 90 cases from a tertiary care center. Int J Dermatol 2016;55(9):1033–9.
8. Joshi TP, Friske SK, Hsiou DA, et al. New Practical Aspects of Sweet Syndrome. Am J Clin Dermatol 2022;23(3):301–18.
9. Moschella SL, Davis M. In: Bolognia JL, Jorizzo JL, Dermatology Rapini RP, editors. Neutrophilic dermatosesVol 1, 2nd edition. Philadelphia: Elsevier; 2008. p. 379.
10. Cohen PR. Sweet's syndrome–a comprehensive review of an acute febrile neutrophilic dermatosis. Orphanet J Rare Dis 2007;2:34.

11. Cohen PR, Hongsmann H, Kurzrock R. Acute febrile neutrophilic dermatosis (Sweet syndrome). In: Goldsmith LA, Katz SI, Gilchrest BA, et al, editors. Fitzpatrick's DermatologyVol 1, 8th edition. New York: McGraw Hill; 2012. p. 362.

12. Hisanaga K, Hosokawa M, Sato N, et al. "Neuro-Sweet disease": benign recurrent encephalitis with neutrophilic dermatosis. Arch Neurol 1999;56(8):1010–3.

13. Kitamura S, Hamauchi A, Ota M. Neuro-Sweet's disease. Int J Dermatol 2016;55(9):e513–4.

14. Bamelis M, Boyden B, Sente F, et al. Sweet's syndrome and acute myelogenous leukemia in a patient who presented with a sudden massive swelling of the tongue. Dermatology 1995;190(4):335–7.

15. Gottlieb CC, Mishra A, Belliveau D, et al. Ocular involvement in acute febrile neutrophilic dermatosis (Sweet syndrome): new cases and review of the literature. Surv Ophthalmol 2008;53(3):219–26.

16. Medenblik-Frysch S, von den Driesch P, Jonas JB, et al. Ocular complications in Sweet's syndrome. Am J Ophthalmol 1992;114(2):230–1.

17. Baartman B, Kosari P, Warren CC, et al. Sight-threatening ocular manifestations of acute febrile neutrophilic dermatosis (Sweet's syndrome). Dermatology 2014;228(3):193–7.

18. Aghazadeh H, Sia D, Ehmann D. Central retinal artery occlusion associated with Sweet syndrome. Can J Ophthalmol 2021;56(3):e103–5.

19. Manglani R, Jilani N, Raji M, et al. Pulmonary Involvement in Sweet's Syndrome. Am J Respir Crit Care Med 2021;204(10):1222–3.

20. Raza S, Kirkland RS, Patel AA, et al. Insight into Sweet's syndrome and associated-malignancy: a review of the current literature. Int J Oncol 2013;42(5):1516–22.

21. Shugarman IL, Schmit JM, Sbicca JA, et al. Easily missed extracutaneous manifestation of malignancy-associated Sweet's syndrome: systemic inflammatory response syndrome. J Clin Oncol 2011;29(24):e702–5.

22. Vanourny J, Swick BL. Sweet syndrome with systemic inflammatory response syndrome. Arch Dermatol 2012;148(8):969–70.

23. Sawicki J, Morton RA, Ellis AK. Sweet syndrome with associated systemic inflammatory response syndrome: an ultimately fatal case. Ann Allergy Asthma Immunol 2010;105(4):321–3.

24. Otheo E, Ros P, Vázquez JL, et al. Systemic inflammatory response syndrome associated with Sweet's syndrome. Pediatr Crit Care Med 2002;3(2):190–3.

25. Vettakkara KMN, Banerjee S, Mittal A, et al. Not so sweet; severe Sweet's syndrome presenting as SIRS and pleural effusion. J Family Med Prim Care 2018;7(6):1584–7.

26. Su WP, Liu HN. Diagnostic criteria for Sweet's syndrome. Cutis 1986;37(3):167–74.

27. von den Driesch P. Sweet's syndrome (acute febrile neutrophilic dermatosis). J Am Acad Dermatol 1994;31(4):535–60.

28. Berro S, Calas A, Sohier P, et al. Sweet's Syndrome Three Weeks after a Severe COVID-19 Infection: A Case Report. Acta Derm Venereol 2021;101(6):adv00486.

29. Taşkın B, Vural S, Altuğ E, et al. Coronavirus 19 presenting with atypical Sweet's syndrome. J Eur Acad Dermatol Venereol 2020;34(10):e534–5.

30. Escanilla C, Goldman Y, Bobadilla F, et al. Sweet syndrome associated with secondary nodular syphilis in an immunocompetent patient. An Bras Dermatol 2021;96(3):319–23.

31. Kürkçüoğlu N, Aksoy F. Sweet's syndrome associated with Helicobacter pylori infection. J Am Acad Dermatol 1997;37(1):123–4.

32. Karadoğan SK, Başkan EB, Alkan G, et al. Generalized Sweet syndrome lesions associated with Behçet disease: a true association or simply comorbidity? Am J Clin Dermatol 2009;10(5):331–5.

33. Arima Y, Namiki T, Ueno M, et al. Histiocytoid Sweet syndrome: a novel association with relapsing polychondritis. Br J Dermatol 2016;174(3):691–4.

34. Fujimoto N, Tajima S, Ishibashi A, et al. Acute febrile neutrophilic dermatosis (Sweet's syndrome) in a patient with relapsing polychondritis. Br J Dermatol 1998;139(5):930–1.

35. Kodama T, Yamazaki Y, Takeo H. Neuro-Sweet disease in a Japanese woman with Sjögren's syndrome. BMJ Case Rep 2019;12(12):e232933.

36. Manzo C, Pollio N, Natale M. Sweet's Syndrome Following Therapy with Hydroxychloroquine in a Patient Affected with Elderly-Onset Primary Sjogren's Syndrome. Medicines (Basel) 2019;6(4):111.

37. Osawa H, Yamabe H, Seino S, et al. A case of Sjögren's syndrome associated with Sweet's syndrome. Clin Rheumatol 1997;16(1):101–5.

38. Flanagan KE, Krueger S, Amano S, et al. Sweet syndrome with perifollicular involvement because of koebnerization from facial hair plucking. J Cutan Pathol 2021;48(9):1189–92.

39. Kluger N, Del Giudice P. First case of Sweet's syndrome after tattooing [published online ahead of print, 2022 Jun 22]. Ann Dermatol Venereol 2022;S0151-9638(22):00033.

40. Satra K, Zalka A, Cohen PR, et al. Sweet's syndrome and pregnancy. J Am Acad Dermatol 1994;30(2 Pt 2):297–300.

41. Pagliarello C, Pepe CA, Lombardi M, et al. Early miscarriage during Sweet's syndrome: uncommon, but probably not coincidental. Eur J Dermatol 2013;23(5):707–8.

42. Corbeddu M, Pilloni L, Pau M, et al. Treatment of Sweet's syndrome in pregnancy. Dermatol Ther 2018;31(4):e12619.

43. Lear JT, Byrne JP. Bullous pyoderma gangrenosum, Sweet's syndrome and malignancy. Br J Dermatol 1997;136(2):296–7.

44. Cohen PR. Subcutaneous Sweet's syndrome: a variant of acute febrile neutrophilic dermatosis that is included in the histopathologic differential diagnosis of neutrophilic panniculitis. J Am Acad Dermatol 2005;52(5):927–8.

45. Ko JS, Fernandez AP, Anderson KA, et al. Morphologic mimickers of Cryptococcus occurring within inflammatory infiltrates in the setting of neutrophilic dermatitis: a series of three cases highlighting clinical dilemmas associated with a novel histopathologic pitfall. J Cutan Pathol 2013;40(1):38–45.

46. Wilson J, Gleghorn K, Kelly B. Cryptococcoid Sweet's syndrome: Two reports of Sweet's syndrome mimicking cutaneous cryptococcosis. J Cutan Pathol 2017;44(5):413–9.

47. Requena L, Kutzner H, Palmedo G, et al. Histiocytoid Sweet syndrome: a dermal infiltration of immature neutrophilic granulocytes. Arch Dermatol 2005;141(7):834–42.

48. Chavan RN, Cappel MA, Ketterling RP, et al. Histiocytoid Sweet syndrome may indicate leukemia cutis: a novel application of fluorescence in situ hybridization. J Am Acad Dermatol 2014;70(6):1021–7.

49. Alegría-Landa V, Rodríguez-Pinilla SM, Santos-Briz A, et al. Clinicopathologic, Immunohistochemical, and Molecular Features of Histiocytoid Sweet Syndrome. JAMA Dermatol 2017;153(7):651–9.

50. Nelson CA, Noe MH, McMahon CM, et al. Sweet syndrome in patients with and without malignancy: A retrospective analysis of 83 patients from a tertiary academic referral center. J Am Acad Dermatol 2018;78(2):303–9.e4.

51. Ghoufi L, Ortonne N, Ingen-Housz-Oro S, et al. Histiocytoid Sweet Syndrome Is More Frequently Associated With Myelodysplastic Syndromes Than the Classical Neutrophilic Variant: A Comparative Series of 62 Patients. Medicine (Baltim) 2016;95(15):e3033.

52. Surovy AM, Pelivani N, Hegyi I, et al. Giant cellulitis-like Sweet Syndrome, a new variant of neutrophilic dermatosis. JAMA Dermatol 2013;149(1):79–83.

53. Kroshinsky D, Alloo A, Rothschild B, et al. Necrotizing Sweet syndrome: a new variant of neutrophilic dermatosis mimicking necrotizing fasciitis. J Am Acad Dermatol 2012;67(5):945–54.

54. Sanchez IM, Lowenstein S, Johnson KA, et al. Clinical Features of Neutrophilic Dermatosis Variants Resembling Necrotizing Fasciitis. JAMA Dermatol 2019;155(1):79–84.

55. Kamimura A, Yanagisawa H, Tsunemi Y, et al. Normolipemic xanthomatized Sweet's syndrome: A variant of Sweet's syndrome with myelodysplastic syndrome. J Dermatol 2021;48(5):695–8.

56. PĂtraȘcu V, Geoloaica LG, Ciurea RN. Recurrent Idiopathic Sweet Syndrome - Case Report and Literature Review. Curr Health Sci J 2020;46(1):90–8.

57. Burke N, Saikaly SK, Motaparthi K, et al. Malignancy-associated Sweet syndrome presenting with simultaneous histopathologic and morphologic variants. JAAD Case Rep 2021;14:104–7.

58. Cohen PR, Kurzrock R. Sweet's syndrome and cancer. Clin Dermatol 1993;11(1):149–57.

59. Costello MJ, Canizares O, Montague M, et al. Cutaneous manifestations of myelogenous leukemia. AMA Arch Derm 1955;71(5):605–14.

60. Shapiro L, Baraf CS, Richheimer LL. Sweet's syndrome (acute febrile neutrophilic dermatosis). Report of a case. Arch Dermatol 1971;103(1):81–4.

61. Merlant M, Lepelletier C, Battistella M, et al. Acute myeloid leukemia and myelodysplastic syndrome-associated Sweet syndrome: A comparative multicenter retrospective study of 39 patients. J Am Acad Dermatol 2021;84(3):838–40.

62. Cohen PR, Holder WR, Tucker SB, et al. Sweet syndrome in patients with solid tumors. Cancer 1993;72(9):2723–31.

63. Sano Y, Moriki M, Yagi H, et al. Photoinduced histiocytoid Sweet's syndrome. J Dermatol 2019;46(10):e378–80.

64. Pai VV, Gupta G, Athanikar S, et al. Photoinduced classic Sweet syndrome presenting as hemorrhagic bullae. Cutis 2014;93(6):E22–4.

65. Verma R, Vasudevan B, Pragasam V, et al. Unusual Presentation of Idiopathic Sweet's Syndrome in a Photodistributed Pattern. Indian J Dermatol 2014;59(2):186–9.

66. Natkunarajah J, Gordon K, Chow J, et al. Photoaggravated Sweet's syndrome. Clin Exp Dermatol 2010;35(3):e18–9.

67. Belhadjali H, Marguery MC, Lamant L, et al. Photosensitivity in Sweet's syndrome: two cases that were photoinduced and photoaggravated. Br J Dermatol 2003;149(3):675–7.

68. Bessis D, Dereure O, Peyron JL, et al. Photoinduced Sweet syndrome. Arch Dermatol 2001;137(8):1106–8.

69. Ollivier L, Renaud E, Gouders D, et al. Sweet syndrome induced by radiations during breast cancer treatment. BMJ Case Rep 2019;12(4):e223938.

70. Dawe SA, Phillips R, Porter W, et al. Sweet's syndrome as a complication of radiotherapy for squamous carcinoma of the pharynx. Br J Dermatol 2003;149(4):884.

71. Vergara G, Vargas-Machuca I, Pastor MA, et al. Localization of Sweet's syndrome in radiation-induced locus minoris resistentae. J Am Acad Dermatol 2003;49(5):907–9.

72. van der Meij EH, Epstein JB, Hay J, et al. Sweet's syndrome in a patient with oral cancer associated with radiotherapy. Eur J Cancer B Oral Oncol 1996;32B(2):133–6.

73. Demitsu T, Tadaki T. Atypical neutrophilic dermatosis on the upper extremity affected by postmastectomy lymphedema: report of 2 cases. Dermatol 1991;183(3):230–3.

74. Bhat AG, Siddappa Malleshappa SK, Pasupula DK, et al. Bullous Variant of Sweet's Syndrome as a Consequence of Radioiodine Contrast Exposure. Cureus 2018;10(10):e3490.

75. Sadhukhan S, Rafi S, Bains A, et al. COVID-19 vaccine-induced Sweet syndrome presenting as fingertip pustules [published online ahead of print, 2022 Nov 15]. J Eur Acad Dermatol Venereol 2022. https://doi.org/10.1111/jdv.18746.

76. Kim MJ, Kim JW, Na JI. Sweet syndrome after the first dose of SARS-CoV-2 vaccine (Pfizer-BioNTech) [published online ahead of print, 2022 Oct 9]. Dermatol Ther 2022;e15915. https://doi.org/10.1111/dth.15915.

77. Pelchat F, Fournier C, Perron E, et al. Sweet syndrome following Moderna COVID-19 vaccine: A case report. SAGE Open Med Case Rep 2022; 10. 2050313X221117884.

78. Ben Salah N, Korbi M, Ben Fadhel N, et al. Sweet Syndrome following SARS-CoV-2 CoronaVac vaccine. J Eur Acad Dermatol Venereol 2022;36(11):e873–5.

79. Darrigade AS, Oulès B, Sohier P, et al. Sweet-like syndrome and multiple COVID arm syndrome following COVID-19 vaccines: 'specific' patterns in a series of 192 patients. Br J Dermatol 2022; 187(4):615–7.

80. Hoshina D, Orita A. Sweet syndrome after severe acute respiratory syndrome coronavirus 2 mRNA vaccine: A case report and literature review. J Dermatol 2022;49(5):e175–6.

81. Kinariwalla N, London AO, Soliman YS, et al. A case of generalized Sweet syndrome with vasculitis triggered by recent COVID-19 vaccination. JAAD Case Rep 2022;19:64–7.

82. Baffa ME, Maglie R, Giovannozzi N, et al. Sweet Syndrome Following SARS-CoV2 Vaccination. Vaccines (Basel) 2021;9(11):1212.

83. Žagar T, Hlača N, Brajac I, et al. Bullous Sweet syndrome following SARS-CoV-2 Oxford AstraZeneca vaccine. Br J Dermatol 2022;186(3):e110.

84. Sechi A, Pierobon E, Pezzolo E, et al. Abrupt onset of Sweet syndrome, pityriasis rubra pilaris, pityriasis lichenoides et varioliformis acuta and erythema multiforme: unravelling a possible common trigger, the COVID-19 vaccine. Clin Exp Dermatol 2022;47(2):437–40.

85. Majid I, Mearaj S. Sweet syndrome after Oxford-AstraZeneca COVID-19 vaccine (AZD1222) in an elderly female. Dermatol Ther 2021;34(6):e15146.

86. Darrigade AS, Théophile H, Sanchez-Pena P, et al. Sweet syndrome induced by SARS-CoV-2 Pfizer-BioNTech mRNA vaccine. Allergy 2021;76(10): 3194–6.

87. Ben Rejeb S, Beltaifa D, Dhaoui A, et al. SARS-CoV-2 vaccine induced Sweet syndrome : a case report. Tunis Med 2021;99(12):1188–91.

88. Itzhaki Gabay S, Samueli B, Test G, et al. Infantile Sweet syndrome following MMRV vaccine [published online ahead of print, 2022 Nov 13]. Pediatr Dermatol 2022. https://doi.org/10.1111/pde.15162.

89. Pedrosa AF, Morais P, Nogueira A, et al. Sweet's syndrome triggered by pneumococcal vaccination. Cutan Ocul Toxicol 2013;32(3):260–1.

90. Tan AW, Tan HH, Lim PL. Bullous Sweet's syndrome following influenza vaccination in a HIV-infected patient. Int J Dermatol 2006;45(10):1254–5.

91. Jovanović M, Poljacki M, Vujanović L, et al. Acute febrile neutrophilic dermatosis (Sweet's syndrome) after influenza vaccination. J Am Acad Dermatol 2005;52(2):367–9.

92. Carpentier O, Piette F, Delaporte E. Sweet's syndrome after BCG vaccination. Acta Derm Venereol 2002;82(3):221.

93. Osband AJ, Laskow DA, Mann RA, et al. Sweet syndrome after kidney transplantation. Transplant Proc 2009;41(5):1954–6.

94. Alkan A, İdemen C, Okçu Heper A, et al. Sweet Syndrome After Autologous Stem Cell Transplant. Exp Clin Transplant 2016;14(1):109–11.

95. Walling HW, Snipes CJ, Gerami P, et al. The relationship between neutrophilic dermatosis of the dorsal hands and Sweet syndrome: report of 9 cases and comparison to atypical pyoderma gangrenosum. Arch Dermatol 2006;142(1):57–63.

96. Strutton G, Weedon D, Robertson I. Pustular vasculitis of the hands. J Am Acad Dermatol 1995;32(2 Pt 1):192–8.

97. Galaria NA, Junkins-Hopkins JM, Kligman D, et al. Neutrophilic dermatosis of the dorsal hands: pustular vasculitis revisited. J Am Acad Dermatol 2000; 43(5 Pt 1):870–4.

98. Cheng AMY, Cheng HS, Smith BJ, et al. Neutrophilic Dermatosis of the Hands: A Review of 17 Cases. J Hand Surg Am 2018;43(2):185.e1. https://doi.org/10.1016/j.jhsa.2017.08.027.

99. Malone JC, Slone SP, Wills-Frank LA, et al. Vascular inflammation (vasculitis) in Sweet syndrome: a clinicopathologic study of 28 biopsy specimens from 21 patients. Arch Dermatol 2002;138(3):345–9.

100. Cohen PR. Skin lesions of Sweet syndrome and its dorsal hand variant contain vasculitis: an oxymoron or an epiphenomenon? Arch Dermatol 2002;138(3):400–3.

101. Neoh CY, Tan AW, Ng SK. Sweet's syndrome: a spectrum of unusual clinical presentations and associations. Br J Dermatol 2007;156(3):480–5.

102. Ramos FS, Ferreira FR, Rabay FMO, et al. Neutrophilic dermatosis of the dorsal hands: response to dapsone monotherapy. An Bras Dermatol 2018; 93(5):730–2.

103. Takahama H, Kanbe T. Neutrophilic dermatosis of the dorsal hands: a case showing HLA B54, the marker of Sweet's syndrome. Int J Dermatol 2010; 49(9):1079–80.

104. Micallef D, Bonnici M, Pisani D, et al. Neutrophilic Dermatosis of the Dorsal Hands: A Review of 123 Cases [published online ahead of print, 2019 Sep 6]. J Am Acad Dermatol 2019;S0190-9622(19):32678–87.

105. Stransky L, Broshtilova V. Neutrophilic dermatosis of the dorsal hands elicited by thermal injury. Contact Dermatitis 2003;49(1):42.

106. Gloor AD, Feldmeyer L, Borradori L. Neutrophilic dermatosis of the dorsal hands triggered by mechanical trauma. J Eur Acad Dermatol Venereol 2021;35(1):e20–1.

107. Aydin F, Senturk N, Yildiz L, et al. Neutrophilic dermatosis of the dorsal hands in a farmer. J Eur Acad Dermatol Venereol 2004;18(6):716–7.

108. Álvarez-Salafranca M, García-García M, de Escalante Yangüela B. Neutrophilic dermatosis of the dorsal hands related to cocaine abuse. An Bras Dermatol 2021;96(5):574–7.

109. Mathieu S, Soubrier M, Tournadre A, et al. Neutrophilic dermatosis of the dorsal hands during thalidomide treatment. Int J Dermatol 2014;53(9):1133–5.

110. Hoverson AR, Davis MD, Weenig RH, et al. Neutrophilic dermatosis (Sweet syndrome) of the hands associated with lenalidomide. Arch Dermatol 2006;142(8):1070–1.

111. Kaur MR, Bazza MA, Ryatt KS. Neutrophilic dermatosis of the dorsal hands treated with indomethacin. Br J Dermatol 2006;155(5):1089–90.

112. Wolf R, Barzilai A, Davidovici B. Neutrophilic dermatosis of the hands after influenza vaccination. Int J Dermatol 2009;48(1):66–8.

113. King BJ, Montagnon CM, Brough K, et al. Neutrophilic dermatosis of the dorsal hands is commonly associated with underlying hematologic malignancy and pulmonary disease: A single-center retrospective case series study [published online ahead of print, 2022 May 23]. J Am Acad Dermatol 2022;S0190-9622(22):00879.

114. Bourke JF, Keohane S, Long CC, et al. Sweet's syndrome and malignancy in the U.K. Br J Dermatol 1997;137(4):609–13.

115. Fett DL, Gibson LE, Su WP. Sweet's syndrome: systemic signs and symptoms and associated disorders. Mayo Clin Proc 1995;70(3):234–40.

116. Cohen PR, Kurzrock R. Sweet's syndrome: a review of current treatment options. Am J Clin Dermatol 2002;3(2):117–31.

117. Hrin ML, Feldman SR, Huang WW. Dapsone as corticosteroid-sparing therapy for Sweet syndrome. J Am Acad Dermatol 2022;86(3):677–9.

118. Suehisa S, Tagami H. Treatment of acute febrile neutrophilic dermatosis (Sweet's syndrome) with colchicine. Br J Dermatol 1981;105(4):483.

119. Suehisa S, Tagami H, Inoue F, et al. Colchicine in the treatment of acute febrile neutrophilic dermatosis (Sweet's syndrome). Br J Dermatol 1983; 108(1):99–101.

120. Maillard H, Leclech C, Peria P, et al. Colchicine for Sweet's syndrome. A study of 20 cases. Br J Dermatol 1999;140(3):565–6.

121. Sullivan TP, King LE Jr, Boyd AS. Colchicine in dermatology. J Am Acad Dermatol 1998;39(6): 993–9.

122. Sanchez MR. Miscellaneous treatments: thalidomide, potassium iodide, levamisole, clofazimine, colchicine, and D-penicillamine. Clin Dermatol 2000;18(1):131–45.

123. Hrin ML, Williams J, Bowers NL, et al. Evaluation of Methotrexate in the Management of Sweet Syndrome. J Cutan Med Surg 2022;26(5):532–3.

124. Jeanfils S, Joly P, Young P, et al. Indomethacin treatment of eighteen patients with Sweet's syndrome. J Am Acad Dermatol 1997;36(3 Pt 1):436–9.

125. DiCaudo DJ, Connolly SM. Neutrophilic dermatosis (pustular vasculitis) of the dorsal hands: a report of 7 cases and review of the literature. Arch Dermatol 2002;138(3):361–5.

126. Wawrzycki B, Chodorowska G, Pietrzak A, et al. Recurrent skin eruption in patient with chronic lymphocytic leukemia and lymphocytic infiltrates of the dermis resembling Sweet's syndrome. G Ital Dermatol Venereol 2011;146(6):487–92.

127. Choi HJ, Chang SE, Lee MW, et al. A case of recurrent Sweet's syndrome in an 80-year-old man: a clue to an underlying malignancy. Int J Dermatol 2006;45(4):457–9.

128. Casarin Costa JR, Virgens AR, de Oliveira Mostro L, et al. Sweet Syndrome: Clinical Features, Histopathology, and Associations of 83 Cases. J Cutan Med Surg 2017;21(3):211–6.

129. Haber R, Dib N, El Gemayel M, et al. Paradoxical neutrophilic dermatosis induced by biologics and immunosuppressive drugs: A systematic review. J Am Acad Dermatol 2021;85(4):1048–9.

130. Martínez Andrés B, Sastre Lozano V, Sánchez Melgarejo JF. Sweet syndrome after treatment with vedolizumab in a patient with Crohn's disease. Rev Esp Enferm Dig 2018;110(8):530.

131. Belvis Jiménez M, Maldonado Pérez B, Argüelles-Arias F. Using Vedolizumab to Treat Severe Sweet's Syndrome in a Patient With Ulcerative Colitis. J Crohns Colitis 2018;12(9):1134–5.

132. Bidinger JJ, Sky K, Battafarano DF, et al. The cutaneous and systemic manifestations of azathioprine hypersensitivity syndrome. J Am Acad Dermatol 2011;65(1):184–91.

From Histiocytoid Sweet Syndrome to Myelodysplasia Cutis
History and Perspectives

Marie-Dominique Vignon-Pennamen, MD[a], Maxime Battistella, MD, PhD[a,b],*

KEYWORDS

- Neutrophilic dermatosis • Sweet syndrome • Histiocytoid sweet syndrome
- Myelodysplastic syndrome • Myelodysplasia cutis • Leukemia cutis • Myeloid dermatoses

KEY POINTS

- Histiocytoid Sweet syndrome (HSS) has been described as a histologic variant of Sweet syndrome composed of immature nonblast myeloid cells. It is frequently associated with myelodysplastic syndrome (MDS).
- Myelodysplasia cutis is an emerging entity among myeloid dermatoses in the spectrum between Sweet syndrome and leukemia cutis, in patients with MDS, with a dermal infiltrate composed of immature nonblast myeloid cells clonally related to myelodysplastic cells in the bone marrow, often responding to treatment of the myeloid clone.
- HSS occurring the context of MDS may be better considered as myelodysplasia cutis.
- Myelodysplasia cutis/HSS can be observed in Vacuoles, E1 enzyme, X-linked, Autoinflammatory, Somatic syndrome and may be the first expression of this syndrome.

INTRODUCTION

Some dates line the history of acute febrile neutrophilic dermatosis. First in 1964, Robert D Sweet reported eight patients with an acute febrile neutrophilic dermatosis, later named Sweet syndrome (SS).[1] In 1973, the first cases of acute myeloid leukemia (AML) occurring in patients with SS were described.[2] In 1990, two patients with a peculiar histologic aspect in myelodysplastic syndrome (MDS)-associated SS were reported. The infiltrates were made of neutrophils with hyposegmentation, as described in the blood and bone marrow under the term "pseudo-Pelger-Huet anomaly."[3] In 2005, a histologic variant of SS called "histiocytoid Sweet syndrome" (HSS) was individualized.[4] Clinically, the patients had SS, but on skin biopsy, the infiltrates were composed of mononuclear cells that resemble histiocytes, expressing myeloperoxidase (MPO), CD33, CD163, CD68, an immunophenotype consistent with myeloid precursors, and myelomonocytic cells. In parallel, we reported a series of nine patients with a relapsing chronic form of SS in which the infiltrates were mostly composed of lymphocytes with few histiocytoid cells and neutrophils, all of them developing MDS.[5] Finally, in 2015, we proposed a new entity among myeloid-associated neutrophilic dermatoses for which we proposed the name of myelodysplasia cutis (MDC) and developed arguments to differentiate MDC from AML-related leukemia cutis (LC).[6]

During these 60 years, many publications have tried to explain the relationship between skin-infiltrating neutrophils and blastic myeloid cells in the context of hemopathy-associated SS.

a Pathology Department, APHP Nord, Hopital Saint-Louis, Université Paris Cité, Paris, France; b INSERM U976 "Human Immunology, Pathophysiology, and Immunotherapy", Paris, France
* Corresponding author. Pathology Department, APHP Nord, Hôpital Saint-Louis, 1 avenue Claude Vellefaux, Paris 75010, France.
E-mail address: maxime.battistella@aphp.fr

Dermatol Clin 42 (2024) 209–217
https://doi.org/10.1016/j.det.2023.08.004
0733-8635/24/© 2023 Elsevier Inc. All rights reserved.

The purpose of this article is to show that classical neutrophilic SS (NSS), HSS, LC, and MDC represent a spectrum of myeloid dermatoses clonally related to bone marrow AML/MDS cells.

Histiocytoid Sweet Syndrome

The presence of histiocytes or cells interpreted morphologically as histiocytes has been described in two series of SS in the 90s.[7,8] Unfortunately, immunohistochemical studies were not done or were missing for MPO. A new histologic variant histiocytoid SS has been proposed in 2005.[4] The investigators reported a series of 41 patients, 26 women, and 15 men. The age ranged from 29 to 79 years. Patients had edematous, erythematous plaques, and nodules in a usual distribution, trunk and limbs. Fever or associated manifestations were not reported. Patients had leukocytosis with neutrophilia, elevated erythrocyte sedimentation rate, and elevated serum C-reactive protein levels. Six patients had an associated malignancy, including myelomonocytic leukemia, lymphoma not otherwise specified, monoclonal gammopathy of undetermined significance, renal carcinoma, breast carcinoma, chronic B-cell lymphocytic leukemia, and multiple myeloma. The follow-up ranged from 12 months to 16 years and no other malignancy was disclosed. A diagnosis of SS was proposed and patients were treated with steroids with resolution of the disease without relapse. The only unusual feature in these patients was the histopathological aspect. Classical features of SS were present: moderate to intense edema of the papillary dermis and an underlying dense, bandlike, inflammatory infiltrate involving the superficial and mid-dermis. However, the infiltrate was predominantly composed of mononuclear cells with elongated twisted or kidney-shaped nuclei. Few mature neutrophils and perivascular lymphocytes were also present. No relationship could be established between the duration of the lesions before biopsy and the composition of the cellular infiltrate. Immunohistochemical studies demonstrated that most cells of the infiltrate had cytoplasmic immunoreactivity for markers indicative of a monocytic–histiocytic lineage: CD68, CD15, CD45, and CD163. These cells were also labeled by MPO, suggesting that they were immature precursors of neutrophils. The specific cutaneous infiltration by AML was excluded by cytologic morphology, absence of expression of blastic markers and absence of development of AML during follow-up.

In the following years, many reports focused on the nature of mononuclear cells infiltrating the dermis in HSS. Some investigators highlighted the frequent association with myeloid neoplasms (MNs), mainly MDS.

Regarding the nature of mononuclear histiocytoid cells observed in the dermis and sometimes in the subcutaneous tissue, two principal theories have been proposed. The first one was that these cells are immature myeloid cells on the granulocyte–monocyte lineage.[4,5,9–11] The immunohistochemical profile showing expression of CD33, CD68, and MPO was considered a major argument to confirm that most of the cells of the cutaneous infiltrate in HSS are immature nonblastic cells, promyelocytes, and myelocytes. In other studies,[12,13] HSS cells were considered to be CD163+ CD68+ macrophages with a nonclassical MPO + phenotype, and expression of myeloid cell nuclear differentiation antigen. All studies corroborated that infiltrating cells in HSS do not represent myeloid blasts. Most of the investigators now consider that mononuclear cells seen in HSS belong to the myeloid lineage.

In parallel, a discussion has been engaged about the association of HSS with MN. In the first description, the investigators indicated that MNs were not more often associated with HSS than with classical NSS. This statement was disclaimed by many case reports and series.[5,12,14–17] In 2006, we showed in a series of nine patients that lymphocytic rich infiltrates in SS could be a predictive marker for MDS.[5] In 2014, five patients with HSS who had underlying myeloid disorders with known mutations, two AML, one chronic myeloid leukemia, and two MDS were studied with fluorescent in situ hybridization (FISH) analysis. Four of those cases manifested chromosomal abnormalities in the cutaneous infiltrates identical to the ones in the bone marrow. The investigators suggested that HSS could represent a form of LC.[14] In 2016, in a retrospective study, classical NSS were compared with HSS.[15] Thirty-six percent of HSS were associated with MN versus 12.5% of NSS, and 31% of HSS had MDS versus 2% of NSS. Relapses were significantly more frequent in patients with HSS than NSS. In NSS, the hematological disease was diagnosed before the cutaneous lesions or at the time of occurrence of skin lesions. Only in some cases of HSS, skin lesions preceded the diagnosis of hematological disorder by about 6 months. In 2018, a retrospective cohort of 83 patients with SS indicated that 55% had hematologic malignancy, most commonly AML (29%), followed by MDS (12%).[17] HSS, some cases with purely subcutaneous involvement, was exclusively observed in the setting of MN. In 2019, a review of literature, confirmed that 40% to 55% of HSS were associated with hematological malignancy, especially MDS (24%–32%).[18]

Finally, in a systematic review on SS performed in PubMed/MEDLINE, Embase and Cochrane Collaboration databases, including 43 publications and 218 patients, about 40% of patients with HSS were subsequently diagnosed with a hematologic or solid cancer versus 21% in NSS, and HSS was more commonly associated with MDS than NSS (46% vs 2,5%).[19] HSS patients had no female predominance, and sometimes showed subcutis involvement only. Besides this indisputable frequent association with MN, HSS has been more rarely described in the setting of autoimmune diseases,[20] relapsing chondritis,[21] and some cases have been considered drug-induced mainly in multiple myeloma treated with bortezomib.[22]

One another essential question has focused on the pathogenic significance of HSS. It is a histologic variant of SS, with about 50% of cases not linked to MN. Some investigators consider that HSS portends the same pathogenic significance as classical idiopathic NSS. When associated with MN, mainly MDS, the interpretation of HSS infiltrates varies among the investigators. For some, HSS is nothing more than LC, as FISH analyses demonstrated similar chromosomal alterations in the bone marrow and the skin.[14]

A clonal relationship between mature neutrophils of NSS and blastic cells of associated MN has been identified with different techniques, that is, FISH[23,24] and targeted next-generation sequencing (NGS) of a gene panel commonly associated with MN.[25] Only two cases of HSS have been studied with NGS technique showing a clonal link between cutaneous and bone marrow infiltrates.[25] The results obtained by these techniques have demonstrated that the neutrophilic dermal infiltration and the malignant myeloid clone share a common clonal progenitor, whether SS was present at initial clinical presentation of MN or arose during the treatment of MN. The occurrence of SS in profoundly neutropenic patients has suggested that the differentiation of myeloid precursors to mature neutrophils occurs in the dermis.[24]

In 2020, a review of the literature has shown that the development of HSS had no prognostic implications in patients with MN on the contrary to LC, the latter being classically associated with poor prognosis.[19] Clinical and pathologic characteristics of HSS are illustrated in **Fig. 1**.

In short, HSS refers to a histopathological pattern corresponding to a heterogeneous group of disorders, among which the association with MN and especially MDS is frequent. The pathophysiological significance of HSS still remains poorly understood, but most of them could represent cutaneous localization of MDS, as discussed afterward. The role of specific MN-related gene mutations in the pathogenesis and the pathogeny of HSS histologic picture outside of MN context need to be investigated.

Myelodysplasia Cutis

The first hypothesis that some forms of SS were linked to MDS has emerged in 2006.[5] In this case series of nine patients, we showed that patients presenting a chronic relapsing SS with abundant mononuclear cells could represent a subgroup especially associated with MDS. All patients were male aged from 55 to 72 years. They had multiple flares of edematous erythematous plaques over the face, trunk, and limbs with often an annular configuration, evocative of SS. All had fever, and sometimes arthralgias. All had elevated sedimentation rate, some of them had leukopenia or anemia. The diagnosis of MDS was established from 2 to 7 years after the onset of skin disease. Follow-up ranged from 3 to 10 years. High-dose oral prednisone provided initial complete remission in all patients. However, the lesions worsened on tapering dosages and 25 mg/d was necessary to control the disease. No significant benefit was obtained with hydroxychloroquine sulfate, dapsone, colchicine, or thalidomide. There was no progression to AML. In these patients, MDS was categorized as low risk and did not justify any specific treatment. Seven patients died of sepsis or vascular complications 3 to 48 months after MDS were diagnosed. Sequential biopsies were studied and two different patterns were observed. At the initial stage, lymphocytic infiltrate was present and suggestive of Jessner lymphocytic infiltrate or lupus erythematosus. The infiltrates were moderate to dense located in the superficial and deep dermis, composed of lymphocytes, histiocytes, and some atypical mononuclear cells with large eccentric elongated twisted or kidney-shaped nuclei. Some cells had pseudo-Pelger-Huet anomaly. The mononucleated cells expressed CD68 and MPO. After many relapses, the nature of the infiltrates changed. Neutrophils predominated and were admixed with the same atypical mononuclear cells observed at the initial stage. The diagnosis of MDS was typically made at a time when the neutrophils were the predominant cells in the skin infiltrates. The atypical mononuclear cells with eccentric elongated twisted or kidney-shaped nuclei and CD68+ MPO + phenotype were suggestive of immature nonblastic myeloid cells.

Some other cases of lymphocytic SS have been described in association with MDS,[26–28] and

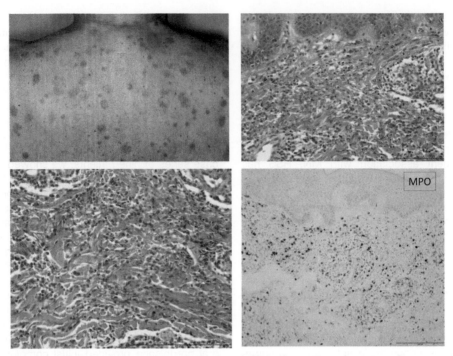

Fig. 1. Clinical and pathologic characteristics of HSS. (*Top left*) Erythematous edematous plaques on the upper trunk; (*top right* and *lower left*) diffuse and interstitial infiltrate of lymphocytes and histiocytoid cells; (*lower right*) some histiocytoid cells express MPO.

patients with chronic relapsing-remitting SS similar to our cases were also described in MDS.[29,30] The concomitant presence of immature myeloid cells and mature neutrophils within the same lesion has also been reported, although the significance of this population of immature myeloid neutrophils in the skin was variably discussed.[31–33] In our opinion, such infiltrates represented the cutaneous component of MDS. Why cutaneous disease seemed from 2 to 7 years before MDS was diagnosed remains unexplained, but this fact is of practical clinical importance and may help in the early diagnosis of MDS and management of patients.

In 2015, our team has proposed the term of MDC. We conducted a comparative study between two groups of patients[6]: 24 patients had MDS with immature nonblastic skin infiltrate, defined as medium-size immature myeloid MPO + cells mixed with mature neutrophils and lymphocytes; 20 had AML with blastic infiltrate defining LC. Most of the MDS patients were tested for bone marrow cytogenetics, and abnormalities were found in six of them. FISH analyses were performed on the skin and showed common cytogenetic abnormalities in the bone marrow and the cutaneous infiltrate in four patients, demonstrating that myeloid cells in the skin were clonally related to the MDS. In the 24 patients with MDS and

nonblastic skin infiltrate, only 20% developed AML, and the median overall survival from skin diagnosis was 62 months, significantly longer than in patients with classical AML-associated LC. We proposed the term of "myelodysplasia cutis" (MDC) to characterize this skin condition in the course of MDS with nonblastic infiltrate and a low risk of progression to AML. In comparison with AML-associated LC, the histopathological discriminant features were the cytologic details, positivity for CD34, CD56, or CD117 in AML-associated LC and the presence of high numbers of CD3+ lymphocytes and a lower Mib-1 (Ki67) proliferative index in MDC. Clinical discriminant features were the presence of nodules for LC and the presence of erythematous plaques with annular pattern, fever, or arthralgias for MDC. Regarding evolution, cutaneous lesions of MDC were often chronic with flares and relapses. In MDC, skin lesions occurred before the bone marrow MDS diagnosis with a mean time of 41 months in 14 patients and occurred during MDS evolution in 10 patients.

The first case of MDC in which NGS analyses was performed in the skin was reported in 2021.[34] A 74 years old man had a diagnosis of MDS with *TET2* mutation. In parallel, he developed a dermatosis, clinically evocative of SS. On biopsy, infiltrate was composed of lymphocytes and immature MPO + myeloid cells. Molecular analyses of a lesional skin biopsy detected the same mutation of *TET2* with high variant allele frequency, consistent with a specific infiltration and favoring the diagnosis of MDC. Azacitidine allowed a dermatologic complete response and a partial hematological response 6 months later. This study confirmed the clonality of the dysplastic myeloid infiltrates both in the marrow and the skin and showed a clinical response of the skin lesions to a myeloid clone-oriented treatment.

A larger study was conducted to validate the concept of MDC using NGS technique in the skin infiltrate.[35] In this work, the following clinicopathological and molecular features were used to define patients with MDC.

1. Diagnosis of MDS according to the WHO 2016 criteria
2. Cutaneous histopathology consistent with "histiocytoid" immature myeloid cells
3. Identical mutation of at least one gene recurrently mutated in MDS in the marrow and skin

This definition ruled out LC and MDS-associated NSS. Seven patients were included (six male, one female), with a median age of 65 years at MDS diagnosis and 68 years at MDC diagnosis. Clinically, two different dermatologic pictures were observed. Four patients had erythematous, edematous papules, and plaques of the head and limbs like in SS. Three patients had diffuse erythematous papules and nodules like in LC.

Histologically, a moderate to dense infiltrate was located in the dermis in a perivascular and periadnexal distribution with sometimes an extensive edema. The infiltrate was composed of lymphocytes, few neutrophils and atypical mononuclear cells identical to cells described in HSS, some of them presenting pseudo-Pelger-Huet anomaly. These immature myeloid cells expressed CD33, CD163, CD68, and MPO but did not express CD34, CD56, and CD117. NGS analysis identified one to five genes identically mutated both in the marrow and the skin showing that the cutaneous immature myeloid cells infiltrate was clonally related to the marrow MDS clone.

Patients received corticosteroid and four of them became steroid-dependent. Azacitidine was introduced in these four patients yielding initial complete remission an all cases. Three patients died of MDS progression within 9 months. In this series of patients, MDC was associated with advanced MDS (higher risk MDS in 6/7 patients).

As it has already been shown, neutrophils in AML-associated SS derive from the leukemic clone, corresponding to differentiation of blasts, suggesting that LC and SS in AML belong to the same disease.[24] Likewise, MDS patients may develop skin involvement by immature myeloid cells defining MDC or infiltration by more mature clonal cells leading to classical NSS.

Formal recognition of MDC entity, for HSS occurring in patients with MDS, is particularly relevant given that the cells in the dermal infiltrate have been shown to be clonally related to MDS in the marrow and blood. MDC seems to describe more specifically the mechanism of disease, and its designation may have important implications for the treatment. Based on the preliminary findings, MDC may respond to hypomethylating agents which are targeted to the neoplastic clone, underscoring the relevance of appropriate diagnostic terminology.

As it has been recently proposed, the spectrum of myeloid dermatoses may include[36]: (1) classical SS represented by an inflammatory dermal infiltration composed primarily of terminally differentiated neutrophils; (2) HSS with morphologically immature nonblast myeloid cell infiltrate; (3) LC, represented by a blast infiltrate in the skin.

MDC represents an emerging entity that falls on this spectrum between HSS and LC with a dermal infiltrate composed of nonblast myeloid cells clonally related to the MDS cells in the marrow. The clinical and pathologic features of MDC are shown in **Fig. 2**.

Vacuoles, E1 Enzyme, X-Linked, Autoinflammatory, Somatic Syndrome

In 2020, Beck and colleagues described a novel adult autoinflammatory syndrome entitled Vacuoles, E1 enzyme, X-linked, Autoinflammatory, Somatic (VEXAS), a newly-discovered disorder that connected previously unrelated inflammatory syndromes.[37] This new syndrome is characterized by a dysregulated innate immune response, manifesting as an adult-onset, treatment-refractory, hyperinflammatory state. More than 150 cases have now been published. According to these case series or case reports, the skin, lungs, blood vessels, and cartilage are the main targets of this syndrome. Other hallmark features include the presence of fever, elevated inflammatory markers, and cytopenias. Disease-related mortality varies between 40% and 63% in different case series but is consistently high with substantial associated morbidity.[38]

In a recent retrospective study, a total of 116 patients with VEXAS syndrome were included.[39] Most patients were male with a median age of 67 years at the onset of symptoms and 71 years at the diagnosis of VEXAS syndrome. The main

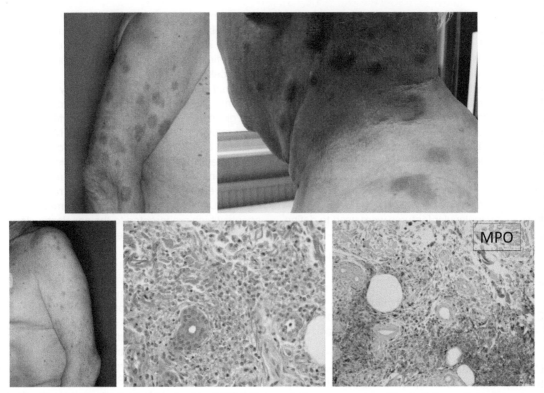

Fig. 2. Clinical and pathologic features of myelodysplasia cutis. (*Upper panels* and *lower left panel*) erythematous edematous plaques on the neck, trunk and arms; (*lower center*) perivascular and interstitial infiltrate in the deep dermis, showing a majority of mononucleated cells with oval or grooved nucleus, with some bilobated nuclei. (*Lower right*) MPO is diffusely expressed in the mononucleated cells.

clinical features were skin lesions, recurrent fever, weight loss, lung involvement, ocular symptoms, relapsing chondritis, unprovoked venous thrombosis, lymph node enlargement, arthralgias, peripheral nervous system involvement, and gastrointestinal involvement. MDS was present in 50% of cases, some of them associated with monoclonal gammopathy of unknown significance. In accordance with other studies, VEXAS syndrome was severe and life-threatening disease with high mortality rates and a 5-year survival rate of 63%. Consensual therapeutic management has not yet been established.

In 2021, clinical and pathologic skin manifestations linked to VEXAS have been described in a multicenter retrospective case series of eight patients.[40] All patients were men, and the median age at the onset of symptoms was 65.5 years. Clinically, patients had erythematous inflammatory plaques and papules, some of them umbilicated, some other purpuric. Livedo racemosa was present in three patients. In five patients, skin involvement seemed before or at the time of other clinical features of VEXAS, with a median delay of 4 months. Other symptoms included

fever (3 of 8), relapsing chondritis (3 of 8), venous thromboembolism (4 of 8), and pulmonary involvement (2 of 8). Cytoplasmic vacuoles involving granulocytic precursors were found in all the marrow aspirates. On skin biopsy, the infiltrates consisted of mature neutrophils with leukocytoclasia, which were admixed with MPO + CD163+ immature myeloid cells with indented nuclei (metamyelocytes and immature band neutrophils), and lymphoid cells in all cases. The infiltrates were typically perivascular and involved the entire dermis and subcutaneous fat in two cases. Infiltration of dermal vessel wall was seen in two patients, one with associated thrombosis without fibrinoid necrosis. One patient had also a typical image of polyarteritis nodosa on the biopsy of a subcutaneous reddish-purple tender nodule. All eight patients had either MDS (6 of 8) or clonal cytopenia of undetermined significance (2 of 8). Two patients also had monoclonal gammopathies, and one had essential thrombocytopenia. Sequencing analysis of paired marrow samples and skin lesion biopsies identified the same loss-of-function *UBA1* variation in both samples for all patients.

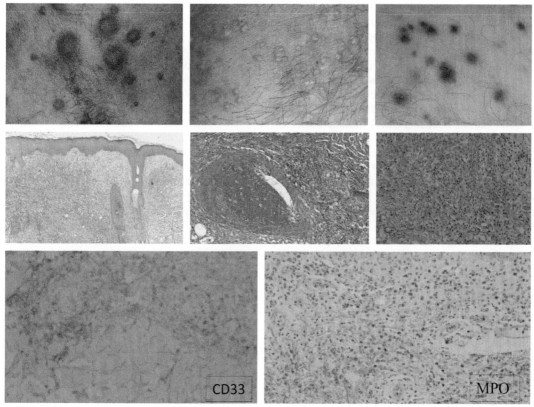

Fig. 3. Clinical and pathologic characteristics of patients with VEXAS syndrome. (*Upper panels*) skin lesions are erythematous edematous and sometimes pupuric plaques or papulo-nodules. (*Middle panels*) histopathology can show superficial and deep perivascular infiltrates and sometimes necrotizing and thrombotic vasculitis close to cutaneous periarteritis nodosa. The infiltrate is made of lymphocyte, mononucleated cells with moderate cytoplasm and grooved incompletely segmented nuclei, and mature neutrophils with leukocytoclasia. (*Lower panels*) immature myeloid cells with indented nuclei express CD33 and MPO.

If the diagnosis of SS or neutrophilic dermatosis had initially been proposed to describe the skin lesions in VEXAS syndrome, it is now recognized that skin infiltrate in VEXAS associate mature neutrophils, immature MPO + myeloid cells as in HSS or MDC, and that VEXAS skin infiltrate shares the same pathogenic mutation as the underlying myeloid clone in the bone marrow.[41] As such, the inflammatory skin manifestations seen in VEXAS syndrome are directly associated with clonal infiltration of the skin rather than a general pro-inflammatory activation state and could fall under the umbrella of MDC. This may have therapeutic consequences, as therapies that target the pathologic clone as well as the pro-inflammatory milieu (corticosteroids, Janus kinase inhibitors, tumor necrosis factor-α, and interleukin 6 antibodies) could be useful to control the disease.[42]

Finally, VEXAS syndrome should be considered in male patients aged more than 60 years with general symptoms, systemic inflammation, and with skin involvement as it has been defined in MDC. Clinical and pathologic characteristics of patients with VEXAS syndrome are shown in **Fig. 3**.

SUMMARY

HSS has historically been defined as a histopathological variant of SS, with the presence of atypical histiocytoid mononuclear cells, later recognized by some investigators as immature myeloid cells, and frequently associated with MN.

MDC is an emerging entity, different from AML-associated LC, in the spectrum of cutaneous manifestations in patients with MN, defined as the skin infiltration by immature nonblastic myeloid cells sharing the same molecular alteration than the bone marrow MDS clone. Reasonably, cases described as HSS occurring in the course of MDS may be better classified as MDC. HSS or

MDC can be a marker of the recently identified VEXAS syndrome. HSS occurring outside of MN context should be studied further, as they do not have clear pathogenic mechanism.

From a practical point of view, pathologists facing a biopsy with an HSS pattern should search for MPO expression by mononuclear cells, and search for MN-defining molecular alterations in the skin infiltrate, including *UBA1* mutation, when techniques such as NGS are accessible. The presence of MN-recurrent mutations in HSS should lead to a diagnosis of MDC and should urge the clinician to explore blood and bone marrow of the patient.

Besides the clonal link between the MDS clone and the skin MDC infiltrate, the pathogenesis of MDC is still poorly known and may imply inflammatory skin-addressing cofactors or specific mutation patterns. MDS is more and more recognized as a disease at the crossroads of immune dysregulation, chronic inflammation, and clonal evolution in myeloid stem cells, and recent advances in targeted and large-scale NGS have helped to illuminate the dynamic genomic landscape in MDS. Likewise, the role of immune dysregulation has been better studied in pathogenesis of MDS leading to refined patient stratification.[43] In general, low-risk MDS is related to a more pro-inflammatory immune response and higher numbers of effector-type cells, and the higher risk disease is characterized by a predominantly immunosuppressive milieu. Around 25% of MDS are associated with systemic inflammatory and autoimmune diseases (SIADs), including neutrophilic dermatoses.[44] A lower marrow blast percentage, and presence of *TET2/IDH*, and *SRSF2* mutations are variables independently associated with SIAD, whereas *UBA1* mutations were present only in 12% of patients with MDS and SIAD.[45] This shows that different mechanisms may drive inflammation in *UBA1*-wild-type MDS patients, including mutations in epigenetic regulators *TET2/IDH* that could potentially promote both the hematological malignancy and the inflammatory disorder by dysregulating T lymphocytes.

DISCLOSURE

Dr M-.D. Vignon-Pennamen and Dr M. Battistella declare no commercial or financial conflicts of interest and no funding sources.

REFERENCES

1. Sweet RD. An acute febrile neutrophilic dermatosis. Br J Dermatol 1964;76:349–56.
2. Matta M, Malak J, Tabet E, et al. Sweet's syndrome: systemic associations. Cutis 1973;12:561–5.
3. Morioka N, Otsuka F, Nogita T, et al. Neutrophilic dermatosis with myelodysplastic syndrome. Nuclear segmentation anomalies in neutrophils in the skin lesion and in peripheral blood. J Am Acad Dermatol 1990;23:247–9.
4. Requena L, Kutzner H, Palmedo G, et al. Histiocytoid Sweet syndrome: a dermal infiltration of immature neutrophilic granulocytes. Arch Dermatol 2005;141:834–42.
5. Vignon-Pennamen MD, Juillard C, Rybojad M, et al. Chronic recurrent lymphocytic Sweet syndrome as a predictive marker of myelodysplasia: a report of 9 cases. Arch Dermatol 2006;142:1170–6.
6. Osio A, Battistella M, Feugeas JP, et al. Myelodysplasia Cutis Versus Leukemia Cutis. J Invest Dermatol 2015;135:2321–4.
7. Delabie J, De Wolf Peters C, Morren M, et al. Histiocytes in Sweet syndrome. Br J Dermatol 1991;124:348–53.
8. Bourke JF, Jones JL, Fletcher A, et al. An immunohistochemical study of the dermal infiltrate and epidermal staining for interleukin 1 in 12 cases of Sweet's syndrome. Br J Dermatol 1996;134:705–9.
9. Alegría-Landa V, Rodríguez-Pinilla SM, Santos-Briz A, et al. Clinicopathologic, Immunohistochemical, and Molecular Features of Histiocytoid Sweet Syndrome. JAMA Dermatol 2017;153:651–9.
10. Chow S, Pasternak S, Green P, et al. Histiocytoid Neutrophilic Dermatoses and Panniculitides: Variations on a Theme. Am J Dermatopathol 2007;29:334–41.
11. Heymann WR. Histiocytoid Sweet syndrome. J Am Acad Dermatol 2009;61:693–4.
12. Magro CM, Momtahen S, Nguyen GH, et al. Histiocytoid Sweet's syndrome: A localized cutaneous proliferation of macrophages frequently associated with myeloproliferative disease. Eur J Dermatol 2015;25:335–41.
13. Peroni A, Colato C, Schena D, et al. Histiocytoid Sweet syndrome is infiltrated predominantly by M2-like macrophages. J Am Acad Dermatol 2015;72:131–9.
14. Chavan RN, Cappel MA, Ketterling RP, et al. Histiocytoid Sweet syndrome may indicate leukemia cutis: A novel application of fluorescent in situ hybridization. J Am Acad Dermatol 2014;70:1021–7.
15. Ghoufi L, Ortonne N, Ingen-Housz-Oro S, et al. Histiocytoid Sweet Syndrome Is More Frequently Associated With Myelodysplastic Syndromes Than the Classical Neutrophilic Variant: A Comparative Series of 62 Patients. Medicine (Baltim) 2016;95:e3033.
16. Bush JW, Wick MR. Cutaneous Sweet syndrome and its relationship to hematological diseases. J Cutan Pathol 2016;43:394–9.

17. Nelson CA, Noe MH, McMahon CM, et al. Sweet syndrome in patients with and without malignancy: A retrospective analysis of 83 patients from a tertiary academic referral center. J Am Acad Dermatol 2018; 78:303–9.

18. Lepelletier C, Bouaziz JD, Rybojad M, et al. Neutrophilic Dermatoses Associated With Myeloid Malignancies. Am J Clin Dermatol 2019;20:325–33.

19. Haber R, Feghali J, El Gemayel M. Risk of malignancy in histiocytoid Sweet syndrome: a systematic review and reappraisal. J Am Acad Dermatol 2020; 83:661–3.

20. Camarillo D, McCalmont TH, Frieden IJ, et al. Two Pediatric Cases of Nonbullous Histiocytoid Neutrophilic Dermatitis Presenting as a Cutaneous Manifestation of Lupus Erythematosus. Arch Dermatol 2008;144:1495–8.

21. Arima Y, Namiki T, Ueno M, et al. Histiocytoid Sweet syndrome: a novel association with relapsing polychondritis. Br J Dermatol 2016;174:677–98.

22. Murase JE, Wu JJ, Theate Y, et al. Bortezomib-induced histiocytoid Sweet syndrome. J Am Acad Dermatol 2009;60:496–7.

23. Van Loon K, Gill RM, McMahon P, et al. 20q– Clonality in a Case of Oral Sweet Syndrome and Myelodysplasia. Am J Clin Pathol 2012;137:310–5.

24. Sujobert P, Cuccuini W, Vignon-Pennamen D, et al. Evidence of differentiation in myeloid malignancies associated neutrophilic dermatosis: a fluorescent in situ hybridization study of 14 patients. J Invest Dermatol 2013;133:1111–4.

25. Passet M, Lepelletier C, Vignon-Pennamen MD, et al. Next-Generation Sequencing in Myeloid Neoplasm-Associated Sweet's Syndrome Demonstrates Clonal Relation between Malignant Cells and Skin-Infiltrating Neutrophils. J Invest Dermatol 2020;140:1873–6.

26. Evans AV, Sabroe RA, Liddell K, et al. Lymphocytic infiltrates as a presenting feature of Sweet's syndrome with myelodysplasia and response to cyclophosphamide. Br J Dermatol 2002;146:1087–90.

27. Browning CE, Dixon JE, Malone JC, et al. Thalidomide in the treatment of recalcitrant Sweet's syndrome associated with myelodysplasia. J Am Acad Dermatol 2005;53:135–8.

28. Yamamoto T, Soejima K, Yokozeki H, et al. Unusual annular erythema associated with myelodysplastic syndrome. Dermatology 2001;202:70–2.

29. Kulasekararaj AG, Kordasti S, Basu T, et al. Chronic relapsing remitting Sweet syndrome – a harbinger of myelodysplastic syndrome. Br J Haematol 2015; 170:649–56.

30. Kakaletsis N, Kaiafa G, Savopoulos C, et al. Initially lymphocytic Sweet's syndrome in male patients with myelodysplasia: a distinguished clinicopathological entity? Case report and systematic review of the literature. Acta Haematol 2014;132:220–5.

31. Tomasini C, Aloi F, Osella-Abate S, et al. Immature Myeloid Precursors in Chronic Neutrophilic Dermatosis Associated With Myelodysplastic Syndrome. Am J Dermatopathol 2000;22:429–33.

32. Piette WW, Trapp JF, O'Donnell MJ, et al. Acute neutrophilic dermatosis with myeloblastic infiltrate in a leukemia patient receiving all-trans-retinoic acid therapy. J Am Acad Dermatol 1994;30:293–7.

33. Magro CM, Kiani B, Li J, et al. Clonality in the setting of Sweet's syndrome and pyoderma gangrenosum is not limited to underlying myeloproliferative disease. J Cutan Pathol 2007;34:526–34.

34. Delaleu J, Battistella M, Rathana K, et al. Identification of clonal skin myeloid cells by next-generation sequencing in myelodysplasia cutis. Br J Dermatol 2021;184:367–9.

35. Delaleu J, Kim R, Zhao LP, et al. Clinical, pathological, and molecular features of myelodysplasia cutis. Blood 2022;139:1251–3.

36. Calvo KR. Skin in the game: the emergence of myelodysplasia cutis. Blood 2022;139:1132–4.

37. Beck DB, Ferrada MA, Sikora KA, et al. Somatic Mutations in *UBA1* and Severe Adult-Onset Autoinflammatory Disease. N Engl J Med 2020;383:2628–38.

38. Sterling D, Duncan ME, Philippidou M, et al. VEXAS syndrome (vacuoles, E1 enzyme, X-linked, autoinflammatory, somatic) for the dermatologist. J Am Acad Dermatol. 2022:S0190-9622(22)00181-5. doi: 10.1016/j.jaad.2022.01.042.

39. Georgin-Lavialle S, Terrier B, Guedon AF, et al. Further characterization of clinical and laboratory features in VEXAS syndrome: large-scale analysis of a multicentre case series of 116 French patients. Br J Dermatol 2022;186:564–74.

40. Zakine E, Schell B, Battistella M, et al. *UBA1* Variations in Neutrophilic Dermatosis Skin Lesions of Patients With VEXAS Syndrome. JAMA Dermatol 2021;157:1349–54.

41. Zakine E, Papageorgiou L, Bourguiba R, et al. Clinical and pathological features of cutaneous manifestations in VEXAS syndrome: a multicenter retrospective study of 59 cases. J Am Acad Dermatol 2023;88:917–20.

42. Bourbon E, Heiblig M, Gerfaud Valentin M, et al. Therapeutic options in VEXAS syndrome: insights from a retrospective series. Blood 2021;137:3682–4.

43. Winter S, Shoaie S, Kordasti S, et al. Integrating the "immunome" in the Stratification of Myelodysplastic Syndrome and Future Clinical Trial Design. J Clin Oncol 2020;38:1723–35.

44. Zhao LP, Boy M, Azoulay C, et al. Genomic landscape of MDS/CMML associated with systemic inflammatory and autoimmune disease. Leukemia 2021;35:2720–4.

45. Zhao LP, Schell B, Sébert M, et al. Prevalence of *UBA1* mutations in MDS/CMML patients with systemic inflammatory and auto-immune disease. Leukemia 2021;35:2731–3.

Neutrophilic Urticarial Dermatosis

Amarachi Orakwue, BS[a], Jeremy Bray, MD[b], Nneka Comfere, MD[c,d],
Olayemi Sokumbi, MD[b,e],*

KEYWORDS

- Neutrophilic urticarial dermatosis • NUD • Classic urticaria • Neutrophilic urticaria
- Urticarial vasculitis • Sweet syndrome • Schnitzler syndrome • Adult-onset Still's disease

KEY POINTS

- Neutrophilic urticarial dermatosis (NUD) commonly coexists with inflammatory systemic diseases, but this association is not obligatory.
- Diagnosis of NUD and its distinct accompanying condition necessitates a meticulous evaluation of the clinical manifestations, histologic features, and laboratory findings.
- Management of NUD depends on the clinical context and associated systemic disease.

INTRODUCTION

Clinically, neutrophilic urticarial dermatosis (NUD) is characterized as pink to reddish urticarial eruption consisting of flat or slightly raised, pruritic or nonpruritic macules, papules, or plaques that resolve within 24 hours.[1,2] Histologically, it is characterized by an intense neutrophilic interstitial and perivascular infiltrate with no blood vessel damage or significant edema.[3] Recently, extension of neutrophils into the epidermis, hair follicles, sweat glands, and sebaceous glands, a term referred to as neutrophilic epitheliotropism, has been identified as a sensitive and specific histopathologic clue for NUD.[3] Its typical extracutaneous signs include fever or arthralgia.[2]

The clinical criteria of NUD are[1].

(1) Recurrent or chronic cutaneous eruptions consisting of macules, papules, or plaques.
(2) Individual lesions resolve within 48 hours.
(3) Pruritic or nonpruritic lesions.

The histologic criteria of NUD are[1].

(1) Diffuse dermal neutrophilic infiltrate with interstitial involvement.
(2) Absence of significant vessel wall alteration (particularly fibrinoid necrosis).
(3) Absence of significant dermal edema.

NUD is typically associated with systemic diseases such as Schnitzler syndrome, adult-onset Still's disease, cryopyrin-associated periodic syndromes, and lupus erythematosus (LE).[4] Since NUDs identification in 2009, there have been reports of its associations with other conditions such as systemic-onset juvenile arthritis, Sjögren syndrome, primary biliary cirrhosis, inflammatory bowel disease, serum sickness-like drug reaction, post-streptococcal rheumatic disease, and acral acquired cutis laxa associated with IgA multiple myeloma.[4] Rarely, the clinical and histologic presentations of NUD can present without associated systemic diseases.[5]

[a] University of Minnesota Medical School, 420 Delaware Street Southeast Suite C607, Minneapolis, MN 55455, USA; [b] Department of Dermatology, Mayo Clinic, 4500 San Pablo Road S, Jacksonville, FL 32224, USA; [c] Department of Dermatology, Mayo Clinic, 200 First Street Southwest, Rochester, MN 55905, USA; [d] Department of Laboratory Medicine & Pathology, Mayo Clinic, 200 First Street Southwest, Rochester, MN 55905, USA; [e] Department of Laboratory Medicine & Pathology, Mayo Clinic, 4500 San Pablo Road S, Jacksonville, FL 32224, USA
* Corresponding author. Departments of Dermatology and Laboratory Medicine & Pathology, Mayo Clinic, 4500 San Pablo Road S Jacksonville, FL 32224.
E-mail address: sokumbi.olayemi@mayo.edu

Dermatol Clin 42 (2024) 219–229
https://doi.org/10.1016/j.det.2023.08.009

DISEASES COMMONLY ASSOCIATED WITH NEUTROPHILIC URTICARIAL DERMATOSIS PATTERN

Schnitzler Syndrome

Schnitzler syndrome is a rare, late-onset, acquired autoinflammatory multisystemic disease.[6,7] It was first described in 1972 by the French dermatologist, Liliane Schnitzler, and there have been around 300 published global cases since then.[2,8] It has a marginal predominance in men, and its mean age of onset is 51 years; the youngest reported patient began experiencing urticaria at 13 years old.[8]

Schnitzler syndrome is defined by monoclonal gammopathy (usually IgM or sometimes IgG) and recurrent, nonpruritic urticarial rash that is neutrophil rich on biopsy, plus at least two of these abnormalities: bone pain, lymphadenopathy, intermittent fever, leukocytosis, hepatomegaly and/or splenomegaly, arthralgias or arthritis, and an elevated erythrocyte sedimentation rate.[6,9] Other abnormalities include peripheral neuropathy, weight loss, headache, elevated inflammatory markers, and fatigue.[7] Patients may also develop lymphoproliferative diseases and amyloid A (AA) amyloidosis may occur in rare instances, if not properly treated.[10] There are two sets of diagnostic criteria called the Lipsker and Strasbourg criteria. However, the Strasbourg criteria as described in **Box 1** are the most recent and its validity has been confirmed.[2,11]

The first clinical presentation of Schnitzler syndrome is recurrent urticarial lesions consisting of red or rose-colored macules or slightly elevated papules and plaques that may become confluent (**Fig. 1**).[6,8] Individual lesions last less than 24 hours and resolve without sequelae.[6] These eruptions are typically nonpruritic, though they can be moderately pruritic.[6,8] They usually occur on the trunk and extremities—sparing the head and neck regions, and angioedema and dermographism are rare.[6,8] There are reports of worsening skin lesion following heat or cold exposure, alcohol consumption, stress, work, or physical exercise.[2,8] Patients may exhibit neurologic symptoms such as vertigo or delirium during the recurrent inflammatory episodes.[12]

The histopathology of urticarial skin lesions in Schnitzler syndrome includes various patterns described as sparse perivascular inflammation, NUD, or leukocytoclastic vasculitis.[6] Histopathology of a plaque in its early stages reveals normal epidermis, dermal neutrophilic infiltrate of variable density, and clusters of neutrophils around sweat ducts.[8] In addition, interstitial neutrophils are distributed along collagen bundles and leukocytoclasia is present.[7]

Box 1
Strasbourg diagnostic criteria of Schnitzler syndrome[2,11]

Obligate criteria

  Chronic urticarial rash and

  Monoclonal IgM or IgG gammopathy

Minor criteria

  Recurrent fever[a]

  Bone morphology anomalies with or without bone pain[b]

  A neutrophilic dermal infiltrate on skin biopsy[c]

  Hyperleukocytosis and/or elevated CRP[d]

Definite diagnosis if

  Two obligate criteria AND at least two minor criteria if IgM and three minor criteria if IgG

Probable diagnosis if

  Two obligate criteria AND at least one minor criteria if IgM and two minor criteria if IgG

[a] Must be greater than 38°C and otherwise unexplained. Occurs usually—but not obligatory—together with the skin rash.

[b] As assessed by bone scintigraphy, MRI or elevation of bone alkaline phosphatase.

[c] Corresponds usually to the entity described as "neutrophilic urticarial dermatosis" (Medicine 2009; 88: 23–31); absence of fibrinoid necrosis and significant dermal edema.

[d] Neutrophils greater than 10,000/mm³ and/or CRP greater than 30 mg/L.

The etiology of Schnitzler syndrome is not established.[6] It is considered an acquired autoinflammatory disorder due to elevated levels of proinflammatory cytokines such as interleukin (IL)-1α, IL-1β, IL-6, and tumor necrosis factor (TNF)-α.[6,8,13] Therefore, drugs targeting the IL-1 pathway are effective therapeutic options.[8] Anakinra is the first drug of choice for Schnitzler syndrome.[14] Alternative therapies such as rilonacept (IL-1 receptor decoy), canakinumab (anti-IL-1β monoclonal antibody), and tocilizumab (anti-IL-6 monoclonal antibody) are also suitable options.[6,13,14] About 15% to 20% of patients with Schnitzler will develop a lymphoproliferative disorder such as Waldenström's macroglobulinemia; thus, regular monitoring for monoclonal gammopathy is crucial.[15]

Adult-Onset Still's Disease

Adult-onset Still's disease (AOSD) is a systemic inflammatory disorder that is often difficult to

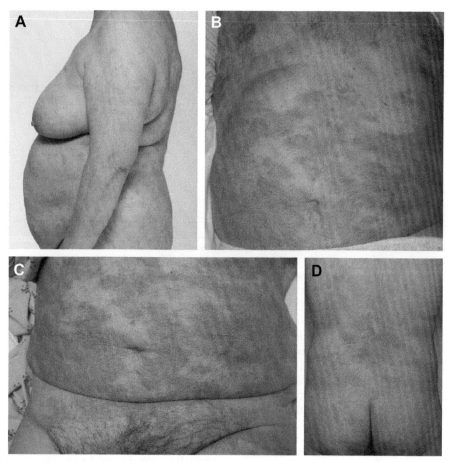

Fig. 1. (*A*) Urticarial papules and plaques on the trunk and upper extremity of a female with Schnitzler syndrome. (*B*) Confluent urticarial plaques on the trunk of an 80-year-old man with 8-month history of recurrent fevers, rashes, lymphadenopathy, arthralgias, confusion, and delirium. (*C*) Urticarial papules on the trunk and extremities of a 56-year-old with recurrent nonpruritic urticaria, elevated ESR/CRP, febrile sensation, and recurrent vertigo. (*D*) Urticarial papules and plaques on the trunk of a male with Schnitzler syndrome.

diagnose. It typically affects young adults around 30 years of age and is slightly more commonly seen in women over men; rarely, it is seen in adults more than 60 years old.[16] The exact etiology of AOSD is unknown; however, there is a connection between genetically predisposed hosts and auto-inflammatory disorders triggered by macrophage cell activation and TH1 cytokines such as IL-1, IL-2, IL-6,IL-18, TNF-α, and interferon-γ.[16]

AOSD is clinically characterized by high-spiking fever, polyarthralgia/arthritis, a salmon-pink evanescent rash, lymphadenopathy, liver dysfunction, and splenomegaly.[17–19] The characteristic salmon-pink evanescent rash is a major diagnostic finding with high sensitivity and specificity as it presents in about 87% of patients with AOSD (**Fig. 2**).[17,20] Some markers of disease activity include elevated levels of ferritin, IL-6, and IL-18.[17,21–25] The histologic findings of the typical evanescent rash reveal a relatively

sparse perivascular mixed inflammatory infiltrate containing neutrophils with little karyorrhexis.[17,19] Acute lesions are more likely to have the perivascular neutrophilic infiltrate, whereas chronic lesions may display keratin whorls in the stratum corneum and dyskeratotic keratinocytes scattered through the epidermis.[17,26,27]

The two most common symptoms in patients with AOSD are recurrent episodes of high-spiking fevers that typically flare in the late afternoon and an asymptomatic macular exanthem that is salmon-pink in color.[17–19] The salmon-pink evanescent rash is most frequently seen on the trunk and extremities and often demonstrates the Koebner phenomenon.[17–19,28] Additional symptoms commonly include arthritis, pharyngitis, lymphadenopathy, liver dysfunction, hepatomegaly, and splenomegaly.[17–19] Specifically, bilateral ankylosing carpal arthritis is a distinctive feature of AOSD.[29]

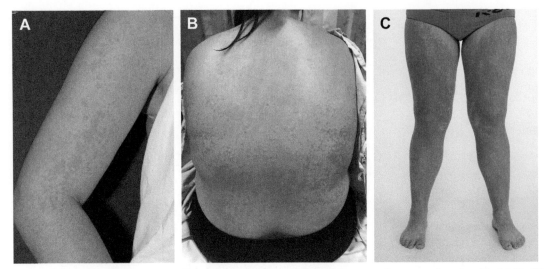

Fig. 2. (*A*) Coalescing urticarial papules and thin plaques on the upper arm of a young female with AOSD. (*B*) Coalescing urticarial papules and plaques on the trunk of a 31-year-ol female with AOSD. (*C*) Confluent urticarial papules and plaques on the lower extremities of a woman with AOSD.

Yamaguchi's criteria for a classification of AOSD include both the major and minor criteria.[17,19] The major criteria consist of the following: (1) fever of ≥39°C, lasting ≥1 week; (2) arthralgia lasting ≥2 weeks; (3) typical rash (ie, macular or maculopapular nonpruritic salmon-pink eruption usually appearing during fever); and (4) leukocytosis (≥10,000/mm3) including 80% more of granulocytes.[19] The minor criteria consist of the following: (1) sore throat; (2) lymphadenopathy and/or splenomegaly; (3) liver dysfunction; and (4) negative rheumatoid factor (RF) and negative antinuclear antibody (ANA).[19] An individual must meet ≥5 criteria including ≥2 major criteria for a diagnosis of AOSD.[19] When considering a diagnosis of AOSD, it is important to exclude other potential causes of the systemic symptoms such as infection (eg, sepsis and infectious mononucleosis), malignancy (eg, malignant lymphoma), and rheumatic disease (eg, polyarteritis nodosa and rheumatoid vasculitis with extra-articular features).[19]

The treatment of AOSD is mostly targeted toward controlling acute systemic symptoms. Many patients respond well to nonsteroidal anti-inflammatory drugs (naproxen 500 mg twice daily) and oral corticosteroids (0.5–1 mg/kg daily).[30–32] Methotrexate and intravenous immunoglobulin can be considered when patients are unable to taper corticosteroids.[30–32] For severe or chronic disease, various biologic agents that inhibit inflammatory signaling pathways such as TNF-α (eg, infliximab, adalimumab, etanercept), IL-1 (eg, anakinra), and IL-6 (eg, tocilizumab) can be helpful.[30–32] In addition, rituximab has been reported to improve refractory disease (**Box 2**).[32]

Cryopyrin-Associated Periodic Syndromes

Cryopyrin-associated periodic syndromes (CAPSs) are rare hereditary autoinflammatory conditions representing a spectrum of disease severity.[2,33,34] They include three clinical phenotypes associated with gain-of-function mutations in the NLRP3 gene (NOD-like receptor family, pyrin domain containing 3) that encodes for cryopyrin—a regulatory protein that forms intracellular protein complexes called inflammasomes.[5,35,36] Defects of the inflammasomes increase its activity and the

---

Box 2
Yamaguchi's criteria for a classification of adult-onset Still's disease[19]

Major criteria

1. Fever of ≥39°C, lasting ≥1 week

2. Arthralgia lasting ≥2 week

3. Typical rash (ie, macular or maculopapular nonpruritic salmon-pink eruption usually appearing during fever)

4. Leukocytosis (≥10,000/mm3) including 80% more of granulocytes

Minor criteria

1. Sore throat

2. Lymphadenopathy and/or splenomegaly

3. Liver dysfunction

4. Negative RF and negative ANA

Classification of AOSD requires ≥5 criteria including ≥2 major criteria.

conversion of inactive IL-1β precursor into active IL-1β.[5,36]

CAPS incidence in the United States is about 1 in 1,000,000 people and it has a prevalence of 300 to 500 individuals.[37] They are inherited in an autosomal-dominant pattern.[33] Its diagnostic criteria as specified in **Box 3** include elevated inflammatory markers (C-reactive protein [CRP]/serum amyloid A [SAA]) plus two or more of CAPS typical symptoms: urticaria-like rash, cold- or stress-triggered episodes, sensorineural hearing loss, musculoskeletal symptoms (arthralgia/arthritis/myalgia), chronic aseptic meningitis, and skeletal abnormalities (epiphyseal overgrowth/frontal bossing).[35]

The three clinical phenotypes of CAPS in order of increasing severity are familial cold autoinflammatory syndrome (FCAS), Muckle–Wells syndrome (MWS), and chronic infantile neurologic cutaneous and articular syndrome/neonatal-onset multisystem inflammatory disease (CINCA/NOMID).[5] They are also called "cryopyrinopathies" and are identified as a continuum of a singular disorder.[37] All three phenotypes present with urticarial rash, NUD, childhood onset, fever, joint pain, persistent neutrophilia, and elevated inflammatory markers (CRP, SAA, and neutrophil protein S100A12).[5,35] Histologically, CAPS lesions reveal a perivascular or perieccrine neutrophilic infiltrate.[37]

FCAS, the mildest CAPS, was first reported in 1940. It presents at birth or during the first 6 months, though there are late-onset cases.[34,37] It is clinically defined by recurrent fever, arthralgia, and an intermittent cold-induced urticaria-like rash.[34,37] The maculopapular and typically non-pruritic (can be itchy and/or painful) rash is usually the first noticeable sign, and it begins one or 2 hours after exposure to cold temperatures.[37]

Histologically, FCAS presents as sparse interstitial neutrophilic infiltrate in the reticular dermis.[37] Common clinical symptoms include conjunctivitis, nausea, and muscle pain, whereas headache, sweating, drowsiness, and amyloidosis are seen in less than 5% of patients.[37]

In 1962, Muckle and Wells first described the intermediate phenotype, MWS.[36] Like FCAS, it is characterized by fever, arthralgia, and an urticaria-like rash.[36,37] However, the urticaria-like rash is also induced by stress or exercise in addition to cold temperatures.[36,37] Sensorineural hearing loss is common as it is associated with 70% of cases, and conjunctivitis in MWS is usually associated with episcleritis and iridocyclitis.[37] Its characteristic AA amyloidosis usually begins with proteinuria and

---

Box 3
Diagnostic criteria of cryopyrin-associated periodic syndrome[35]

Mandatory criteria

Raised inflammatory markers (CRP/SAA)

Plus ≥ 2 of 6 CAPS typical signs/symptoms:

Urticaria-like rash

Cold/stress-triggered episodes

Sensorineural hearing loss

Musculoskeletal symptoms (arthralgia/arthritis/myalgia)

Chronic aseptic meningitis

Skeletal abnormalities (epiphyseal overgrowth/frontal bossing)

Box 4
Systemic lupus international collaborating clinics criteria[42]

Clinical Criteria

Acute cutaneous lupus

Chronic cutaneous lupus

Oral/nasal ulcers

Nonscarring alopecia

Synovitis

Serositis

Renal

Neurologic

Anemia

Leukopenia/lymphopenia

Thrombocytopenia

Immunologic Criteria

ANA

Anti-dsDNA antibody

Anti-Smith antibody

Antiphospholipid antibodies

Lupus anticoagulant

Anticardiolipin

Beta-2-glycoprotein

Low complement

Definite diagnosis if

Fulfillment of at least four criteria (at least one clinical criterion and one immunologic criterion),

OR

Lupus nephritis is present with ANA or anti-dsDNA antibodies

leads to the most serious complication of renal dysfunction in about 25% of patients.[37] MWS symptoms are typically chronic and last for 2 to 3 days.[37]

In the early 1980s, Prieur, Giscelli, Hassink, and Goldsmith first described the most severe phenotype, CINCA/NOMID.[38,39] This syndrome emerges due to de novo mutations.[36] The main feature of CINCA/NOMID is a neonatal onset of cutaneous symptoms, along with end-organ damage and a triad of arthropathy, chronic urticaria, and central nervous system (CNS) abnormalities.[36] These CNS abnormalities range from hearing loss to chronic aseptic meningitis and results in mental retardation.[36,37] Related symptoms include chronic headaches, irritability in young children, vomiting, and papilledema on fundoscopy.[37] Premature birth is common and one-third of children have early stages of amyloidosis that worsens with age and atypical facies—frontal prominence, facial hypoplasia, and saddle nose.[37] Patients with CINCA/NOMID can develop osteoarthropathy mainly of the large joints and overgrowth of epimetaphyseal cartilage mainly of the long bones.[37] Osseocartilaginous overgrowth in the patella and

distal femur is a distinct feature and supports a diagnosis of CINCA/NOMID when present.[37]

There are no fixed distinctions between FCAS, MWS, and CINCA/NOMID as they share similar features.[37] Their clinical manifestations can be significantly improved by the inhibition of Il-1β.[33] The three effective treatments for CAPS include anakinra (IL-1 receptor antagonist), rilonacept (soluble IL-1 decoy receptor), and canakinumab (anti-IL-1β monoclonal antibody).[37] Patients who are unable to tolerate daily injections of anakinra can use rilonacept or canakinumab due to their longer half-lives.[37]

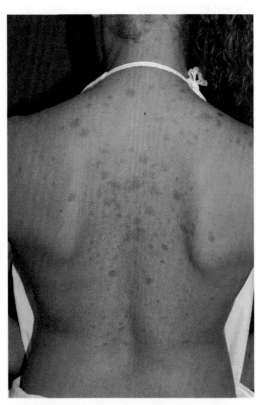

Fig. 3. Young woman with lupus erythematosus who presented with urticarial papules and NUD on histopathology.

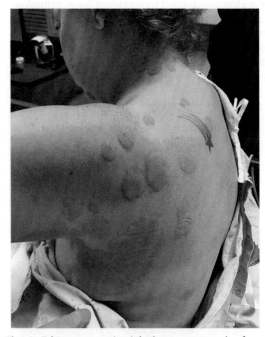

Fig. 4. Edematous urticarial plaques on trunk of patient with common urticaria.

Lupus Erythematosus

LE is a chronic, polygenic, autoimmune inflammatory disease characterized by various clinical manifestations and the production of humoral antibodies against parts of cell nucleus.[5,40,41] Systemic LE is typically diagnosed using the systemic lupus international collaborating clinics criteria.[42] As depicted in **Box 4**, it requires a fulfillment of at least four criteria: one clinical criteria and one immunologic criteria or a sole criteria of lupus nephritis in the presence of ANA or anti-double-stranded DNA (dsDNA) antibodies.[42]

Patients present clinically with widely distributed rose or red macules or slightly elevated papules (**Fig. 3**).[43] These lesions are mostly present on the trunk and rarely involve the face and limbs.[2,43] The histologic findings of LE is similar to that of NUD—marked neutrophilic interstitial and perivascular infiltrate with leukocytoclasia, but no significant edema or fibrinoid necrosis of blood vessels.[2,43]

Sometimes, mild vacuolization of the basement membrane and a lupus band may be present which can lead to a missed NUD diagnosis.[2]

The laboratory findings of NUD in a setting of LE are the same as those usually seen in LE and they include elevated erythrocyte sedimentation rate (ESR), hypergammaglobulinemia, antinuclear antibodies, and anti-dsDNA, anti-Sjögren syndrome antigen A (Ro/SSA), and anti-Sjögren syndrome antigen B (La/SSB) antibodies.[2] An elevated CRP without serositis, thromboembolic events, or infection is a rare sign in LE.[2]

NUD occurs before the diagnosis or during the course of LE.[5] In patients with LE, NUD typically presents with fever and joint pain.[5,43] Other associated symptoms include paresthesia, sore throat, abdominal pain, and episcleritis.[2] Koebner phenomenon may occur in remarkably rare instances.[2] The triad symptoms of a rash, fever, and joint pain are usually misdiagnosed as a classic lupus flare and thus treated with ineffective

Table 1
Histopathology of urticarial dermatosis[1,2,4,6,45,47–50]

Dermatosis	Clinical Findings	Histopathologic Findings
Classic urticaria	• Urticarial plaques are typically red and pruritic • Lesions can recover in 2–3 h and usually without residual pigmentation • Lesions respond to antihistamines • Angioedema may be present	• Perivascular, mainly mononuclear cell inflammation, with/without eosinophils (**Fig. 5**) • Dermal edema
Neutrophilic urticaria	• Individual urticarial lesions may be present for 24 h or less, several days, or more	• Vascular and perivascular neutrophilic inflammation, with/without eosinophils (**Fig. 6**) • Dermal edema
Neutrophilic urticarial dermatosis	• Pink to reddish urticarial eruptions consisting of flat or slightly raised, pruritic or nonpruritic macules, papules, or plaques • Individual lesions resolve within 24 h • Probable association with dermographism • May present with a burning sensation in the skin • Associated with fever or arthralgia	• Perivascular and interstitial neutrophilic inflammation with/without eosinophils (**Fig. 7**) • Leukocytoclasia
Urticarial vasculitis (leukocytoclastic vasculitis)	• Painful, pruritic, or burning lesions • Lesions persist more than 24 h • May include palpable purpura and angioedema • Residual hyperpigmentation following resolution	• More perivascular than interstitial neutrophilic inflammation, with/without eosinophils (**Fig. 8**) • Leukocytoclasia • Fibrinoid necrosis of small vessels • Endothelial swelling • Hemorrhage
Sweet syndrome	• Erythematous or purplish papules and nodules • Raised plaques • Edematous lesions • May be associated with fever, joint pains, or episcleritis	• Significant dermal edema • Intense neutrophilic infiltrate typically in the superficial dermis

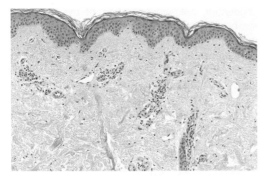

Fig. 5. Dermal edema, perivascular lymphocytes, neutrophils and eosinophils. Intraluminal neutrophils present. (Hematoxylin-eosin stain; X20).

immunosuppressive therapies.[5,43] The treatment of choice includes neutrophil migration inhibitors such as dapsone and colchicine.[5,43,44]

RECOMMENDED LABORATORY TESTS IF NEUTROPHILIC URTICARIAL DERMATOSIS IS DIAGNOSED

A diagnosis of NUD must be followed by a screening for systemic disease (**Box 5**).[2] However, there are rare instances in which NUD occurs in isolation.[2] Screening for systemic diseases associated with NUD should be performed at initial diagnosis and if the disease worsens,[2] although it can arise during the course of an existing systemic disease.[2]

DIFFERENTIAL DIAGNOSIS OF NEUTROPHILIC URTICARIAL DERMATOSIS

It is important to differentiate between NUD, classic urticaria, neutrophilic urticaria, urticarial vasculitis/leukocytoclastic vasculitis, and Sweet syndrome as NUD is usually associated with inflammatory disorders.[4] Classic urticarial plaques

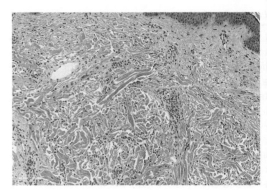

Fig. 7. Neutrophilic perivascular and interstitial infiltrate with leukocytoclasia; there is no vasculitis (Hematoxylin-eosin stain; X20).

are typically red and pruritic (**Fig. 4**).[45] The clinical lesions resolve without residual pigmentation, may be associated with angioedema, and respond to antihistamines.[45] However, NUD does not respond to antihistamine therapy and may present with a burning sensation in the skin.[4] Histologically, they both feature a lymphocytic, neutrophilic, or a mixed dermal infiltrate.[1,4]

Neutrophilic urticaria has a defined histologic entity, but its clinical aspects have been poorly understood.[46] Unlike NUDs individual lesions which resolve in 24 hours, neutrophilic urticaria presents with urticarial lesions that resolve in 24 hours or less, several days, or more.[46,47] It has a strong association with dermographism as compared with NUD.[46,47] Along with NUD, they both feature a neutrophil-rich perivascular infiltrate.[4,6] However, neutrophilic urticaria lacks the interstitial inflammation and leukocytoclasia seen in NUD.[4,6]

Urticarial vasculitis consists of long-lasting urticarial rashes.[48] It may present with angioedema and fever similar to NUD, but may be associated with palpable purpura which is not seen in NUD.[49] NUD is different from urticarial vasculitis due to its absence

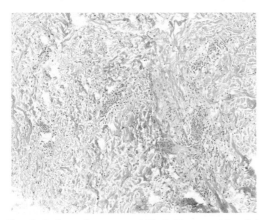

Fig. 6. Perivascular neutrophilic infiltrate with minimal interstitial spread and without leukocytoclasia (Hematoxylin-eosin stain; X20).

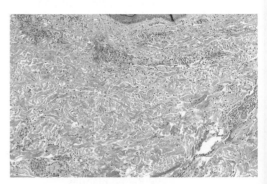

Fig. 8. Leukocytoclasia, perivascular and interstitial neutrophils, fibrinoid necrosis of vessel walls, hemorrhage, and edema of dermis (Hematoxylin-eosin stain; X20).

of fibrinoid necrosis of small vessels, endothelial cell swelling, and extravasation of erythrocytes.[6]

Sweet syndrome, also called acute febrile neutrophilic dermatosis, is a distinct entity but with many similarities to NUD.[2,50] Clinically, Sweet syndrome's lesions are more edematous and raised than NUD.[2] Its papules and nodules are erythematous or purplish and consist of raised plaques.[2] Like NUD, it may present with fever or joint pains.[2] Sweet syndrome is histologically different from NUD primarily by the presence of edema in its superficial dermis and its denser neutrophilic infiltrate (Table 1).[2]

SUMMARY

NUDs etiology is not well established and its association with several systemic diseases suggests a link to autoinflammation.[5] Diagnosis of NUD and its accompanying condition requires a rigorous analysis of clinical, histologic, and laboratory findings.[5] Its treatment is determined by the clinical symptoms and underlying disease.[5] Neutrophil migration inhibitors and IL-1 antagonists are found to be effective therapies against NUD.[5] Further histopathological analysis of cases identified as "urticaria vasculitis" will likely reveal more patients presenting with NUD.[2]

FUNDING/SUPPORT

This research did not receive any specific grant from funding agencies in the public, commercial, or not-for-profit sectors.

FINANCIAL DISCLOSURES

The authors have no relevant financial or nonfinancial interests to disclose.

CLINICS CARE POINTS

- Screening for neutrophilic urticarial dermatosis (NUD) at initial onset via a rigorous analysis of the clinical presentation, histopathologic features, and laboratory results determines the specific therapeutic management. Antihistamines should at least be used initially, though they are usually ineffective.

- In patients with Schnitzler syndrome or cryopyrin-associated periodic syndrome, interleukin-1 antagonists such as anakinra, rilonacept, or canakinumab are the most effective treatments.

- Anakinra or tocilizumab is preferred in severe or chronic states of adult-onset Still's disease over first-line therapy nonsteroidal antiinflammatory drugs, corticosteroids, or methotrexate.

- In NUD associated with lupus erythematosus, antineutrophilic agents such as dapsone and colchicine are treatments of choice as immunosuppressants are ineffective and result in multiple adverse effects.

REFERENCES

1. Kieffer C, Cribier B, Lipsker D. Neutrophilic Urticarial Dermatosis: A Variant of Neutrophilic Urticaria Strongly Associated With Systemic Disease. Report of 9 New Cases and Review of the Literature. Medicine 2009;88(1).
2. Gusdorf L, Lipsker D. Neutrophilic urticarial dermatosis: A review. Ann Dermatol Venereol 2018; 145(12):735–40.
3. Salam A, Papalexopoulou N, White JM, et al. Neutrophilic urticarial dermatosis: a novel association with poststreptococcal rheumatic disease. Clin Exp Dermatol 2018;43(3):311–4.
4. Gusdorf L, Lipsker D. Neutrophilic urticarial dermatosis: an entity bridging monogenic and polygenic autoinflammatory disorders, and beyond. J Eur Acad Dermatol Venereol 2020;34(4):685–90.
5. Gillihan R, Farahbakhsh N, Motaparthi K. Neutrophilic Urticarial Dermatosis Without Underlying Systemic Disease. J Clin Aesthet Dermatol 2020;13(3): 20–1.
6. Sokumbi O, Drage LA, Peters MS. Clinical and histopathologic review of Schnitzler syndrome: the Mayo Clinic experience (1972-2011). J Am Acad Dermatol 2012;67(6):1289–95.
7. Al-Hakim A, Mistry A, Savic S. Improving Diagnosis and Clinical Management of Acquired Systemic Autoinflammatory Diseases. J Inflamm Res 2022; 15:5739–55.
8. Lipsker D. The Schnitzler syndrome. Orphanet J Rare Dis 2010;5:38.
9. Ryan JG, De Koning HD, Beck LA, et al. IL-1 blockade in Schnitzler syndrome: ex vivo findings correlate with clinical remission. J Allergy Clin Immunol 2008;121(1):260–2.
10. Efthimiou P, Petryna O, Nakasato P, et al. New insights on multigenic autoinflammatory diseases. Ther Adv Musculoskelet Dis 2022;14. 1759720x221 117880.
11. Gusdorf L, Asli B, Barbarot S, et al. Schnitzler syndrome: validation and applicability of diagnostic criteria in real-life patients. Allergy 2017;72(2): 177–82.
12. Tolkachjov SN, Wetter DA. Schnitzler Syndrome With Delirium and Vertigo: The Utility of Neurologic Manifestations in Diagnosis. J Drugs Dermatol JDD 2017; 16(6):625–7.
13. Bhutani M, Shahid Z, Schnebelen A, et al. Cutaneous manifestations of multiple myeloma and other

plasma cell proliferative disorders. Semin Oncol 2016;43(3):395–400.

14. Kano Y, Sugihara M. Schnitzler Syndrome Presenting as a Fever of Unknown Origin with Elevated Alkaline Phosphatase Levels. Intern Med 2023; 62(9):1361–4.

15. van Leersum FS, Potjewijd J, van Geel M, et al. Schnitzler's syndrome - a novel hypothesis of a shared pathophysiologic mechanism with Waldenström's disease. Orphanet J Rare Dis 2019;14(1): 151.

16. Gerfaud-Valentin M, Maucort-Boulch D, Hot A, et al. Adult-onset Still disease: manifestations, treatment, outcome, and prognostic factors in 57 patients. Medicine (Baltim) 2014;93(2):91–9.

17. Lee JY, Yang CC, Hsu MM. Histopathology of persistent papules and plaques in adult-onset Still's disease. J Am Acad Dermatol 2005;52(6): 1003–8.

18. Bywaters EG. Still's disease in the adult. Ann Rheum Dis 1971;30(2):121–33.

19. Yamaguchi M, Ohta A, Tsunematsu T, et al. Preliminary criteria for classification of adult Still's disease. J Rheumatol 1992;19(3):424–30.

20. Ohta A, Yamaguchi M, Tsunematsu T, et al. Adult Still's disease: a multicenter survey of Japanese patients. J Rheumatol 1990;17(8):1058–63.

21. Schwarz-Eywill M, Heilig B, Bauer H, et al. Evaluation of serum ferritin as a marker for adult Still's disease activity. Ann Rheum Dis 1992;51(5):683–5.

22. Rooney M, David J, Symons J, et al. Inflammatory cytokine responses in juvenile chronic arthritis. Br J Rheumatol 1995;34(5):454–60.

23. Scheinberg MA, Chapira E, Fernandes ML, et al. Interleukin 6: a possible marker of disease activity in adult onset Still's disease. Clin Exp Rheumatol 1996;14(6):653–5.

24. Hoshino T, Ohta A, Yang D, et al. Elevated serum interleukin 6, interferon-gamma, and tumor necrosis factor-alpha levels in patients with adult Still's disease. J Rheumatol 1998;25(2):396–8.

25. Kawaguchi Y, Terajima H, Harigai M, et al. Interleukin-18 as a novel diagnostic marker and indicator of disease severity in adult-onset Still's disease. Arthritis Rheum 2001;44(7):1716–7.

26. Lübbe J, Hofer M, Chavaz P, et al. Adult-onset Still's disease with persistent plaques. Br J Dermatol 1999;141(4):710–3.

27. Suzuki K, Kimura Y, Aoki M, et al. Persistent plaques and linear pigmentation in adult-onset Still's disease. Dermatology 2001;202(4):333–5.

28. Joy M, Wittner L, Ellis S. A challenging diagnosis of adult-onset Still's disease in the setting of raised anti-streptolysin O titres. Rheumatol Adv Pract 2019;3. © The Author(s) 2019. Published by Oxford University Press on behalf of the British Society for Rheumatology.

29. Mitrovic S, Fautrel B. Clinical Phenotypes of Adult-Onset Still's Disease: New Insights from Pathophysiology and Literature Findings. J Clin Med 2021;10(12).

30. Giampietro C, Ridene M, Lequerre T, et al. Anakinra in adult-onset Still's disease: long-term treatment in patients resistant to conventional therapy. Arthritis Care Res 2013;65(5):822–6.

31. Ortiz-Sanjuán F, Blanco R, Calvo-Rio V, et al. Efficacy of tocilizumab in conventional treatment-refractory adult-onset Still's disease: multicenter retrospective open-label study of thirty-four patients. Arthritis Rheumatol 2014;66(6):1659–65.

32. Belfeki N, Smiti Khanfir M, Said F, et al. Successful treatment of refractory adult onset Still's disease with rituximab. Reumatismo 2016;68(3):159–62.

33. Levy R, Gérard L, Kuemmerle-Deschner J, et al. Phenotypic and genotypic characteristics of cryopyrin-associated periodic syndrome: a series of 136 patients from the Eurofever Registry. Ann Rheum Dis 2015;74(11):2043–9.

34. Shinkai K, McCalmont TH, Leslie KS. Cryopyrin-associated periodic syndromes and autoinflammation. Clin Exp Dermatol 2008;33(1):1–9.

35. Kuemmerle-Deschner JB, Ozen S, Tyrrell PN, et al. Diagnostic criteria for cryopyrin-associated periodic syndrome (CAPS). Ann Rheum Dis 2017;76(6): 942–7.

36. Yu JR, Leslie KS. Cryopyrin-associated periodic syndrome: an update on diagnosis and treatment response. Curr Allergy Asthma Rep 2011;11(1):12–20.

37. Miyamae T. Cryopyrin-associated periodic syndromes: diagnosis and management. Paediatr Drugs 2012;14(2):109–17.

38. Prieur AM, Griscelli C. Arthropathy with rash, chronic meningitis, eye lesions, and mental retardation. J Pediatr 1981;99(1):79–83.

39. Hassink SG, Goldsmith DP. Neonatal onset multisystem inflammatory disease. Arthritis Rheum 1983;26(5):668–73.

40. Mok C, Lau C. Pathogenesis of systemic lupus erythematosus. J Clini Pathol 2003;56(7):481–90.

41. Kuhn A, Ruzicka T. Classification of Cutaneous Lupus Erythematosus. In: Kuhn A, Lehmann P, Ruzicka T, editors. Cutaneous lupus erythematosus. Berlin, Heidelberg: Springer; 2005.

42. Tiao J, Feng R, Carr K, et al. Using the American College of Rheumatology (ACR) and Systemic Lupus International Collaborating Clinics (SLICC) criteria to determine the diagnosis of systemic lupus erythematosus (SLE) in patients with subacute cutaneous lupus erythematosus (SCLE). J Am Acad Dermatol 2016;74(5):862–9.

43. Gusdorf L, Bessis D, Lipsker D. Lupus erythematosus and neutrophilic urticarial dermatosis: a retrospective study of 7 patients. Medicine 2014;93(29).

44. Lipsker D, Saurat J-H. Neutrophilic cutaneous lupus erythematosus. Dermatology 2008;216(4):283.

45. Kayiran MA, Akdeniz N. Diagnosis and treatment of urticaria in primary care. North Clin Istanb 2019;6(1):93–9.
46. Toppe E, Haas N, Henz BM. Neutrophilic urticaria: clinical features, histological changes and possible mechanisms. Br J Dermatol 1998;138(2):248–53.
47. Peters MS, Winkelmann RK. Neutrophilic urticaria. Br J Dermatol 1985;113(1):25–30.
48. Kolkhir P, Grakhova M, Bonnekoh H, et al. Treatment of urticarial vasculitis: A systematic review. J Allergy Clini Immunol 2019;143(2):458–66.
49. Venzor J, Lee WL, Huston DP. Urticarial vasculitis. Clin Rev Allergy Immunol 2002;23(2):201–16.
50. Cohen PR. Sweet's syndrome - A comprehensive review of an acute febrile neutrophilic dermatosis. Orphanet J Rare Dis 2007;2(1):34.

Characterization and Management of Amicrobial Pustulosis of the Folds, Aseptic Abscess Syndrome, Behçet Disease, Neutrophilic Eccrine Hidradenitis, and Pyostomatitis Vegetans – Pyodermatitis Vegetans

Giang Huong Nguyen, MD, DPhil[a,*], Michael J. Camilleri, MD[a,b], David A. Wetter, MD[a]

KEYWORDS

- Amicrobial pustulosis of the folds • Aseptic abscess syndrome • Behçet disease
- Neutrophilic dermatosis • Neutrophilic eccrine hidradenitis • Pyodermatitis vegetans
- Pyostomatitis vegetans

KEY POINTS

- Although neutrophilic dermatoses such as Sweet syndrome and pyoderma gangrenosum are relatively more prevalent, clinicians should be familiar with less-common entities such as amicrobial pustulosis of the folds, aseptic abscess syndrome, Behçet disease, neutrophilic eccrine hidradenitis, and pyostomatitis vegetans–pyodermatitis vegetans.
- Given the varied characteristics of neutrophilic dermatoses, particularly subtypes that are less frequently observed in routine outpatient or hospital practices, clinicians should have a high index of suspicion to correctly diagnose these entities.
- Evaluations for associated inflammatory, autoimmune, or malignant conditions should be considered for patients with suspected or confirmed neutrophilic dermatoses, depending on the clinical presentation and findings from the review of systems.

INTRODUCTION

Neutrophilic dermatoses encompass a diverse group of inflammatory skin disorders. Patients often seek care because of marked morbidity, and the varying presentations can make diagnosis challenging. Treatments for Behçet disease (BD) have been assessed in clinical trials, but for other dermatoses, management approaches may be anecdotal at best. Here, the authors describe 5

[a] Department of Dermatology, Mayo Clinic, 200 First Street Southwest, Rochester, MN 55905, USA;
[b] Department of Laboratory Medicine and Pathology, Mayo Clinic, 200 First Street Southwest, Rochester, MN 55905, USA
* Corresponding author.
E-mail address: nguyen.giang2@mayo.edu

Dermatol Clin 42 (2024) 231–245
https://doi.org/10.1016/j.det.2023.12.003
0733-8635/24/© 2023 Elsevier Inc. All rights reserved.

neutrophilic dermatoses and review their characteristics and current management.

AMICROBIAL PUSTULOSIS OF THE FOLDS
Epidemiology

Initially described by Crickx and colleagues,[1] amicrobial pustulosis of the folds (APF) is characterized by chronically relapsing, pustular eruptions that predominantly affect cutaneous folds. Only about 70 cases have been reported in the literature to date. APF mostly affects women, and the age of onset is typically around 30 years.[2]

Pathogenesis

The underlying cause of APF remains unknown, but autoinflammation is a hypothesized trigger.[3] APF skin biopsies show overexpression of various inflammatory cell markers and cytokines,[4] and APF is associated with inflammatory conditions (Box 1).[1–3] A recent report described 2 sisters with APF who had the human leukocyte antigen (HLA) DRB1*08 allele,[5] a genetic marker of other autoimmune diseases.

Medications also may have a triggering role. Tumor necrosis factor α (TNF-α) inhibitors (eg, infliximab, adalimumab) have been implicated in the initiation of APF because an increase in the concentration of interferon α affects neutrophil recruitment and chemotaxis.[6] In a series, patients with inflammatory bowel disease (IBD) treated with TNF-α inhibitors had APF develop, but their skin condition improved with discontinuation of the inhibitor.[7] Another report indicated that amlodipine was a putative cause of APF.[8]

Clinicopathologic Features

Patients with APF often report the sudden appearance of symmetric, painful papulopustular lesions on skin folds and periorificial regions (eg, nostrils) that eventually coalesce into plaques (Fig. 1). Nonscarring alopecia, palmoplantar involvement, and onychodystrophy are rare.[6,9,10] Systemic compromise (besides the skin) is uncommon, and fever has been described.[10] The disease tends to have a chronic course, with periods of remission and frequent relapses.

Although APF may be associated with autoimmune disease, it is not associated with activity of the underlying disease.[2] Most patients have strong evidence of antinuclear factors or soluble extractable nuclear antibodies without autoimmune disease, and many have increased acute-phase reactants such as herpes simplex virus and C-reactive protein.[2]

Cultures of the pustules are negative for microbes, but secondary bacterial colonization is frequent. Histopathologic analysis shows intraepidermal neutrophilic spongiosis or subcorneal pustules with a predominantly neutrophilic dermal infiltrate but no evidence of vasculitis (Fig. 2). The direct immunofluorescent lupus band test may be positive.[2]

Diagnosis and Management

APF is diagnosed by considering clinical and histopathologic findings and comorbid conditions. Diagnostic criteria are shown in Table 1; patients must fulfill all 3 major plus 1 minor criteria. From its clinical appearance alone, APF may be difficult to distinguish from other conditions (Box 2).

Because APF is rare, no evidence-based therapy guidelines have been established to date. Anecdotally, systemic corticosteroids are often used as the first-line therapy. Prednisone (0.5–1 mg/kg daily) is associated with rapid improvement, but APF may recur after the dose is reduced or discontinued. Topical corticosteroids were effective for 2 of 4 patients with APF seen at our institution.[9] Many treatments have been reported (Box 3).[2,3]

Box 1
Diseases associated with amicrobial pustulosis of the folds

Adenocarcinoma of the lung

Antiphospholipid syndrome

Autoimmune hepatitis

Celiac disease

Grave disease

Hashimoto thyroiditis

Hodgkin lymphoma

Idiopathic thrombocytopenic purpura

Immunoglobulin A nephropathy

Inflammatory bowel disease

Juvenile idiopathic arthritis

Myasthenia gravis

Palindromic rheumatism

Rheumatoid arthritis

Sharp syndrome

Sjögren syndrome

Systemic lupus erythematosus

Undifferentiated connective tissue disease

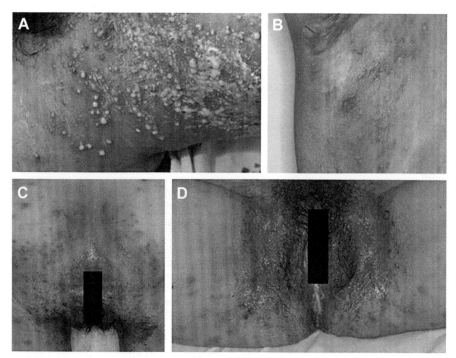

Fig. 1. Amicrobial Pustulosis of the Folds. (*A* and *B*) A 54-year-old woman presented with generalized pustules involving the neck (*A*) and axilla (*B*). (*C* and *D*) The patient was a 30-year-old woman with pustules on the gluteal cleft, perianal, and vulvar regions (*C*) and macerated pustular plaques involving inguinal folds and vulvar regions (*D*). Black bar–covered skin was clinically similar to the surrounding areas. (*From* Wang et al[9]; used with permission.)

ASEPTIC ABSCESS SYNDROME
Epidemiology

Aseptic abscess (AA) syndrome is a rare inflammatory disorder, initially described in 1995, that is characterized by multiple internal abscesses, mostly in the spleen. The first reported case was a 25-year-old man with multiple sterile abdominal

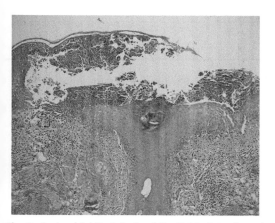

Fig. 2. Amicrobial Pustulosis of the Folds. Intradermal and diffuse dermal neutrophils (hematoxylin-eosin, original magnification × 100).

abscesses that developed several years before Crohn disease was diagnosed.[11] Because Crohn disease also was identified in subsequent cases, AA syndrome was hypothesized to be an extraintestinal manifestation of Crohn disease.[12]

AA syndrome can affect patients of any age. For patients with co-occurring IBD, the mean age at AA onset is 34.5 years. The mean age for patients without IBD is 26.9 years. AA syndrome shows a slight male predominance.[13]

Pathogenesis

The pathogenesis of AA syndrome is unknown, although autoimmunity is postulated to have a role.[14] Recently, a novel *LPIN2* variant was identified and linked to numerous autoinflammatory diseases.[15]

Clinicopathologic Features

Patients often report a history of fever, abdominal pain, and weight loss. Extensive laboratory studies show elevated inflammatory markers but no infectious causes. Skin manifestations are common (20%–49% of patients)[12–14] and are mainly cutaneous abscesses, but other presentations can include oral aphthosis, erythema nodosum,

Table 1
Diagnostic criteria for amicrobial pustulosis of the folds

Diagnostic Criteria[a]	Comment
Major criteria	
Pustulosis	Involving $\geq$1 large folds, $\geq$1 small folds, and/or anogenital region
Histopathologic findings	Intraepidermal spongiform pustules Predominately neutrophilic dermal infiltrate
Microbial culture	Negative cultures with material from intact pustules
Minor criteria	
Autoimmune or autoinflammatory condition	Associated with $\geq$1 autoimmune or autoinflammatory conditions (see **Box 1**)
Histopathologic findings	Positive for antinuclear factor antibodies, titers $\geq$1:160 Positive for $\geq$1 of the following autoantibodies: anti—extractable nuclear antigen, anti-dsDNA, antihistone, antiphospholipid, anti—smooth muscle, antimitochondrial, antiendomysial, anti—gastric parietal mucosal cell

[a] Diagnosis is confirmed if patients meet all 3 major and 1 minor criteria.

pustulosis, pyoderma gangrenosum (PG), and Sweet syndrome.[16–18] Lesions eventually evolve into deep ulcers, similar to those of PG. However, all AAs begin as subcutaneous nodules, and no type of PG follows such a path. Systemic neutrophilic presentations can also occur (eg, meningitis, pleural effusion, myocarditis, ascites).[19]

Most early cases had a history of intra-abdominal abscesses, and thus, the current diagnostic criteria exclude patients with only skin manifestations. Trefond and colleagues[19] have suggested that patients with only skin abscesses (no systemic symptoms) tend to have a different disease course than patients with abscesses in deep locations. Regarding the classical presentation, AA syndrome commonly affects the spleen, but reports have described AAs in the liver, lungs, pancreas, ear-nose-throat system, kidneys, brain, breasts, testicles, vagina, prostate, pituitary gland, lymph nodes, and muscle.[19] AA syndrome initially was believed to be exclusively associated with Crohn disease, but recent studies have shown its association with other diseases (**Box 4**). IBD, if present, can develop months to years before, concurrently with, or after an AA syndrome diagnosis.[19]

For patients with AA syndrome, serial aerobic and anaerobic cultures of abscess aspirate do not identify any organisms. Histopathology shows a spongiotic but slightly acanthotic epidermis, with focal abscesses extending to the deep dermis, and intraepidermal and dermal neutrophils and multinuclear giant cells. Skin and internal lesions have the same histopathologic findings. Although AA syndrome classically presents as a neutrophilic dermatosis, AAs can be surrounded by granulomas, an atypical finding.

Diagnosis and Management

The diagnostic criteria for AA syndrome (**Box 5**) were proposed in 2007.[12] The diagnosis is considered after excluding other diseases in the differential diagnosis, such as polyarteritis nodosa, disseminated tuberculous abscess, ecthyma gangrenosum, ecthyma, PG, deep mycosis, atypical mycosis, and syphilitic gumma.

AA syndrome might be rarely diagnosed because patients with solely cutaneous AA are excluded by the current diagnostic criteria.

Box 2
Diseases clinically resembling amicrobial pustulosis of the folds

Acute generalized exanthematous pustulosis

Folliculitis

Immunoglobulin A pemphigus

Impetigo

Pemphigus foliaceus

Pemphigus vegetans

Pustular psoriasis

Subcorneal pustular dermatosis

Symmetric drug-related intertriginous and flexural erythema

Box 3
Treatments reported for amicrobial pustulosis of the folds

Acitretin

Anakinra

Azathioprine

Colchicine

Cyclosporine

Dapsone

Doxycycline

Hydroxychloroquine

Levamisole

Methotrexate

Mycophenolate mofetil

Tumor necrosis factor α inhibitors (adalimumab, infliximab)

Ustekinumab

UV-A

Others (cimetidine, ascorbic acid, zinc)

Box 5
Diagnostic criteria for aseptic abscess syndrome

Abscess is observed radiographically

Histopathologic analysis shows neutrophilic features

Blood cultures and infectious evaluation are negative for microbes

Antibiotic therapy is ineffective (>2 wk of therapy or 3 mo if tuberculosis is suspected)

Rapid improvement with corticosteroid treatment

Additionally, the disease is not well known, and patients often may be misdiagnosed for months to years. Because AA syndrome is rare, evidence-based treatment guidelines do not exist. Almost all patients described in the literature had first-line treatment with broad-spectrum antibiotics, but the disease remained uncontrolled. Patients frequently had a dramatic response to systemic corticosteroids (0.5–1 mg/kg) but relapsed after corticosteroids were discontinued. Given the high rate of recurrence, splenectomy and corticosteroid-sparing agents (**Box 6**) are frequently trialed.[19]

BEHÇET DISEASE
Epidemiology

BD, described in 1937 as a 3-symptom complex of recurrent oral ulcers, genital ulcers, and uveitis, is a rare systemic vasculitis disease.[20] Also termed "*Silk Road disease*," BD has a distinct geographic distribution, with Turkey having the highest prevalence.[21] Typically, BD develops in the third and fourth decade of life, and it affects both sexes equally. The cause is unknown, but risk factors for a more severe disease course are male sex, earlier age at onset, and ethnic origin in the Middle East or Far East Asia.[21]

Box 4
Diseases associated with aseptic abscess syndrome

Behçet disease

Crohn disease

Erythema elevatum diutinum

Gammopathies

Inflammatory bowel disease

Mesenteric panniculitis

Myeloproliferative syndrome

Polyarthritis nodosa

Pyoderma gangrenosum

Relapsing polychondritis

Rheumatoid arthritis

Spondylarthritis

Ulcerative colitis

Box 6
Noncorticosteroid treatments for aseptic abscess syndrome

Colchicine

Cyclosporine

Interleukin 1β blockage

Interleukin 6 inhibitors

Mesalamine

Methotrexate

Mycophenolate mofetil

Tumor necrosis factor α inhibitors (adalimumab, infliximab)[a]

[a] Showed high rates of complete clinical responses, considered first-line therapy.[19,55]

Pathogenesis

The pathogenesis of BD is unknown, but one hypothesis is that it is caused by an irregular immune response, attributable to environmental and/or autoantigen triggers, in genetically susceptible individuals. The disease prevalence is associated with HLA-B51, with carriers having a 5.78-fold increased risk of BD development.[22,23] Recent studies have described involvement of the nuclear factor—κB pathway, as well as microRNAs and DNA methylation of cytoskeletal remodeling genes.[24]

Clinicopathologic Features

Most patients have recurrent, painful, oral aphthous ulcerations, commonly on nonkeratinizing mucosal surfaces (eg, lips, buccal mucosa, ventral and lateral surface of the tongue, floor of the mouth, soft palate) (**Fig. 3**). Although genital ulceration is less frequent, those lesions tend to be larger and have irregular margins. Multiple genital ulcers can develop, and scarring is common. For men, ulcers can affect the penis shaft, glans, and, rarely, the meatal urethra. For women, ulcers can involve the labium, vulva, vagina, and, rarely, the cervix. They may cause bloody, purulent discharge when present in deeper locations, making diagnosis challenging. Complications such as bladder, urethral, or rectal fistula have been reported.[25,26]

Ulcers may develop on other anatomic locations, such as the axilla, thigh, breast, neck, inguinal region, and between the toes.[25] These lesions tend to heal with scars. Ocular involvement such as uveitis, defined as panuveitis and retinal vasculitis, affects 10% to 20% of patients.[20] Without proper recognition and treatment, blindness could result. BD can manifest with other

Box 7
Additional cutaneous findings of Behçet disease[a]
Acne-like sterile pustules
Acral pruritic papulonodular lesions
Erythema nodosum—like lesions
Folliculitis
Necrotizing vasculitis
Palpable purpura
Pernio
Polyarteritis nodosa
Pyoderma gangrenosum
Superficial thrombophlebitis
Sweet syndrome—like lesions
[a] Oral and genital ulcers are most common.

cutaneous findings (**Box 7**). Extracutaneous findings are thought to arise from systemic inflammation associated with vasculitis.[25] Histopathologic findings are nonspecific, with mixed dermal inflammatory infiltrates and lymphocytic or neutrophilic vasculitis (affecting all sizes of vessels) that more commonly involve the venous side of circulation.

Diagnosis and Management

BD is diagnosed on the basis of clinical findings, by using the scoring system from the International Criteria for BD (**Table 2**).[27] The recurrent oral and genital ulcers of BD resemble those of other conditions (**Box 8**).

Given the heterogeneity of BD, treatment can vary greatly, depending on the involved organs, the severity and duration of involvement, the frequency of attacks, and the patient's age and sex. A coordinated, multidisciplinary approach, often led by a rheumatologist, is necessary to suppress inflammatory exacerbations and prevent permanent organ damage. Clinical trials are limited to the treatment of mucocutaneous, articular, and ocular manifestations.

For localized oral and genital ulcers, first-line therapies are antiseptics, antibiotics, antimicrobial agents, nonsteroidal anti-inflammatory drugs, and topical or intralesional corticosteroids. **Table 3** summarizes outcomes of select clinical trials assessing topical interventions. The efficacy of triamcinolone, sucralfate, pentoxifylline, pimecrolimus, and low-level laser therapy (eg, carbon dioxide, diode, and neodymium-doped yttrium aluminum garnet lasers) also has been proven.[28,29]

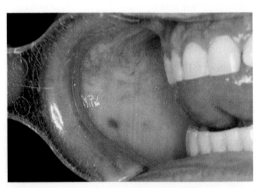

Fig. 3. Behçet Disease. A 42-year-old woman with a long-term history of Behçet disease presented with a 2-mm oral ulceration on the right buccal mucosa.

Table 2
International criteria for Behçet disease

Sign or Symptom	Points[a]
Genital aphthosis	2
Ocular lesions	2
Oral aphthosis	2
Neurologic manifestations	1
Skin lesion	1
Vascular manifestations	1
Positive pathergy test	1[b]

[a] A score ≥4 indicates a definitive diagnosis of Behçet disease.
[b] A positive skin pathergy test has been associated with Behçet disease. It is a nonspecific hypersensitivity reaction after a needle puncture. This test is optional, and the scoring system does not account for it. However, if the test is conducted and has a positive result, 1 point is added to the score.
From International Team for the Revision of the International Criteria for Behçet's Disease.[27]

For severe and refractory mucocutaneous lesions, systemic therapies are necessary. First-line treatments are colchicine, systemic corticosteroids, and apremilast (**Table 4**). Many systemic immunosuppressant therapies have shown varying response rates and control of mucocutaneous symptoms (see **Table 4**). Ongoing clinical trials are investigating other treatment modalities (**Table 5**).

Biologic agents (eg, tocilizumab, alemtuzumab, anakinra, canakinumab, ustekinumab) have shown various degrees of efficacy in controlling mucocutaneous symptoms.[28,29] More recently, Janus kinase inhibitors were reported to have

Box 8
Differential diagnosis of recurrent oral and genital ulcers

Complex aphthosis

Deficiency of iron, vitamin B$_{12}$, and folic acid

Erythema multiforme

Fixed drug eruption

Herpes simplex

Inflammatory bowel syndrome

Mouth and genital ulcers with inflamed cartilage (MAGIC syndrome)

Recurrent aphthous stomatitis

Reiter syndrome

Sweet syndrome

efficacy in treating recalcitrant BD; future research will likely focus on Janus kinase inhibition.[30]

NEUTROPHILIC ECCRINE HIDRADENITIS
Epidemiology

Neutrophilic eccrine hidradenitis (NEH) is a prototypical neutrophilic dermatosis of the eccrine sweat glands. It is characterized by inflamed papules or plaques on the trunk or extremities and mostly is seen with patients receiving chemotherapy. The first known case, described in 1982, was a patient with acute myeloid leukemia who received treatment with cytarabine and doxorubicin.[31] NEH has been observed with other malignancies, including lymphomas and solid tumors, but it rarely can also be idiopathic. The disease can occur in children and older adults.[32]

The incidence and cause of NEH are unknown, although it is associated with many medications (**Box 9**).[33] NEH is thought to have a noninfectious origin, but many infectious agents are linked with NEH, most recently coronavirus disease 2019 (COVID-19).[34] When pediatric patients have NEH without malignancy, heat damage is a suspected cause. In the context of malignancy, the direct cytotoxic effects of chemotherapy may be a trigger.[35] This hypothesis helps explain why NEH often develops after 1 course of chemotherapy.

Clinicopathologic Features

In its classical presentation, NEH presents as painless, erythematous to violaceous, edematous papules or plaques on the trunk or extremities. Patients typically have hematologic malignancy, and NEH can present as early as 2 days to 2 years after initiating chemotherapy (**Fig. 4**). Most patients will have fever and neutropenia. The palmoplantar variant is typically seen in healthy children.[36] Lesions may be painful, single or multiple, have a linear or annular shape, and may be papules or pustules. Rarely, NEH presents as hyperpigmented plaques, annular lesions, and sclerodermoid changes.[37,38] When NEH involves the face, it can resemble cellulitis.[39–41]

The defining histopathologic finding is the necrotic eccrine glands (**Fig. 5**). For patients with severe neutropenia, neutrophils may be rare or absent, but necrosis of eccrine glands is always prominent. Dense neutrophilic infiltrates typically are seen within and around the eccrine glands. Other features include apocrine gland necrosis, squamous syringometaplasia, dermal hemorrhage, epidermal and dermal spongiosis, basilar vacuolization, focal necrotic keratinocytes, mucin deposits, mild and superficial panniculitis, and leukocytoclastic vasculitis.[31]

Table 3
Summary of clinical trials assessing topical interventions for oral and genital symptoms of Behçet disease

Topical Intervention[a]	No. of Patients	Duration of Treatment	Results
Triamcinolone 0.1% ointment vs phenytoin syrup	60	1 wk	Triamcinolone was more effective for OU
Sucralfate vs placebo	30	12 wk	Decreased the frequency, healing time, and pain of OU Decreased healing time and pain of GU
Pimecrolimus vs placebo	45	4 wk	Decreased healing time of GU
Pimecrolimus + colchicine vs colchicine	38	4 wk	Pimecrolimus + colchicine had less pain and severity of GU
Pentoxifylline + colchicine vs colchicine	21	2 wk	Pentoxifylline + colchicine had less pain and decreased healing time for OU
Interferon alfa vs placebo	84 30	12 wk 24 wk	No beneficial effects for OU (both trials)
Cyclosporine vs placebo	24	8 wk	No beneficial effects
Diode laser vs triamcinolone 0.1% cream	50	5 d	Diode laser decreased pain and frequency of OU

Abbreviations: GU, genital ulcers; OU, oral ulcers.
[a] Dosages for specific medications were as follows: pentoxifylline, 1000 mg/d; colchicine, 1 to 2 g/d; cyclosporine, 5 to 10 mg/kg per day.

Diagnosis and Management

A biopsy is often needed to confirm the diagnosis, and the final diagnosis depends on clinical and histopathologic correlation. NEH is part of a broad differential diagnosis (**Box 10**). After NEH is confirmed, patients should undergo a preliminary evaluation for possible hematologic malignancy and infection.

Given the self-limited presentation of NEH, first-line therapy is supportive care to manage fever and pain. Topical corticosteroids and systemic antibiotics are often prescribed, especially when infection is suspected. Lesions self-resolve without scarring, within days to weeks. Patients should be informed that relapse is common with subsequent chemotherapy, but treatment of the underlying malignancy is essential and should not be interrupted. Systemic colchicine (0.6–1.8 mg) may be administered in these settings.[42] One case report described administering dapsone (100–200 mg) for prophylaxis.[43] The benefit of systemic corticosteroids is debatable, and they should be used with caution in the setting of neutropenia.

PYOSTOMATITIS VEGETANS–PYODERMATITIS VEGETANS
Epidemiology

Initially described in 1898, pyostomatitis vegetans–pyodermatitis vegetans (PSV-PDV) is a rare, chronic mucocutaneous disorder. Characterized by large, verrucous plaques with elevated borders and multiple pustules affecting the mucosal skin,[44] it has been attributed to bacterial infection in immunocompromised individuals.[45–47] PDV has a cutaneous presentation that is distinct from the oral presentation of PSV, but several authors recently supported the notion that they are essentially the same disease, with similar histopathologic features.[48,49] The disease has been associated with IBD and primary sclerosing cholangitis (PSC), as well as many other conditions (**Box 11**), and it can affect adults and children.

Pathogenesis

The pathogenesis of PSV-PDV is poorly understood. Postulated causes include abnormal inflammatory reactions in immunocompromised patients, as well as bacterial and fungal infection.[50] Several case reports describe circulating autoantibodies mimicking autoimmune blistering disease.[51,52] Another report of 2 patients described oral and skin manifestations with corresponding positive direct immunofluorescence findings and immunoglobulin (Ig) A and IgA/IgG pemphigus.[52] This finding was considered an epiphenomenon induced by epidermal damage, but autoantibodies might also contribute to PSV-PDV pathogenesis

Table 4
Summary of clinical trials assessing systemic interventions for mucocutaneous manifestations of Behçet disease

Systemic Intervention[a]	No. of Patients	Duration of Treatment	Results
First-line treatment			
Apremilast vs placebo	222	12 wk	Decreased pain and the number of OUs (both trials)
	204	12 wk	
Colchicine vs placebo	28	36 wk	Decreased frequency of EN-like lesions
	82	24 mo	Decreased frequency of GU, EN-like lesions, arthritis
	282	8 mo	Decreased frequency and activity of OU, GU, PPL, EN-like lesions
Colchicine + benzathine penicillin vs colchicine	154	32 mo	Combination treatment decreased frequency and duration of OU and EN-like lesions; decreased GU frequency and articular involvement
Methylprednisolone vs placebo	76	27 wk	Decreased frequency of EN-like lesions (women)
Second-line treatment			
Azathioprine vs placebo	75	24 mo	Reduced frequency of OU, GU, and arthritis
Cyclosporine vs colchicine	96	16 wk	Cyclosporine reduced frequency and severity of OU, GU, and PPL
Cyclosporine vs corticosteroid, azathioprine	76	6 mo	Cyclosporine was more effective on OU, GU, TP, cutaneous lesions, and arthritis
Cyclosporine vs combination (corticosteroid, chlorambucil)	40	24 mo	Cyclosporine was more effective for ocular symptoms, but the combination was more effective for OU, GU, and arthritis
Dapsone vs placebo	20	3 mo	Reduced number of OU, GU, EN, and PPL; decreased arthritis
Interferon alfa-2a vs placebo	222	12 wk	Reduced the number of OU and decreased pain (both trials)
	204	12 wk	
Isotretinoin vs placebo	60	3 mo	Reduced disease activity, index of OU, and cutaneous findings
Levamisole vs placebo	47	8 wk	Improved OU, GU, arthritis, and uveitis
Mycophenolate sodium vs placebo	10	2–4 mo	Reduced activity of all skin lesions
Rebamipide vs placebo	25	12–24 wk	Reduced number of OU and decreased pain

(continued on next page)

Table 4
(continued)

Systemic Intervention[a]	No. of Patients	Duration of Treatment	Results
Thalidomide vs placebo	95	24 wk	Reduced frequency of OU, GU, and PPL but increased EN-like lesions
Zinc sulfate vs placebo	27	6 mo	Reduced clinical activity index
Biologic Agent			
Daclizumab vs placebo	17	6 mo	No benefit
Etanercept vs placebo	40	4 wk	Reduced frequency of OU, nodular skin lesions, and PPL
Rituximab vs cytoxic combination	20	6 mo	Rituximab showed improvement in disease activity index
Secukinumab vs placebo	118	Early termination	No benefit
Ustekinumab	15	52 wk	Reduced the number of OU and GU

Abbreviations: EN, erythema nodosum; GU, genital ulcer; OU, oral ulcer; PPL, papulopustular lesions; TP, thrombophlebitis.

[a] Dosages for specific medications were as follows: apremilast, 30 mg, twice a day; azathioprine, 2.5 mg/kg per day; cyclophosphamide, 1 g/m^2 per month; colchicine, 1 to 2 mg/d; cyclosporine, 5 to 10 mg/kg per day; daclizumab, 1 mg/kg every 2 wk; dapsone, 100 mg/d; etanercept, 50 mg/mo; isotretinoin, 20 mg/d; levamisole, 3 × 50 mg, 2 d/wk; mycophenolate sodium, 2 g/d; rebamipide, 300 mg/d; secukinumab, 150 to 300 mg/mo; thalidomide, 100 mg/d; zinc sulfate, 300 mg/d; ustekinumab, 90 mg every 3 mo.

Table 5
Selected clinical trials targeting oral and genital symptoms of Behçet disease

Study	Intervention	No. of Patients	Study Design	Status
NCT04528082	Apremilast Pediatric Study in Children With Active Oral Ulcers Associated With Behçet's Disease (BEAN)	60	Randomized control	Recruiting
NCT04186559	Topical Pentoxifylline Gel on Behçet's Disease Genital Ulcers	60	Randomized	Unknown
NCT03888846	Topical Pentoxifylline Gel on Behçet's Disease Oral Ulcers	60	Randomized	Unknown
NCT05032248	Uses of Tacrolimus in Behçet Disease (oral ulcer)	40	Randomized	Completed
NCT03771768	Diode Laser vs Topical Corticosteroids in Management of Oral Ulcers	38	Randomized	Completed
NCT05449548	Lenalidomide in the Treatment of Mucosal Behçet's Syndrome	42	Single group	Recruiting

Box 9
Medications associated with neutrophilic eccrine hidradenitis

Acetaminophen

Anthracyclines

Antineoplastic agents

Antiretroviral medication (stavudine, zidovudine)

Azathioprine

BRAF inhibitors

Carbamazepine

Cetuximab (epidermal growth factor receptor inhibitor)

Cyclophosphamide

Folinic acid, fluorouracil, and oxaliplatin

Granulocyte colony-stimulating factor

Imatinib (tyrosine kinase inhibitor)

Infliximab

Methotrexate

Minocycline

Pegfilgrastim

Ticagrelor (antiplatelet agent)

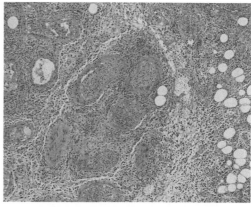

Fig. 5. Neutrophilic Eccrine Hidradenitis. Neutrophilic inflammation surrounding eccrine sweat glands, with eccrine gland necrosis (hematoxylin-eosin, original magnification × 1000).

Box 10
Differential diagnosis of neutrophilic eccrine hidradenitis

Drug eruption

Erythematous multiforme

Hand-foot syndrome

Graft-vs-host disease

Leukemia cutis

Palmoplantar eccrine hidradenitis[a]

Pyoderma gangrenosum

Sweet syndrome

Toxic erythema of chemotherapy

Urticarial vasculitis

[a] A subtype (variant) of neutrophilic eccrine hidradenitis.

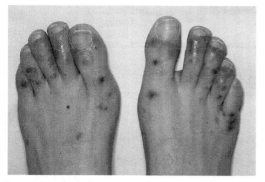

Fig. 4. Neutrophilic Eccrine Hidradenitis. A 20-year-old man presented with multiple painful, erythematous, and edematous papules on the dorsal feet. He had a history of acute lymphocytic leukemia that was treated with cytarabine and 6-mercaptopurine.

Box 11
Conditions associated with pyostomatitis vegetans—pyodermatitis vegetans

Diffuse T-cell lymphoma

Inflammatory bowel disease (notably ulcerative colitis)

Lupus nephritis

Myelodysplastic syndrome

Myeloid leukemia

Primary immunodeficiency disorders

Primary sclerosing cholangitis

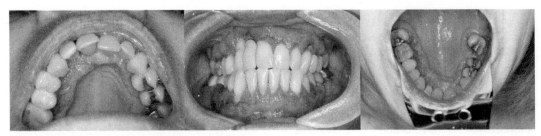

Fig. 6. Pyostomatitis Vegetans. A 61-year-old woman had a 5-month history of painful gingiva, marked swelling, and hypertrophy that was accompanied by erythema and erosion.

by epitope exposure and mucosal damage that causes an autoimmune reaction.

Clinicopathologic Features

PSV-PDV is characterized by vesicular, pustular, exudative, and vegetating plaques (termed *pyodermatitis*) that commonly involve the scalp, face, axillae, and genital regions. Confluent, erythematous, and small pustules and erosions on mucosal surfaces can create the typical "snail tracks" appearance. Symptoms can be associated with or preceded by bowel involvement by several years.[52] The most common sites of oral symptoms are the gingiva, buccal mucosa, and upper and/or lower mucosal lip (**Fig. 6**).

Histopathologic analysis shows epidermal hyperplasia with focal acantholysis and intraepithelial and dermal neutrophilic and eosinophilic microabscesses (**Fig. 7**). Recently, PSV-PDV was hypothesized to mimic an IgA variant of pemphigus vegetans because the 2 share many features.[52]

Diagnosis and Management

Clinical and histologic findings from a thorough assessment must be considered to diagnose

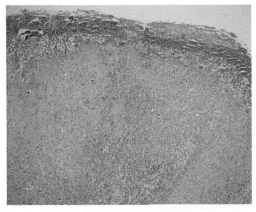

Fig. 7. Pyostomatitis Vegetans. Subcorneal neutrophilic spongiform pustule and diffuse neutrophilic dermal inflammation (hematoxylin-eosin, original magnification × 100).

Box 12
Amicrobial pustulosis of the folds

- Rare disease, characterized by aseptic pustular lesions involving skin folds
- Associated with autoimmune disease
- Topical and systemic corticosteroids appear most effective

Aseptic abscess syndrome

- Rare disease, characterized by multiple sterile abdominal abscesses
- Associated with autoimmune disease, especially inflammatory bowel disease
- Systemic corticosteroids appear most effective

Behçet disease

- Recurrent oral and genital ulcers might precede other organ involvement, with systemic presentation caused by systemic vasculitis
- New therapeutic agents include apremilast and tumor necrosis factor α inhibitors
- Multidisciplinary care is necessary

Neutrophilic eccrine hidradenitis

- Characterized by erythematous, edematous papules or plaques on the trunk or extremities
- Associated with chemotherapeutic agents
- Often self-resolves, but topical corticosteroids, dapsone, and colchicine can be considered

Pyostomatitis vegetans–pyodermatitis vegetans

- Rare, chronic mucocutaneous disorder
- Associated with inflammatory bowel disease and others
- Topical and systemic corticosteroids are first-line therapies

PSV-PDV. Peripheral eosinophilia is reported in 90% of cases. The differential diagnosis includes autoimmune bullous diseases, such as pemphigus vegetans, IgA pemphigus, and dermatitis herpetiformis.

Given the rarity of PSV-PDV, treatment approaches generally are anecdotal. Various therapeutic strategies and variable responses are reported. The most common first-line therapies are topical and systemic corticosteroids. Other medications, such as dapsone (100–200 mg), azathioprine (2 mg/kg), mycophenolate mofetil (2–3 g), cyclosporine (3–5 mg/kg), adalimumab (40 mg, subcutaneous, every other week), golimumab (50 mg every 30 days), and infliximab (5 mg/kg every 4–10 weeks), have been used as second-line agents, with varying success.[53] Recently, 5-aminosalicylic acid was reported as helpful. Subtotal and total colectomy have been performed when PSV-PDV is associated with ulcerative colitis.[54]

SUMMARY

Neutrophilic dermatoses are inflammatory disorders that can have heterogenous cutaneous and systemic symptoms and varying approaches to management. **Box 12** summarizes salient details about the 5 disorders described in this review. Large, multi-institutional, and collaborative studies are urgently needed to address the unmet needs of patients with these challenging, rare conditions.

DISCLOSURE

No conflicts of interest to disclose. No funding to disclose.

REFERENCES

1. Crickx B, Diego M, Guillevin L, et al. Pustulose amicrobienne et lupus érythémateux systémique. Journées Dermatol Paris 1991;6.
2. Schissler C, Velter C, Lipsker D. Amicrobial pustulosis of the folds: Where have we gone 25years after its original description? Ann Dermatol Venereol 2017;144(3):169–75.
3. Boms S, Gambichler T. Review of literature on amicrobial pustulosis of the folds associated with autoimmune disorders. Am J Clin Dermatol 2006;7(6):369–74.
4. Marzano AV, Tavecchio S, Berti E, et al. Cytokine and chemokine profile in amicrobial pustulosis of the folds: evidence for autoinflammation. Medicine (Baltim) 2015;94(50):e2301.
5. Gallo-Pineda G, Jimenez-Anton A, Navarro-Navarro I, et al. HLA-DR8 expression in two sisters with amicrobial pustulosis of the folds. Australas J Dermatol 2023;64(2):e199–201.
6. Zirwas M, Dobkin HE, Krishnamurthy S. Amicrobial pustulosis of the folds and palmoplantar pustulosis simultaneously induced by different tumor necrosis factor-alpha inhibitors: Demonstration of a shared pathophysiology. JAAD Case Rep 2017;3(5):401–3.
7. Marzano AV, Tavecchio S, Berti E, et al. Pustular skin reaction to tumor necrosis factor alpha antagonists in patients with inflammatory bowel diseases. Inflamm Bowel Dis 2015;21(11):E26–7.
8. Inamura E, Yamaguchi Y, Fujimura Y, et al. A case of drug-induced amicrobial pustulosis of the folds. J Dtsch Dermatol Ges 2021;19(3):430–3.
9. Wang MZ, Camilleri MJ, Guo R, et al. Amicrobial pustulosis of the folds: Report of 4 cases. J Cutan Pathol 2017;44(4):367–72.
10. Marzano AV, Ramoni S, Caputo R. Amicrobial pustulosis of the folds. Report of 6 cases and a literature review. Dermatology 2008;216(4):305–11.
11. Andre M, Aumaitre O, Marcheix JC, et al. Aseptic systemic abscesses preceding diagnosis of Crohn's disease by three years. Dig Dis Sci 1995;40(3):525–7.
12. Andre M, Aumaitre O, Papo T, et al. Disseminated aseptic abscesses associated with Crohn's disease: a new entity? Dig Dis Sci 1998;43(2):420–8.
13. Andre MFJ, Piette JC, Kemeny JL, et al. Aseptic abscesses: a study of 30 patients with or without inflammatory bowel disease and review of the literature. Medicine (Baltim) 2007;86(3):145–61.
14. Andre M, Aumaitre O. [Aseptic abscesses syndrome]. Rev Med Interne 2011;32(11):678–88. Le syndrome des abces aseptiques.
15. Marzano AV, Ortega-Loayza AG, Ceccherini I, et al. LPIN2 gene mutation in a patient with overlapping neutrophilic disease (pyoderma gangrenosum and aseptic abscess syndrome). JAAD Case Rep 2018;4(2):120–2.
16. Agirgol S, Ustaoglu E, Demir FT, et al. Aseptic abscess syndrome with severe skin involvement: case report. Indian J Dermatol 2020;65(5):434–6.
17. Szwebel TA, Casadevall M, Chosidow O, et al. [Atypical recurrent aseptic cutaneous abscesses as the presenting manifestation of Crohn's disease]. Rev Med Interne 2010;31(10):705–8. Abces cutanes aseptiques recidivants atypiques revelateurs d'une maladie de Crohn.
18. von Tirpitz C, Buchwald HJ, Lang GK, et al. Simultaneous onset of pyoderma gangrenosum and bitemporal abscesses of the upper eyelids during a flare of ulcerative colitis. Inflamm Bowel Dis 1998;4(2):98–100.
19. Trefond L, Frances C, Costedoat-Chalumeau N, et al. Aseptic abscess syndrome: clinical characteristics, associated diseases, and up to 30 years' evolution data on a 71-patient series. J Clin Med 2022;11(13). https://doi.org/10.3390/jcm11133669.

20. Davatchi F, Chams-Davatchi C, Shams H, et al. Behcet's disease: epidemiology, clinical manifestations, and diagnosis. Expert Rev Clin Immunol 2017; 13(1):57–65.

21. Verity DH, Marr JE, Ohno S, et al. Behcet's disease, the Silk Road and HLA-B51: historical and geographical perspectives. Tissue Antigens 1999; 54(3):213–20.

22. Alpsoy E, Bozca BC, Bilgic A. Behcet disease: an update for dermatologists. Am J Clin Dermatol 2021;22(4):477–502.

23. de Menthon M, Lavalley MP, Maldini C, et al. HLA-B51/B5 and the risk of Behcet's disease: a systematic review and meta-analysis of case-control genetic association studies. Arthritis Rheum 2009;61(10):1287–96.

24. Wu J, Ding J, Yang J, et al. MicroRNA Roles in the Nuclear Factor Kappa B Signaling Pathway in Cancer. Front Immunol 2018;9:546.

25. Yazici Y, Hatemi G, Bodaghi B, et al. Behcet syndrome. Nat Rev Dis Primers 2021;7(1):67.

26. Kural-Seyahi E, Fresko I, Seyahi N, et al. The long-term mortality and morbidity of Behcet syndrome: a 2-decade outcome survey of 387 patients followed at a dedicated center. Medicine (Baltim) 2003;82(1):60–76.

27. International Team for the Revision of the International Criteria for Behcet's Disease. The International Criteria for Behcet's Disease (ICBD): a collaborative study of 27 countries on the sensitivity and specificity of the new criteria. J Eur Acad Dermatol Venereol 2014;28(3):338–47. https://doi.org/10.1111/jdv.12107.

28. Alpsoy E, Leccese P, Emmi G, et al. Treatment of Behcet's Disease: An Algorithmic Multidisciplinary Approach. Front Med 2021;8:624795.

29. Hatemi G, Christensen R, Bang D, et al. 2018 update of the EULAR recommendations for the management of Behcet's syndrome. Ann Rheum Dis 2018;77(6):808–18.

30. Liu J, Hou Y, Sun L, et al. A pilot study of tofacitinib for refractory Behcet's syndrome. Ann Rheum Dis 2020;79(11):1517–20.

31. Harrist TJ, Fine JD, Berman RS, et al. Neutrophilic eccrine hidradenitis. A distinctive type of neutrophilic dermatosis associated with myelogenous leukemia and chemotherapy. Arch Dermatol 1982; 118(4):263–6.

32. Cohen PR. Neutrophilic dermatoses occurring in oncology patients. Int J Dermatol 2007;46(1): 106–11.

33. Bassas-Vila J, Fernandez-Figueras MT, Romani J, et al. Infectious eccrine hidradenitis: a report of 3 cases and a review of the literature. Actas Dermosifiliogr 2014;105(2):e7–12.

34. Barrera-Godinez A, Mendez-Flores S, Gatica-Torres M, et al. Not all that glitters is COVID-19: a case series demonstrating the need for histopathology when skin findings accompany SARS-CoV-2 infection. J Eur Acad Dermatol Venereol 2021; 35(9):1865–73.

35. Templeton SF, Solomon AR, Swerlick RA. Intradermal bleomycin injections into normal human skin. A histopathologic and immunopathologic study. Arch Dermatol 1994;130(5):577–83.

36. Salik D, Kolivras A, Sass U, et al. [Palmoplantar neutrophilic eccrine hidradenitis with general extension in a child in remission after acute lymphoblastic leukemia]. Ann Dermatol Venereol 2014;141(4): 285–9. Hidradenite eccrine neutrophilique palmoplantaire avec extension generalisee chez un enfant en remission d'une leucemie aigue lymphoblastique.

37. Headley CM, Ioffreda MD, Zaenglein AL. Neutrophilic eccrine hidradenitis: a case report of an unusual annular presentation. Cutis 2005;75(2):93–7.

38. Yasukawa K, Kato N, Aikawa K, et al. Neutrophilic eccrine hidradenitis with sclerodermoid change heralding the relapse of acute myelogenous leukemia: is this a paraneoplastic phenomenon? Dermatology 2007;215(3):261–4.

39. Bardenstein DS, Haluschak J, Gerson S, et al. Neutrophilic eccrine hidradenitis simulating orbital cellulitis. Arch Ophthalmol 1994;112(11):1460–3.

40. Srivastava M, Scharf S, Meehan SA, et al. Neutrophilic eccrine hidradenitis masquerading as facial cellulitis. J Am Acad Dermatol 2007;56(4):693–6.

41. Ostlere LS, Wells J, Stevens HP, et al. Neutrophilic eccrine hidradenitis with an unusual presentation. Br J Dermatol 1993;128(6):696–8.

42. Shear NH, Knowles SR, Shapiro L, et al. Dapsone in prevention of recurrent neutrophilic eccrine hidradenitis. J Am Acad Dermatol 1996;35(5 Pt 2):819–22.

43. Belot V, Perrinaud A, Corven C, et al. [Adult idiopathic neutrophilic eccrine hidradenitis treated with colchicine]. Presse Med 2006;35(10 Pt 1): 1475–8. Hidradenite eccrine neutrophilique idiopathique de l'adulte d'evolution prolongee traitee par colchicine.

44. Hallopeau H. "Pyodermite végétante", ihre Beziehungen zur Dermatitis herpetiformis und dem Pemphigus vegetans. Archiv für Dermatologie und Syphilis 1898; 43(1):289–306.

45. Brown CS, Kligman AM. Mycosis-like pyoderma. AMA Arch Derm 1957;75(1):123–5.

46. Potekaev NS, Iurin OG, Gorbacheva ZS, et al. [Pyoderma vegetans as an early sign of HIV infection]. Ter Arkh 1991;63(11):78–80. Vegetiruiushchaia piodermiia kak rannii priznak VICh-infektsii.

47. Katz TM, Katz AM. Idiopathic pyostomatitispyodermatitis vegetans with nasal obstruction: A case report. SAGE Open Med Case Rep 2023;11. https://doi.org/10.1177/2050313X231160909. 2050313X231160909.

48. Hegarty AM, Barrett AW, Scully C. Pyostomatitis vegetans. Clin Exp Dermatol 2004;29(1):1–7.

49. Nigen S, Poulin Y, Rochette L, et al. Pyodermatitis-pyostomatitis vegetans: two cases and a review of the literature. J Cutan Med Surg 2003;7(3):250–5.

50. Adisen E, Tezel F, Gurer MA. Pyoderma vegetans: a case for discussion. Acta Derm Venereol 2009; 89(2):186–8.

51. Ahn BK, Kim SC. Pyodermatitis-pyostomatitis vegetans with circulating autoantibodies to bullous pemphigoid antigen 230. J Am Acad Dermatol 2004; 50(5):785–8.

52. Clark LG, Tolkachjov SN, Bridges AG, et al. Pyostomatitis vegetans (PSV)-pyodermatitis vegetans (PDV): A clinicopathologic study of 7 cases at a tertiary referral center. J Am Acad Dermatol 2016; 75(3):578–84.

53. Gheisari M, Zerehpoosh FB, Zaresharifi S. Pyodermatitis-pyostomatitis vegetans: a case report and review of literature. Dermatol Online J 2020;26(5).

54. Hobbs LK, Zufall A, Khalil S, et al. Treatment of pyodermatitis-pyostomatitis vegetans: a systematic review and meta-analysis. SKIN The Journal of Cutaneous Medicine 2021;5(4):333–46. https://doi.org/10.25251/skin.5.4.1.

55. Elessa D, Thietart S, Corpechot C, et al. TNF-alpha antagonist infliximab for aseptic abscess syndrome. Presse Med 2019;48(12):1579–80.

Hidradenitis Suppurativa-Related Autoinflammatory Syndromes

An Updated Review on the Clinics, Genetics, and Treatment of Pyoderma gangrenosum, Acne and Suppurative Hidradenitis (PASH), Pyogenic Arthritis, Pyoderma gangrenosum, Acne and Suppurative Hidradenitis (PAPASH), Synovitis, Acne, Pustulosis, Hyperostosis and Osteitis (SAPHO), and Rarer Forms

Carlo Alberto Maronese, MD[a,b,1], Chiara Moltrasio, PhD[b,1],
Angelo Valerio Marzano, MD[a,b,*]

KEYWORDS

- Hidradenitis suppurativa • Autoinflammatory syndromes
- Hidradenitis suppurativa-related autoinflammatory syndromes • Classification • Clinics
- Pathogenesis • Treatments

KEY POINTS

- There is still no consensus on the nosology of hidradenitis suppurativa-related autoinflammatory syndromes.
- The pathogenic scenario of these rare conditions is fragmentary and a robust genotype–phenotype correlation is lacking.
- A great-unmet need exists in terms of effective treatments in this clinical setting.
- The effort of researchers must be directed toward the discovery of new biomarkers and molecular pathways with the goal of providing faster development of novel, patient-tailored therapeutic approaches.

---

[a] Department of Pathophysiology and Transplantation, Università degli Studi di Milano, Via Pace, 9, Milan 20122, Italy; [b] Dermatology Unit, Fondazione IRCCS Ca' Granda Ospedale Maggiore Policlinico, Via Pace, 9, Milan 20122, Italy
[1] These authors contributed equally to this study and share first authorship.
* Corresponding author. Dermatology Unit, Fondazione IRCCS Ca' Granda Ospedale Maggiore Policlinico, Via Pace, 9, Milan 20122, Italy.
E-mail address: angelo.marzano@unimi.it

Dermatol Clin 42 (2024) 247–265
https://doi.org/10.1016/j.det.2023.12.004

INTRODUCTION: THE RELATIONSHIP WITH PYOGENIC ARTHRITIS, PYODERMA GANGRENOSUM AND ACNE (PAPA) AND THE CONUNDRUM OF CLASSIFICATION

Hidradenitis suppurativa (HS) is an autoinflammatory skin disorder of the terminal hair follicle, manifesting with painful nodules, abscesses, draining tunnels, and hypertrophic scarring, typically occurring in apocrine gland bearing skin. Besides common comorbidities, in a few patients, HS may occur in association with specific immune-mediated autoinflammatory diseases or inherited conditions, defining the setting of "syndromic" HS (sHS). Among these cases, HS-related autoinflammatory syndromes represent a unique group that is simultaneously classified within neutrophilic dermatoses[1] and is hallmarked by the refractoriness to standard management strategies.[2–4]

The term encompasses the following entities: pyoderma gangrenosum (PG), acne and HS (PASH); PG, acne, pyogenic arthritis and HS (PAPASH); psoriatic arthritis (PsA), PG, acne and HS (PsAPASH); pustular psoriasis, arthritis, PG, synovitis, acne and HS (PsAPSASH); PG, acne, HS and ankylosing spondylitis (PASS); PsA, PG, HS and Crohn disease (PsAPSC); vasculitis with PASH (VPASH); synovitis, acne, pustulosis, hyperostosis, osteitis (SAPHO; **Fig. 1**).

Notwithstanding recent advances, their nosologic framing is still subject of debate because there is a wide range of monogenic and polygenic conditions increasingly associated with HS, complicating the diagnosis and classification of these complex phenotypes.

A provisional classification of sHS was first provided by Gasparic and colleagues,[5] distinguishing 3 main categories based on the possible pathomechanisms: (1) sHS associated with a genetic condition; (2) sHS associated with follicular keratinization disorders or follicular occlusion syndrome; and (3) sHS associated with autoinflammatory diseases, both monogenic and polygenic. Since the publication of our adaptation of Gasparic's initial proposal,[3] new associations have been described, particularly with pachyonychia congenita[6] and Smith-Magenis syndrome.[7]

Defects held responsible for each of these provisional categories affect key steps in the natural history of HS, facilitating disease progression and self-maintenance (**Fig. 2**).

An alternative grouping/terminology, that is, PAPA spectrum disorders, has been proposed due to the similarity of many of these entities with PAPA (pyogenic arthritis, PG, and acne) and also due to historical reasons. This spectrum of disorders is somewhat wider, including PG, acne, and

ulcerative colitis (PAC) and other intermediate/mixed phenotypes. PAPA syndrome is a rare, autosomal dominant disease determined by pathogenic variants in the proline-serine-threonine phosphatase-interacting protein (PSTPIP1) gene, also known as CD2 (cluster of differentiation 2)-binding protein 1, which is located on chromosome 15q24.3.[8] Its first description dates back to 1997 when Lindor and colleagues[8] identified a family that manifested the defining clinical triad across 3 generations. The causative gene, PSTPIP1, was identified in the same year; however, culprit pathogenic variants were characterized only in the early 2000s.[9] The first 2 reported pathogenic variants (NM_003978.5 (PSTPIP1):c.688 G > A;p. Ala230Thr and c.748 G > A; p.Glu250Lys)[9] were functionally related to the exacerbation of pyrin-mediated IL-1β release and neutrophil-mediated inflammation. Subsequently, several other mutations in different domains of PSTPIP1 with a consequent impairment of other functions (eg, podosome formation) have been described, underlying the variable expression of PSTPIP1 causative variants.[10]

Importantly, PAPA-like clinical phenotypes have been identified also in individuals that did not carry pathogenic variants in PSTPIP1; a proportion of these cases may in fact correspond to HS-related autoinflammatory syndromes. Recently, Stone and colleagues[11] found an elevation of total serum IL-18 in treated PAPA syndrome patients at levels well above those found in most patients with Familial Mediterranean Fever (FMF). This elevation may have practical relevance, aiding the diagnosis of true PAPA cases from mimickers with somewhat similar clinical features.[11] Increasing evidence shows that PAPA syndrome also exists on a spectrum with other PSTPIP1-associated inflammatory diseases (PAIDs).[12] Among these, PSTPIP1-associated myeloid-related proteinemia inflammatory, a PAID specifically associated with de novo mutations in PSTPIP1-:c.748 G > A; p.Glu250Lys and c.769 G > A; p.Glu257Lys, seems to include heterogeneous nephropathies within its clinical spectrum. Interestingly, renal involvement was reported also in a PAPA patient whose phenotype was driven by the aforementioned p.Glu250Lys mutation.[13]

Missense variants in the SH3 domain of PSTPIP1 have been reported also in HS. According to a study on 117 patients with HS collected across 3 different dermatologic centers, SH3 domain variants were present in about 6% of enrolled individuals.[14] All these findings highlight how a range of different clinical phenotypes affecting multiple tissues, both with and without HS, can result from different PSTPIP1 variants

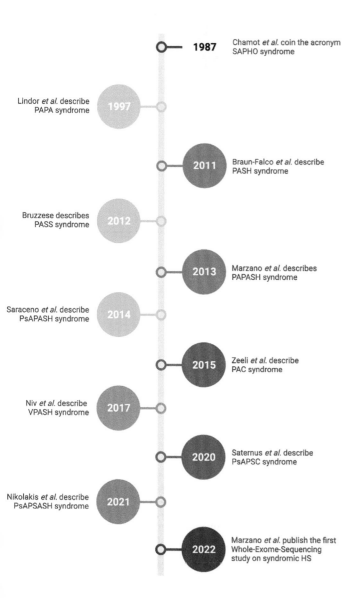

Fig. 1. Timeline of the discovery of HS-related autoinflammatory syndromes. PAC, PG, acne, and ulcerative colitis; PAPA, pyogenic arthritis, PG, and acne; PAPASH, pyogenic arthritis, PG, acne, HS; PASH, PG, acne, HS; PASS, PG, acne, HS and ankylosing spondylitis; PsAPASH, PsA, PG, acne and HS; PsAPSASH, pustular psoriasis, arthritis, PG, synovitis, acne and HS; PsAPSC, PsA, PG, HS and CD; SAPHO, synovitis, acne, pustulosis, hyperostosis, osteitis; VPASH, PASH with leukocytoclastic vasculitis. (Created with BioRender.com.)

Timeline entries:

- **1987** — Chamot *et al.* coin the acronym SAPHO syndrome
- **1997** — Lindor *et al.* describe PAPA syndrome
- **2011** — Braun-Falco *et al.* describe PASH syndrome
- **2012** — Bruzzese describes PASS syndrome
- **2013** — Marzano *et al.* describes PAPASH syndrome
- **2014** — Saraceno *et al.* describe PsAPASH syndrome
- **2015** — Zeeli *et al.* describe PAC syndrome
- **2017** — Niv *et al.* describe VPASH syndrome
- **2020** — Saternus *et al.* describe PsAPSC syndrome
- **2021** — Nikolakis *et al.* describe PsAPSASH syndrome
- **2022** — Marzano *et al.* publish the first Whole-Exome-Sequencing study on syndromic HS

and underlie the challenges to finding a satisfactory classification for these forms.

Besides *PSTPIP1* mutations, a pathogenic variant in *MEFV* (Mediterranean Fever) gene has recently been reported to underlie a case of PAPA with recurrent PG, arthritis, and extensive acne. Genetic assessment proved instrumental to successfully manage the patient, shifting from anakinra to colchicine. Indeed, there exists some degree of genetic overlap between PAPA and FMF, suggesting a common druggable pathway.[15] This underscores the importance of defining the exact genetic substrate in each patient and is also noteworthy as FMF is tightly linked to HS. Indeed, epidemiologic evidence from a case-control study documented an increased prevalence of FMF (0.7% vs 0.1% in controls) in a cohort of 4417 patients with HS, suggesting a close association between these 2 conditions. Patients with HS-FMF also carried heterozygous pathogenic variants in the *MEFV* gene, highlighting an increased prevalence of *MEFV* mutations in patients with complex HS clinical phenotypes and reinforcing the importance of an autoinflammatory component in the pathogenesis of moderate-severe HS and related syndromic forms.[16]

Although many features are shared between PAPA and HS-related autoinflammatory syndromes, as stated above, the following paragraphs will focus on the latter, providing critical insights into their clinics, genetics, and medical management.

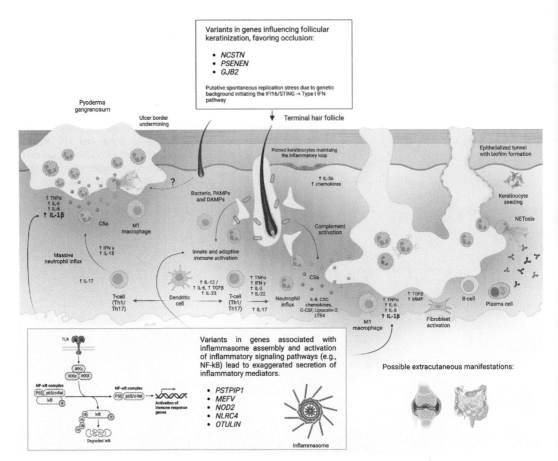

Fig. 2. PG and syndromic HS pathogenesis. Variants in genes related to keratinization pathway including, among others, *NCSTN*, favor follicular occlusion that precedes an inflammatory response. The inflammatory scenario between the follicular epithelium, infiltrating T cell, neutrophils, monocytes and dendritic cells is sustained by the secretion and overexpression of several cytokines such as TNF-a, IL-6, IL-8, IL-12, IL-15, IL-17, and IL-1β. IL-1β is considered the key driver of inflammation, released following the activation of inflammatory signaling pathways such as NF-kB and assembly/activation of inflammasome (eg, NLRP3). Variants in genes such as *PSTPIP1*, *MEFV*, *NOD2*, *NLRC4*, and *OTULIN* are responsible for an exaggerated inflammatory response. CXC, C-X-C motif chemokine; G-CSF, granulocyte colony-stimulating factor; *GJB2*, gap junction protein beta 2; IL, interleukin; INF, interferon; LTB4, leukotriene B4; *MEFV*, Mediterranean fever; MMP, matrix metalloproteinase; *NCSTN*, nicastrin; NF-kB, nuclear factor kappa-light-chain-enhancer of activated B cells; *NLRC4*, NLR family CARD domain containing 4; *NOD2*, nucleotide-binding oligomerization domain-containing protein 2; *OTULIN*, otulin; *PSENEN*, presenilin enhancer; *PSTPIP1*, proline-serine-threonine phosphatase interacting protein 1; TGF, transforming growth factor; Th, T helper cells; TLR, Toll-like receptor; TNF, tumor necrosis factor. (Created with BioRender.com.)

PYODERMA GANGRENOSUM, ACNE, AND HIDRADENITIS SUPPURATIVA

PASH syndrome is an autoinflammatory polygenic disorder typified by the triad of PG, acne, and HS, and constitutes the prototype of HS-related auto-inflammatory syndromes. Its first description dates back to 2011 with the important 2-patient case series published by Braun-Falco and colleagues.[17] However, as noted by the authors, at least 3 cases with the classic triad had been reported previously by Ah-Weng and colleagues,[18] and many more may have gone undiagnosed.[19]

Genetics

The genetic variants described in PASH patients are summarized in **Table 1**.

In the first 2 patients, hemi-allelic increase of the $(CCTG)_n$ microsatellite motif was reported in the promoter region of *PSTPIP1* gene.[17] After this first evidence, 2 other patients with PASH were found to be heterozygotes for $(CCTG)_5$ and $(CCTG)_8$ repeats in the *PSTPIP1* promoter region.[20] However, PSTPIP1 expression does not seem to be modulated by the $(CCTG)_n$ motif; moreover, longer forms of the PSTPIP1 have also been reported in patients

Table 1
List of variants of uncertain significance, likely pathogenic and pathogenic variants described in PASH, PAPASH, SAPHO, and PASH/SAPHO overlapping syndrome

Gene	Exon/Intron	Variant	Protein	ACMG Classification	Kind of Mutations	Variant Segregation	Ethnicity	References
NCSTN	3	NM_015331.3: c.278del	p.Pro93LeufsTer15	Pathogenic	Frameshift	Sporadic SAPHO	Han Chinese	Li et al,[94] 2018
NCSTN	4	NM_015331.3: c.344_351del	p.Thr115 fs	Pathogenic	Frameshift	PASH (in 2 familial and one sporadic subjects)	Not reported	Duchatelet et al,[20] 2015
NCSTN	5	NM_015331.3: c.482delA	p.Ile162Yfs*57	Unpreviously reported, validation ongoing	Frameshift	PASH/SAPHO	Italian	Marzano et al,[33] 2022
NCSTN	9	NM_015331.3: c.1140_1141del	p.D381fs*7	Unpreviously reported, validation ongoing	Frameshift	Sporadic PAPASH	Italian	Marzano et al,[33] 2022
NCSTN	14	NM_015331.3: c.1635 C > G	p.Tyr545*	Pathogenic	Nonsense	Familial PASH	Iranian	Faraji Zonooz et al,[28] 2016
PSENEN	4	NM_172341.4: c. c.228_229insCACC	p.Ile77Hisfs*45	Likely pathogenic	Frameshift	Familial PASH	Han Chinese	Zhang et al,[30] 2020
MEFV	10	NM_000243.2: c.2080A > G	p.Met694Val	Pathogenic	Missense	Sporadic PAPASH and FMF	Armenian	Marzano et al,[22] 2014
MEFV	10	NM_000243.2: c.2177 T > C	p.Val726Ala	Pathogenic	Missense	Sporadic PAPASH and FMF	Armenian	Marzano et al,[22] 2014
MEFV	10	NM_000243.2: c.2080A > G	p.Met694Val	Pathogenic	Missense	Sporadic PAPASH	Spanish	Monte Serrano et al,[73] 2021
NOD2	8	NM_022162.3 : c.2722 G > C	p.Val908Leu	VUS with pathogenic evidence	Missense	Sporadic PASH	Italian	Marzano et al,[22] 2014;Marzano et al,[33] 2022

(continued on next page)

Table 1
(continued)

Gene	Exon/Intron	Variant	Protein	ACMG Classification	Kind of Mutations	Variant Segregation	Ethnicity	References
NOD2	11	NM_022162.3: c.3017dupC	p.L1007Pfs*2	VUS with pathogenic evidence	Frameshift	Sporadic PASH	Italian	Marzano et al,[33] 2022
NOD2		NM_022162.3: c.2104 C > T	p.Arg702Trp	VUS with pathogenic evidence	Missense	Sporadic PASH	Italian	Marzano et al,[33] 2022
PSTPIP1	11	NM_003978.5: c.748del	p.Glu250 fs	Likely pathogenic	Missense	Sporadic PAPASH	Not reported	Kotzerke et al,[70] 2021
PSTPIP1	11	NM_003978: c.831 G > T	p.Glu277Asp	Likely pathogenic	Missense	Sporadic PAPASH and FMF	Armenian	Marzano et al,[68] 2018
PSTPIP1	14	NM_003978.5: c.1034 A > G	p.Tyr345Cys	VUS with pathogenic evidence	Missense	Familial PASH	Japanese	Saito et al,[29] 2018
PSTPIP1	15	NM_003978.5: c.1213 C > T	p.Arg405Cys	VUS with pathogenic evidence	Missense	PASH	Spanish	Calderón-Castrat et al,[27] 2016
IL1RN	4	NM_173842.3: c.106 A > T	p.Ala140Thr	VUS with pathogenic evidence	Missense	Sporadic PAPASH and FMF	Armenian	Marzano et al,[22] 2014
NLRC4	8	NM_021209.4: c.541 C > T	p.Arg181*	VUS with pathogenic evidence	Missense	Sporadic PAPASH	Italian	Marzano et al,[33] 2022
NLRC4	8	NM_021209.4: c.2668 T > C	p.Cys890Arg	VUS with pathogenic evidence	Missense	Sporadic PASH/SAPHO	Italian	Marzano et al,[33] 2022
OTULIN	2	NM_138348.6: c.209 T > C	p.Ile70Thr	VUS with pathogenic evidence	Missense	Sporadic PASH	Italian	Marzano et al,[33] 2022

Gene								
OTULIN	2	NM_138348. 6c.345 G > T	p.Gln115His	VUS with pathogenic evidence	Missense	Sporadic PASH	Italian	Marzano et al,[33] 2022
GJB2	2	NM_004004.6: c.35delG	p.Gly12 fs	Pathogenic	Frameshift	Sporadic PASH	Italian	Marzano et al,[33] 2022

Abbreviations: GJB2, gap junction protein beta 2; IL1RN, interleukin 1 receptor antagonist; MEFV, Mediterranean fever; NCSTN, nicastrin; NLRC4, NLR family CARD domain containing 4; NOD2, nucleotide-binding oligomerization domain-containing protein 2; OTULIN, otulin; PAPASH, pyogenic arthritis, pyoderma gangrenosum, acne, suppurative hidradenitis; PASH, pyoderma gangrenosum, acne, suppurative hidradenitis; PSENEN, presenilin enhancer; PSTPIP1, proline-serine-threonine phosphatase interacting protein 1; SAPHO, synovitis, acne, pustulosis, hyperostosis, osteitis; VUS, variant of uncertain significance.

with aseptic abscess syndrome, Crohn disease as well as in healthy subjects,[17] implying that this genetic imbalance may not be functionally related to PASH phenotype.

In 2015, Duchatelet and colleagues[20] described a PASH patient harboring a mutation in exon 4 of the NCSTN (nicastrin) gene (NM_015331.3: c.344_351del; p.Thr115 fs); this genetic change refers to an 8-nucleotide deletion that results in a premature stop codon with loss-of-function of the encoded protein. NCSTN encodes a type I transmembrane glycoprotein belonging to the gamma-secretase complex, a highly conserved membrane-embedded protease complex that carries out essential functions in cell and developmental biology. Pathogenic variants in NCSTN are mainly related to the familial form of HS and this mutation did not allow to distinguish it from the previously reported HS causative variants, thus supporting a common genetic background between sporadic HS and PASH syndrome.[21]

Subsequently, in 3 patients with PASH and 1 with PASH/SAPHO overlap syndrome, a targeted sequencing approach was performed to unravel potential disease-causing mutations in 10 candidate inflammatory genes.[22] In the first patient with PASH, a variant in nucleotide-binding oligomerization domain-containing protein 2 (NOD2; (NM_022162.3:c.2104 C > T; p.Arg702Trp) was reported; the same patient also carried a variant in MEFV (NM_000243.3: c.1772 T > C; p.Ile591Thr) gene. This is consistent with aforementioned evidence on the association between FMF and HS.[16]

Based on guidelines from the American College of Medical Genetics and Genomics (ACMG) and the Association for Molecular Pathology,[23] the latter are now predicted as likely benign variants, not causative of disease. In the second patient with PASH, a variant of uncertain significance (VUS) in NOD2 gene (NM_022162.3: c.2722 G > C; p.Val908Leu) was retrieved, together with a missense variant (NM_001243133.2: c.2107 C > A; p.Gln703Lys) in NLRP3 (NOD-like receptor family, pyrin domain containing 3) gene. The latter variant is now considered to be both clinically unremarkable and disease causing with a reduced penetrance without any functional effect on the inflammasome basal activity.[24] However, both variants reported in the NOD2 gene have shown significant association with Crohn disease (CD), possibly highlighting a link between CD and HS pathogenesis.[25] In the third patient with PASH, no pathogenic variants were found, whereas in the patient with PASH/SAPHO, overlap syndrome a point mutation in PSMB8 (proteasome 20S subunit beta 8; NM_148919.4: c.22 G > A; p.Gly8Arg) gene was

reported. No functional data are available on the latter.

In the same study,[22] the expression of cytokines, chemokines, and other effector molecules was analyzed both in lesional skin and serum of these patients, unraveling the overexpression of interleukin (IL)-1β and its receptors in the skin, likely due to deregulated inflammasome signaling. Furthermore, in skin biopsies from ulcerative lesions of PG, an increased expression of tumor necrosis factor (TNF)-α, IL-17, and their receptors was also reported. Notably, serum levels of these cytokines were within the normal range, suggesting a "confined" inflammation in the skin. This is in line with evidence on cytokines levels in sporadic HS.[26] Finally, several chemokines involved in neutrophilic activation and transendothelial migration such as IL-8 (interleukin-8), CXCL (C-X-C motif ligand) 1/2/3 e 16, and RANTES (Regulated upon Activation, Normal T Cell Expressed and Presumably Secreted) were also overexpressed.[22]

In 2016, Calderon and colleagues,[27] described a patient showing clinical features compatible with PASH syndrome in the presence of a mutation in exon 15 of the PSTPIP1 gene (NM_003978.5:c.1213 C > T; p.Arg405Cys). This variant was previously validated only in sporadic PG, thus expanding the phenotypic spectrum associated with the PSTPIP1 diseases.

Subsequently, Faraji and colleagues,[28] first reported a multigenerational Iranian family (24 affected and 32 unaffected subjects) presenting with manifestations of PASH in an autosomal dominant inheritance pattern. The authors found a recurrent heterozygous pathogenic variant in NCSTN gene (NM_015331.3:c.1635 C > G; p.Tyr545*), confirming the causative role of gamma-secretase complex proteins in the pathogenesis of both familial and syndromic HS.

In 2018, a novel PSTPIP1 heterozygous mutation (NM_003978.5:c.1034 A > G; p.Tyr345Cys) was described in a 37-year-old Japanese woman and in their affected relatives.[29] Of note, her mother suffered from HS/acne while 1 sister presented with only manifestations of acne, underlying the incomplete penetrance and variable expression of this condition.

Two years later, Zhang and colleagues[30] first reported a likely pathogenic variant in PSENEN (presenilin enhancer, gamma-secretase subunit; NM_172341.4:c.228_229insCACC; p.Ile77Hisfs* 45) gene in a PASH Chinese family. PSENEN is another essential subunit of the gamma-secretase complex that modulates both endoproteolysis of presenilin and gamma-secretase activity. The above-mentioned mutation refers to a frameshift that causes a premature stop codon with the loss of normal function of its protein product.

Through a novel whole exome sequencing (WES) approach, Brandao and colleagues[31] identified altered keratinization as a potential pathogenetic pathway in PASH syndrome, supporting the concept of HS-related autoinflammatory syndromes belonging to the group of autoinflammatory keratinization diseases.[32]

Finally, Marzano and colleagues[33] described 3 different variants in *NOD2* (NM_022162.3:c.2104 C > T; c.3017dupC and c.2722 G > C) that act as susceptibility and risk factors for inflammatory bowel disease (IBD) in a cohort of patients with PASH, also presenting with gut inflammation. Furthermore, 2 VUS in *OTULIN* (NM_138348.6:c.209 T > C and c.345 G > T) gene were retrieved as well as a pathogenic variant in *GJB2* (gap junction protein beta 2; NM_004004.6:c.35del; p.Gly12 fs). Mutations in *OTULIN* gene are associated to OTULIN-related autoinflammatory syndrome, an autosomal recessive autoinflammatory disease affecting multiple organs including the skin,[34] supporting a possible contribution of this gene to skin and gut inflammation. *GJB2* is a key gene involved in epidermal and hair follicle keratinization, further confirming that genetically disrupted keratinization may play a significant role in the pathogenesis of syndromic HS.

Three PASH/SAPHO overlap patients, who had joint inflammation, showed 3 different variants in *NCSTN* (NM_015331.3: c.482delA; p.Ile162Yfs *57), *NLRC4* (NLR family CARD domain containing 4; NM_001199138.2: c.2668 T > C; p.Cys890Arg), and *WDR1* (WD Repeat Domain 1; NM_017491.5: c.323 A > G; p.His108Arg), respectively. Both *NLRC4* and *WDR1* play essential roles in innate immune response and inflammation and, when mutated, they may contribute to the onset of autoinflammatory conditions[35,36] (**Table 1**).

The same groups[37] also reported the potential causative role of absent in melanoma-2 (*AIM2*) in susceptibility to develop syndromic forms of HS, highlighting the prominence of the IL-1β pathway in the complex pathogenetic scenario of these rare entities. Indeed, AIM2 is a key component of the innate immune system that after detecting the presence of foreign DNA as well as damaged self-DNA in the cytosol, triggers the assembly of the AIM2 inflammasome, which in turn leads to both the secretion of IL-1β and IL-18.

Finally, Brandao and colleagues,[38] through a variant enrichment analysis workflow, identified signaling pathways related to neutrophil and endothelial cells homeostasis/activations, hypothesizing that dysregulated neutrophil transendothelial migration could induce increased neutrophil infiltration and tissue damage.

Clinical

Clinically, PASH manifests with a temporal progression that is partly similar to what is seen in PAPA. Onset occurs very early in adolescence with severe acne, which is typically followed by HS and somewhat later by PG. It is important to underscore that the triad may not be complete or not have become so at the time of evaluation. Indeed, in a large single center case series spanning over 9 years and including 130 cases of PG, 14% of studied subjects had comorbid HS with no clear mention concerning acne status. This likely indicates a possible, hidden proportion of undiagnosed PASH cases.[39]

The role of acne has been much speculated on.[40] Indeed, it has been argued that genetic predisposition to autoinflammation could translate into an enhanced expression of this common dermatosis. Thus, acne may not represent a true manifestation of this spectrum of disease, but rather an epiphenomenon.[41] The clinical picture is generally very severe, with nodulocystic lesions being a constant. Onset occurs during adolescence as in acne vulgaris but onset with acne *fulminans* is much more common than in the general population.[40] Sometimes, especially in older individuals, only residual scarring may be seen.[27]

Similar to acne, HS is very severe in patients with PASH and often proves refractory to standard treatment options. Differently from acne and PG, a certain degree of HS activity is maintained throughout life, with complete remission being of much rarer occurrence. PG typically presents in its classic ulcerative or vegetative form; however, multilesional, devastating cases are not the rule. It may prove challenging to discern whether PG-like lesions in the context of PASH represent true PG or rather an atypical expression of HS.[42,43] In a similar way, a proportion of acne-like lesions may represent ectopic HS.

Triggering factors such as bowel bypass surgery have been recorded.[44] Isolated case reports have proposed possible associations with testicular cancer[45] and polycystic ovary syndrome[46]; however, at the moment, the actual relationship of PASH with these entities remains to be elucidated. As HS has been described in SAPHO (see later discussion), observations of bone disease have also been published in PASH, including osteopoikilosis[47] and destruction of the coccyx by direct extension of HS.[48]

Treatment

A wide array of antibiotics, conventional immunomodulating/immunosuppressive agents as well as biologics has been tried in PASH, with diverse outcomes.

Although a growing body of evidence supports the classification of PASH as a polygenic autoinflammatory disorder, some authors advocated for a targeted antibiotic therapy as a possible beneficial approach.[49] It is worth mentioning that nontargeted antibiotics have resulted in sustained remission of both PG and HS.[50]

Since its original description, combination approaches have been deemed necessary by many authors to achieve adequate disease control.[47] Staub and colleagues achieved complete disease control via a regimen consisting of cyclosporine, dapsone, and infliximab.[51] Huang and colleagues reported success with combined prednisone, thalidomide, colchicine, and doxycycline in a 20-year-old man who had proved refractory to a variety of conventional regimens.[52]

Although data on the response to biologics is conflicting and plagued by the use of heterogeneous outcome measures, anti-TNF agents are still regarded as a first choice in PASH management. Indeed, TNF inhibition currently represents the cornerstone for the management of both sporadic HS and PG cases.[53,54] Moreover, refractory acne has shown response to anti-TNF agents.[41] Weight-based infliximab regimens, particularly, have shown success also after the failure of other anti-TNF agents.[51]

Critical reevaluation of available reports reveals several issues with response assessment. As an example, some complete remissions with adalimumab were assessed after only a brief follow-up time, as short as 8 weeks in some cases.[55] However, the typical patient journey is longer and much more complicated than that, with loss of response being a common event.[56]

Moreover, lack of description of treatment outcomes impairs clinical guidance on isotretinoin and biologic use to address acne lesions.[41] Reasonably, acitretin should be regarded as a first option, due to its effectiveness in HS, however, traditionally, isotretinoin has been preferred.[41]

In stark contrast with patients with PAPA, IL-1 inhibition often results in a lack of response in many of those affected by PASH. Although some positive responses have been noted,[57] Jun and colleagues, reported failure with canakinumab in 2 individuals with an incomplete expression of the disease, that is, presenting only with PG and HS.[58] Moreover, incomplete responses with standard dose anakinra have been documented,[17] underscoring the importance of weight-based, dose-intensified regimens when opting for this medication.[59]

Targeting the IL-23 axis may also be a viable strategy in PASH, as suggested by 2 recent yet isolated reports.[60,61] Curiously, this conflicts with the possible placing of IL-23 inhibition in the treatment of sporadic HS, where 2 major phase II trials failed to meet their respective endpoints.[62,63] Adequate patient selection as well as longer therapeutic courses may constitute a means to overcome this.[64]

As a substantial degree of metabolic dysregulation may concur, a multidisciplinary approach may be required in order to obtain optimal patient management.[65] This is in keeping with the increasingly recognized need to incorporate phase-appropriate would care and to screen for relevant comorbidities in sporadic HS and PG.[66] Moreover, because a proportion of PASH cases may be latent, that is, one of the components may not yet be clinically evident, caution is advised when surgically approaching either HS or PG cases especially in individuals with a history of severe acne, due to the possibility of the so-called pathergy phenomenon.[67]

RARER PHENOTYPES

Several alternative phenotypes have been described, including PAPASH, PsAPASH, and PAC. Although a proportion of the former may actually represent true, separate forms, these diseases should be regarded as part of the same spectrum. It is thought provoking that although many different clinical phenotypes coalesce under the umbrella term of SAPHO, the nosology of HS-related or PG-related autoinflammatory syndromes has evolved in the direction of extreme fragmentation.

Pyoderma Gangrenosum, Acne, Pyogenic Arthritis, and Hidradenitis Suppurativa

PAPASH may be regarded as the sum of the clinical phenotypes seen in PAPA and PASH, with only 11 cases described to date.[33,57,68–74]

Marzano and colleagues[68] first characterized this syndrome, reporting the case of a 16-year-old girl with pyogenic arthritis, PG, acne, and HS. Molecular genetic analysis of *PSTPIP1* gene detected a likely pathogenic missense variant (NM_003978.5: c.831 G > T; p.Glu277 fs) in the exon 11 of this gene. Subsequently, in the same patient, pathogenic variants in *IL1RN* (interleukin 1 receptor antagonist; NM_173842.3:c.106 A > T; p.Ala140Thr) and in *MEFV* gene (NM_000243.2:c.2177 T > C; p.Val726Ala and c.2080A > G; p.Met694Val) were also described.[22] Of note, this patient was also affected by FMF and *MEFV* mutations were mainly attributed to the latter phenotype.[33]

In 2020, Kotzerke and colleagues[70] described a previously unreported missense variant in *PSTPIP1* gene (NM_003978.5:c.748del; p.Glu250 fs), functionally associated with decreased inhibition of the inflammasome.

Interestingly, Monte-Serrano and colleagues[73] first reported a patient with PAPASH harboring a pathogenic variant in *MEFV* gene (NM_000243.2: c.2080A > G; p.Met694Val) in the absence of concomitant FMF, although this is still to be validated.

More recently, Marzano and colleagues[33] found a novel, likely pathogenic *NCSTN* variant (NM_015331.3:c.1141_1142del; p.Asp381 fs) in a patient with PAPASH and a likely pathogenic variant in *NLRC4* gene (NM_001199138.2:c. c.541 C > T; p.Arg181*) in another patient with PAPASH with both gut and joint inflammation (see **Table 1**).

Concerning PAPASH treatment, both partial[57] and complete[33] responses have been documented with anakinra, whereas relatively good disease control has been observed under anti-TNF agents.[72] It is thought-provoking that notwithstanding TNF inhibition, the patient with PAPASH reported by Garzorz showed marked IL17 production both at the skin and at a systemic level, suggesting a role for anti-IL17 agents in the management of this specific form.[72]

Pyoderma Gangrenosum, Acne, and Ulcerative Colitis

Although PAC has been proposed as a separate form, reconsideration of its current nosology may be supported from evidence on PG comorbidities and from IBD often being a concomitant diagnosis of patients with PG and HS.[65,66,75–79]

Although some degree of nonspecific intestinal inflammation was noticed in 2 patients with PASS,[74] IBD has further proved as a recurrent feature of this spectrum of disorders in a WES study on 10 patients with sHS, of whom 2 had CD and one had ulcerative colitis (UC).[33]

Further supporting the association of IBD, and of UC particularly, with HS-related autoinflammatory syndromes, rather than confining its presence to a separate form are the observations of 2 PASH[33,43] and 2 PAPASH patients with a concurrent intestinal picture consistent with UC.[69,71]

Indeed, approximately 14% of patients with PASH (6 out of 44)[33,43,58,80] and 27% of those with PAPASH (3 out of 11)[33,69,71] had a concomitant diagnosis of either CD or UC, which is similar to what is seen in sporadic PG (9.3%-14.02%-23.8%-34%)[66,75–77] but lower than in sporadic HS.[65,78,79]

Careful consideration should be given before introducing an IL-17 inhibitor across the spectrum of HS-related autoinflammatory syndromes because this class of medications, especially IL-17A inhibitors, may trigger an underlying IBD.[81,82]

Psoriatic Arthritis, Pyoderma Gangrenosum, Hidradenitis Suppurativa, and Crohn Disease

A unique combination of PsA, PG, HS, and CD in a 52-year-old female led to another provisional entity being proposed, that is, PsA, PG, HS, and Crohn disease (PsAPSC).[83] Curiously, the patient lacked acne and demonstrated a paradoxic response to adalimumab, which resulted in worsening of psoriasis vulgaris and appearance of PG.

No genetic details of this patient have been reported.

Psoriatic Arthritis, Pyoderma Gangrenosum, Acne and Pyoderma Gangrenosum, Hidradenitis Suppurativa

PsAPASH, first described by Saraceno and colleagues,[84] represents a clinical variant of PASH syndrome in the presence of PsA. To date, no genetic determinant has been described.

Pustular Psoriasis, Arthritis, Pyoderma Gangrenosum, Synovitis, Acne, and Hidradenitis Suppurativa

A patient with a peculiar, almost unique combination of clinical manifestations, consisting of pustular psoriasis, arthritis, PG, synovitis, acne and HS, whose genetic background is unknown, has been reported to show a favorable response to the anti-IL-17-A agent secukinumab, after failing to respond to adalimumab.[85] Of note, this phenotype could also be considered a variant of SAPHO syndrome.

Pyoderma Gangrenosum, Acne, Hidradenitis Suppurativa, and Ankylosing Spondylitis

PASS syndrome has been introduced by Bruzzese and colleagues to indicate the constellation of PG, acne conglobata, HS and ankylosing spondylitis.[86]

Since its original description in 2012, only 11 cases have been reported,[74,83,86–89] of whom only 2[86,89] were found to be HLA-B27 positive. Curiously, either frank sternoclavicular joint involvement or chest arthralgias were recorded in 3,[74,87,88] with 7 subjects having also nonpalmoplantar pustulosis.[74,89] These observations indicate possible overlaps with SAPHO syndrome, as discussed in later discussion.

In the largest series reported to date, consisting of 6 cases, TNF inhibitors, namely infliximab and adalimumab, resulted in a satisfactory control of the cutaneous picture, either in high-dose or combination regimens with conventional immunomodulating agents.[74] On the contrary, etanercept failed to determine a response in 2 out of /2 cases.[86,88]

Leuenberger and colleagues[88] reported dramatic improvement of both skin lesions and articular manifestations with IL-1 antagonism; however, it must be underscored that follow-up duration was rather limited and that sporadic HS cases treated with anakinra tend to lose response few months after drug initiation.[90] This is also consistent with the report of a PASS case losing response to anakinra 200 mg die after 8 months and requiring infliximab to achieve sustained remission.[87] Finally, a case of primary failure with anakinra has also been observed.[74]

Recently, the IL-17A inhibitor secukinumab proved as a valid treatment option in this setting, with an almost complete response at 2 years of follow-up in a patient that had previously failed conventional immunomodulating agents.[89]

Vasculitis with Pyoderma Gangrenosum, Acne, and Hidradenitis Suppurativa

Leukocytoclastic vasculitis with C3 deposits on direct immunofluorescence has been observed in association with a case of PASH, leading the authors to coin the acronym VPASH.[91] Although both PG and vasculitis responded well to dapsone, presence of a monoclonal gammopathy of unknown significance and lack of known genetic variants weakens the reported association, which may stem from immunocomplex formation in the context of uncontrolled inflammation. Of note, MPO-ANCA-[71] and PR3-ANCA-[69] positivity without vasculitis were found in 2 patients with PAPASH with colitis.

Synovitis, Acne, Pustulosis, Hyperostosis, Osteitis

Synovitis, acne, pustulosis, hyperostosis, osteitis (SAPHO) syndrome is a rare disorder, whose acronym was coined in 1987 to group together different inflammatory osteocutaneous pictures of unclear etiopathogenesis with ill-defined disease associations.[92]

HS can rarely be associated with SAPHO, however clear epidemiologic data are lacking. Interestingly, some authors[92] casted doubt on the strength of the association between HS or dissecting cellulitis and true SAPHO because most reports lacked features such as palmoplantar pustulosis.[93–98] The same authors proposed a new subclassification of SAPHO ideally to disentangle the different entities that had coalesced under this umbrella term. They proposed a separate category for HS-associated spondyloarthropathy to encompass cases generally regarded as HS-

SAPHO.[92] More research will be needed to validate this proposal.

Weighing in on the complex relationship between HS and SAPHO from a dermatologic perspective, it is important to underscore that a considerable proportion of patients with HS presents with or will develop osteoarticular manifestations—less than a third according to a French study.[99] As about 1 out of 10 patients with HS will have true arthritis, clinicians should always consider screening for this comorbidity.[65] However, a diagnosis of SAPHO syndrome has been reached in less than 2% of the aforementioned French cohort, highlighting the relative rarity of such association.[99]

Genetics

So far, no specific pathogenic variants have been found, even though the familial character of SAPHO syndrome highlights the possibility of potential genetic determinants. The involvement of putative autoinflammatory genes such as NOD2 and PSTPIP2 (proline-serine-threonine phosphatase interacting protein 2)—an important paralog of PSTPIP1 gene—is debatable.[100]

In 2018, Li and colleagues[94] described a 44-year-old Chinese Han male patient with SAPHO syndrome presenting with HS. Genetic examination revealed a heterozygous single-nucleotide deletion in NCSTN gene (NM_015331.3:c.278del; p.Pro93LeufsTer15), which caused a frameshift with consequent loss-of-function of the encoded protein (see **Table 1**). Since HS, PASH and SAPHO syndrome are all linked to a degree to the NCSTN gene, the authors hypothesized a common genetic background for all these entities, with a central role of gamma-secretase genes.

Recently, an interesting association was established between copy number variations of the genes CSF2RA (colony stimulating factor 2 receptor subunit alpha), NOD2, MEGF6 (multiple EGF like domains 6), ADAM5 (ADAM metallopeptidase domain 5), and the predisposition to SAPHO syndrome.[101] Specifically, CSF2RA copy number was found to be significantly reduced in patients with SAPHO, resulting in a decrease in its interaction with granulocyte-macrophage colony-stimulating factor (GM-CSF) and its receptor, thus leading to an accumulation of GM-CSF in the peripheral blood of these patients. GM-CSF plays a key role in inflammation pathways and its aberrant expression was documented in several disorders including synovitis,[102] where it may promote joint inflammation through an increased secretion of proinflammatory cytokines such as IL-1β. SAPHO syndrome has been shown to partly depend on genetically encoded overproduction of IL-1β,[103] thus leading the authors to assume that a decreased expression of CSF2RA might be considered as the major cause of SAPHO syndrome onset.

Subsequently, through an association study conducted on 71 Chinese patients with SAPHO syndrome, Guo and colleagues[104] revealed that 3 single nucleotide polymorphism (SNP) sites (rs10889677, rs2201841, and rs7517847) of *IL-23R* and the variant rs2243248 of *IL-4* showed strong association with SAPHO syndrome. In addition, patients carrying the haplotype A-G-C-G-T, comprising 5 SNPs of the *IL-23R* gene were more likely to develop SAPHO syndrome.

Finally, a genome-wide association study conducted by Cai and colleagues[105] identified 2 genetically disrupted pathways: (1) Rap1 signaling pathway which exerts several functions in the control of cell adhesion and cell junction, migration, polarization, and proliferation and (2) bacterial invasion of epithelial cells. These findings suggest that a pathogen infection or allergic reaction might lead to the overexpression of proinflammatory mediators, which in turn increase the permeability of skin barrier or endothelial cells, thus increasing dermatologic complications of SAPHO syndrome.

Treatment

According to a systematic review on biologic use in SAPHO syndrome that included a total of 66 patients, anti-TNF-α agents had a response rate of 93.3% and 72.4% on osteoarticular and skin manifestations, respectively. The number of patients treated with biologics other than anti-TNF-α drugs was generally low, with 7 on IL-1 blockers and 13 on therapeutics targeting the IL-23/IL-17 axis. IL-1 antagonism or inhibition, although active on the musculoskeletal component of the syndrome, lacked effect on cutaneous lesions. Conversely, ustekinumab and anti-IL17 agents seem to perform well in both.[106] Wang and colleagues reported longer term data describing a 4-patient cohort of secukinumab-treated subjects experiencing sustained remission at 24 weeks of follow-up; it must be underscored however that only pustulosis was considered.[107] This is in line with the dramatic response on joint symptoms and palmoplantar pustulosis that was obtained in just 3 months in a patient with SAPHO treated with secukinumab[108] and in 1 patient treated with ixekizumab.[109] IL-23 inhibition with tildrakizumab also proved successful in the setting of a patient with osteoarticular manifestations and palmoplantar pustulosis who had lost response to adalimumab, leading to complete remission in just 4 weeks.[110]

Although Janus Kinase (JAK) inhibitors are regarded as a possible therapeutic option for many cognate conditions, published experiences of their use in SAPHO is still rather limited. Substantial improvement in pain, disease activity, and inflammatory markers was observed during a study on 12 female patients receiving 5 mg tofacitinib twice daily. Interestingly, cutaneous lesions also improved in 7 out of 8 patients but no further details were provided.[111] Analogously, upadacitinib, a relatively selective JAK1 inhibitor, proved effective in a patient with SAPHO with mild palmoplantar pustulosis and joint symptoms.[112]

As previously stated, the major issue with response evaluation in SAPHO is the great heterogeneity of pictures included under the same terminology.

Considering HS-SAPHO cases exclusively, use of anti-TNF agents seems to translate into substantial improvement both on the cutaneous and on the articular manifestations in most reports.[33,95–98,113–116] However, the majority of reported HS-SAPHO cases lacked palmoplantar pustulosis.[93–98,113–115,117–120] Evidence on other biologic classes is scant; however, the dramatic response to risankizumab documented in an anti-TNF-refractory patient with HS-SAPHO is of interest.[121]

Tofacitinib was beneficial in an HS-SAPHO case but unfortunately no details were available on HS course.[122]

MTX has often been used either as an adjuvant or in monotherapy and seems the preferred immunomodulating agent in this setting. Alternative regimens with tetracyclines or retinoids generally showed little effect. A variety of other approaches has been described including lesion-directed treatment, such as intralesional CS injections, or use of endocrine modulators, that is, metformin[114] or finasteride.[119] Although the latter may be considered on a case-by-case fashion, there is insufficient evidence to support their use.

Combined treatment approaches involving cutaneous surgery may prove advantageous,[114] in keeping with evidence in sporadic HS.[123]

FUTURE PERSPECTIVES

More than 10 years after the original description of PASH, a reliable genotype–phenotype correlation still eludes us. Research endeavors will need to be directed toward increasing -omics studies (eg, genomics and transcriptomics) to identify novel causative variants and biological signaling pathways possibly involved and druggable in sHS. This will allow us to draw a robust genotype–phenotype correlation and, by translating the -omic findings into functional models, to develop personalized therapy for each patient.

Although considerable advances have been made in the management of either sporadic HS or PG, no trials are currently addressing the syndromic setting. As syndromic forms represent the prototype of refractory HS, new approaches may be needed to adequately treat these patients. Although anti-TNF agents and, to a lesser degree, dose-intensified anakinra represent the best-supported therapeutic options in HS-related autoinflammatory syndromes, the encouraging results obtained in isolated reports with off-label biologics may foreshadow a change in the therapeutic landscape. Indeed, a great-unmet need exists in terms of truly effective treatments in this setting.[124] The heterogeneous drug response could also be due to the genetic and immunologic background of each patient; therefore, unraveling the disease's pathogenesis, by broadening subcategorization of patients with sHS, is of paramount importance for endotype-directed therapies development.[125] Moreover, in the future, combination regimens associating biologics and small molecules may be assessed in this group of disorders, where they could possibly substitute the combinations of conventional immunosuppressant and immuno-modulating agents that had traditionally been used.[126]

Hopefully, evidence on sporadic and syndromic HS will shape each other in a mutual manner, so that new acquisitions in one can be the basis for advancing our understanding in the other.

Finally, critical rethinking of available reports probably indicates that, aside from research purposes, unnecessary nosologic fragmentation should be avoided. The newly proposed terminology HS-related autoinflammatory syndromes could be used to encompass the various phenotypes hitherto described. In fact, although it is important not to lose clinical details and subtle nuances, it is similarly important to avoid separating cases in a myriad of different unique entities.

CLINICS CARE POINTS

- HS-related autoinflammatory syndromes encompass the following entities: PASH, PA-PASH, PsAPASH, PsAPSASH, PASS, PsAPSC, VPASH, and SAPHO.
- The nosology of this group of disorders has not yet reached a consensus, and a wide range of monogenic and polygenic conditions is increasingly associated with HS.
- No clinical trials are currently addressing the setting of HS-related autoinflammatory syndromes.

- To date, TNF-α and IL-1β inhibitors represent the best-supported therapeutic strategies in HS-related autoinflammatory syndromes.
- Other off-label biologics are paving the way for novel pathogenic and therapeutic scenarios.
- Combination regimens associating biologics and small molecules may be assessed in HS-related autoinflammatory syndromes, potentially capable of replacing traditionally used combinations of conventional immunosuppressive and immunomodulatory agents.
- Further research is needed to discover novel biomarkers of response and biological pathways potentially druggable in HS-related autoinflammatory syndromes.

DISCLOSURE

The authors declare no competing interests.

REFERENCES

1. Marzano AV, Borghi A, Wallach D, et al. A Comprehensive Review of Neutrophilic Diseases. Clin Rev Allergy Immunol 2018;54:114–30.
2. Cugno M, Borghi A, Marzano AV. PAPA, PASH and PAPASH Syndromes: Pathophysiology, Presentation and Treatment. Am J Clin Dermatol 2017;18:555–62.
3. Garcovich S, Genovese G, Moltrasio C, et al. PASH, PAPASH, PsAPASH, and PASS: The autoinflammatory syndromes of hidradenitis suppurativa. Clin Dermatol 2021;39:240–7.
4. Marzano AV, Borghi A, Meroni PL, et al. Pyoderma gangrenosum and its syndromic forms: evidence for a link with autoinflammation. Br J Dermatol 2016;175:882–91.
5. Gasparic J, Theut Riis P, Jemec GB. Recognizing syndromic hidradenitis suppurativa: a review of the literature. J Eur Acad Dermatol Venereol 2017;31:1809–16.
6. Pavlovsky M, Peled A, Sarig O, et al. Coexistence of pachyonychia congenita and hidradenitis suppurativa: more than a coincidence. Br J Dermatol 2022;187:392–400.
7. McKenzie SA, Ni CS, Hsiao JL. Hidradenitis Suppurativa in a Patient with Smith-Magenis Syndrome: A Case Report. Cureus 2019;11:e4970.
8. Lindor NM, Arsenault TM, Solomon H, et al. A new autosomal dominant disorder of pyogenic sterile arthritis, pyoderma gangrenosum, and acne: PAPA syndrome. Mayo Clin Proc 1997;72:611–5.
9. Wise CA, Gillum JD, Seidman CE, et al. Mutations in CD2BP1 disrupt binding to PTP PEST and are

responsible for PAPA syndrome, an autoinflammatory disorder. Hum Mol Genet 2002;1:961–9.

10. Starnes TW, Bennin DA, Bing X, et al. The F-BAR protein PSTPIP1 controls extracellular matrix degradation and filopodia formation in macrophages. Blood 2014;123:2703–14.

11. Stone DL, Ombrello A, Arostegui JI, et al. Excess Serum Interleukin-18 Distinguishes Patients With Pathogenic Mutations in PSTPIP1. Arthritis Rheumatol 2022;74:353–7.

12. Boursier G, Piram M, Rittore C, et al. Phenotypic Associations of PSTPIP1 Sequence Variants in PSTPIP1-Associated Autoinflammatory Diseases. J Invest Dermatol 2021;141:1141–7.

13. Zhao R, Novice T, Konda S. Renal involvement as a potential feature of pyogenic arthritis, pyoderma gangrenosum, and acne syndrome with E250K mutation of PSTPIP1 gene. JAAD Case Rep 2022; 32:48–51.

14. Morales-Heil DJ, Cao L, Sweeney C, et al. Rare missense variants in the SH3 domain of *PSTPIP1* are associated with hidradenitis suppurativa. HGG Adv 2023;4:100187.

15. Maggio MC, Ceccherini I, Grossi A, et al. PAPA and FMF in two siblings: possible amplification of clinical presentation? A case report. Ital J Pediatr 2019;45:111.

16. Vural S, Gündoğdu M, Gökpınar İli E, et al. Association of pyrin mutations and autoinflammation with complex phenotype hidradenitis suppurativa: a case-control study. Br J Dermatol 2019;180:1459–67.

17. Braun-Falco M, Kovnerystyy O, Lohse P, et al. Pyoderma gangrenosum, acne, and suppurative hidradenitis (PASH)–a new autoinflammatory syndrome distinct from PAPA syndrome. J Am Acad Dermatol 2012;66:409–15.

18. Ah-Weng A, Langtry JA, Velangi S, et al. Pyoderma gangrenosum associated with hidradenitis suppurativa. Clin Exp Dermatol 2005;30:669–71.

19. Hsiao JL, Antaya RJ, Berger T, et al. Hidradenitis suppurativa and concomitant pyoderma gangrenosum: a case series and literature review. Arch Dermatol 2010;146:1265–70.

20. Duchatelet S, Miskinyte S, Join-Lambert O, et al. First nicastrin mutation in PASH (pyoderma gangrenosum, acne and suppurative hidradenitis) syndrome. Br J Dermatol 2015;173:610–2.

21. Pink AE, Simpson MA, Brice GW, et al. PSENEN and NCSTN mutations in familial hidradenitis suppurativa (Acne Inversa). J Invest Dermatol 2011;131:1568–70.

22. Marzano AV, Ceccherini I, Gattorno M, et al. Association of pyoderma gangrenosum, acne, and suppurative hidradenitis (PASH) shares genetic and cytokine profiles with other autoinflammatory diseases. Medicine (Baltim) 2014;93:e187.

23. Richards S, Aziz N, Bale S, et al. Standards and guidelines for the interpretation of sequence variants: a joint consensus recommendation of the American College of Medical Genetics and Genomics and the Association for Molecular Pathology. Genet Med 2015;17:405–24.

24. Theodoropoulou K, Wittkowski H, Busso N, et al. Increased Prevalence of *NLRP3* Q703K Variant Among Patients With Autoinflammatory Diseases: An International Multicentric Study. Front Immunol 2020; 11:877.

25. Zhang M, Chen QD, Xu HX, et al. Association of hidradenitis suppurativa with Crohn's disease. World J Clin Cases 2021;9:3506–16.

26. Saraç Öztürk G, Ergun T, Peker Eyüboğlu İ, et al. Serum high-sensitivity C-reactive protein, tumor necrosis factor-α, interleukin (IL)-1β, IL-17A and IL-23 levels in patients with hidradenitis suppurativa. Cytokine 2021;144:155585.

27. Calderón-Castrat X, Bancalari-Díaz D, Román-Curto C, et al. PSTPIP1 gene mutation in a pyoderma gangrenosum, acne and suppurative hidradenitis (PASH) syndrome. Br J Dermatol 2016;175: 194–8.

28. Faraji Zonooz M, Sabbagh-Kermani F, Fattahi Z, et al. Whole Genome Linkage Analysis Followed by Whole Exome Sequencing Identifies Nicastrin (NCSTN) as a Causative Gene in a Multiplex Family with γ-Secretase Spectrum of Autoinflammatory Skin Phenotypes. J Invest Dermatol 2016;136: 1283–6.

29. Saito N, Minami-Hori M, Nagahata H, et al. Novel PSTPIP1 gene mutation in pyoderma gangrenosum, acne and suppurative hidradenitis syndrome. J Dermatol 2018;45:e213–4.

30. Zhang X, He Y, Xu H, et al. First PSENEN mutation in PASH syndrome. J Dermatol 2020;47: 1335–7.

31. Brandao L, Moura R, Tricarico PM, et al. Altered keratinization and vitamin D metabolism may be key pathogenetic pathways in syndromic hidradenitis suppurativa: a novel whole exome sequencing approach. J Dermatol Sci 2020;99:17–22.

32. Nomura T. Hidradenitis Suppurativa as a Potential Subtype of Autoinflammatory Keratinization Disease. Front Immunol 2020;11:847.

33. Marzano AV, Genovese G, Moltrasio C, et al. Whole-Exome Sequencing in 10 Unrelated Patients with Syndromic Hidradenitis Suppurativa: A Preliminary Step for a Genotype-Phenotype Correlation. Dermatology 2022;238:860–9.

34. Damgaard RB, Elliott PR, Swatek KN, et al. OTULIN deficiency in ORAS causes cell type-specific LUBAC degradation, dysregulated TNF signalling and cell death. EMBO Mol Med 2019;11:e9324.

35. Canna SW, de Jesus AA, Gouni S, et al. An activating NLRC4 inflammasome mutation causes autoinflammation with recurrent macrophage activation syndrome. Nat Genet 2014;46:1140–6.

36. Kile BT, Panopoulos AD, Stirzaker RA, et al. Mutations in the cofilin partner Aip1/Wdr1 cause autoinflammatory disease and macrothrombocytopenia. Blood 2007;110:2371–80.

37. Moltrasio C, Cagliani R, Sironi M, et al. Autoinflammation in Syndromic Hidradenitis Suppurativa: The Role of AIM2. Vaccines (Basel) 2023;11:162.

38. Brandão LAC, Moura RR, Marzano AV, et al. Variant Enrichment Analysis to Explore Pathways Functionality in Complex Autoinflammatory Skin Disorders through Whole Exome Sequencing Analysis. Int J Mol Sci 2022;23:2278.

39. Fischer AH, Jourabchi N, Khalifian S, et al. Spectrum of diseases associated with pyoderma gangrenosum and correlation with effectiveness of therapy: New insights on the diagnosis and therapy of comorbid hidradenitis suppurativa. Wound Repair Regen 2022;30:338–44.

40. Baroud S, Wu J, Zouboulis CC. Acne Syndromes and Mosaicism. Biomedicines 2021;9:1735.

41. Maitrepierre F, Marzano AV, Lipsker D. A Unified Concept of Acne in the PAPA Spectrum Disorders. Dermatology 2021;237:827–34.

42. Turcu G, Ioana Nedelcu R, Teodora Nedelcu I, et al. Pyoderma gangrenosum and suppurative hidradenitis association, overlap or spectrum of the same disease? Case report and discussion. Exp Ther Med 2020;20:38–41.

43. Murphy B, Morrison G, Podmore P. Successful use of adalimumab to treat pyoderma gangrenosum, acne and suppurative hidradenitis (PASH syndrome) following colectomy in ulcerative colitis. Int J Colorectal Dis 2015;30:1139–40.

44. Marzano AV, Ishak RS, Colombo A, et al. Pyoderma gangrenosum, acne and suppurative hidradenitis syndrome following bowel bypass surgery. Dermatology 2012;225:215–9.

45. Maione V, Perantoni M, Caravello S, et al. A case of PASH syndrome associated to testicular cancer. Dermatol Ther 2021;34:e14763.

46. Zivanovic D, Masirevic I, Ruzicka T, et al. Pyoderma gangrenosum, acne, suppurative hidradenitis (PASH) and polycystic ovary syndrome: Coincidentally or aetiologically connected? Australas J Dermatol 2017;58:e54–9.

47. Gracia-Cazaña T, Frias M, Roselló R, et al. PASH syndrome associated with osteopoikilosis. Int J Dermatol 2015;54:e369–71.

48. McCarthy S, Foley CC, Dvorakova V, et al. PASH syndrome with bony destruction. Clin Exp Dermatol 2019;44:918–20.

49. Join-Lambert O, Duchatelet S, Delage M, et al. Remission of refractory pyoderma gangrenosum, severe acne, and hidradenitis suppurativa (PASH) syndrome using targeted antibiotic therapy in 4 patients. J Am Acad Dermatol 2015;73:S66–9.

50. Lamiaux M, Dabouz F, Wantz M, et al. Successful combined antibiotic therapy with oral clindamycin and oral rifampicin for pyoderma gangrenosum in patient with PASH syndrome. JAAD Case Rep 2017;4:17–21.

51. Staub J, Pfannschmidt N, Strohal R, et al. Successful treatment of PASH syndrome with infliximab, cyclosporine and dapsone. J Eur Acad Dermatol Venereol 2015;29:2243–7.

52. Huang J, Tsang LS, Shi W, et al. Pyoderma Gangrenosum, Acne, and Hidradenitis Suppurativa Syndrome: A Case Report and Literature Review. Front Med 2022;9:856786.

53. Zouboulis CC, Desai N, Emtestam L, et al. European S1 guideline for the treatment of hidradenitis suppurativa/acne inversa. J Eur Acad Dermatol Venereol 2015;29:619–44.

54. Maronese CA, Pimentel MA, Li MM, et al. Pyoderma Gangrenosum: An Updated Literature Review on Established and Emerging Pharmacological Treatments. Am J Clin Dermatol 2022;23: 615–34.

55. De Wet J, Jordaan HF, Kannenberg SM, et al. Pyoderma gangrenosum, acne, and suppurative hidradenitis syndrome in end-stage renal disease successfully treated with adalimumab. Dermatol Online J 2017;23. 13030/qt82d4m2zw.

56. Burlando M, Fabbrocini G, Marasca C, et al. Adalimumab Originator vs. Biosimilar in Hidradenitis Suppurativa: A Multicentric Retrospective Study. Biomedicines 2022;10:2522.

57. Faleri S, Feichtner K, Ruzicka T. Schwere Akne bei Autoinflammationskrankheiten [Severe acne in autoinflammatory diseases]. Hautarzt 2016;67: 897–901.

58. Sun NZ, Ro T, Jolly P, et al. Non-response to Interleukin-1 Antagonist Canakinumab in Two Patients with Refractory Pyoderma Gangrenosum and Hidradenitis Suppurativa. J Clin Aesthet Dermatol 2017;10:36–8.

59. Jennings L, Molloy O, Quinlan C, et al. Treatment of pyoderma gangrenosum, acne, suppurative hidradenitis (PASH) with weight-based anakinra dosing in a Hepatitis B carrier. Int J Dermatol 2017;56: e128–9.

60. Marletta DA, Barei F, Moltrasio C, et al. A case of PASH syndrome treated with guselkumab. Int J Dermatol 2023;62(11):e585–7.

61. Kok Y, Nicolopoulos J, Varigos G, et al. Tildrakizumab in the treatment of PASH syndrome: A potential novel therapeutic target. Australas J Dermatol 2020;61(3):e373–4. https://doi.org/10.1111/ajd. 13285.

62. Kimball AB, Prens EP, Passeron T, et al. Efficacy and Safety of Risankizumab for the Treatment of Hidradenitis Suppurativa: A Phase 2, Randomized,

Placebo-Controlled Trial. Dermatol Ther 2023;13: 1099–111.

63. Kimball AB, Podda M, Alavi A, et al. Guselkumab for the treatment of patients with moderate-to-severe hidradenitis suppurativa: A phase 2 randomized study. J Eur Acad Dermatol Venereol 2023;37(10):2098–108.

64. Flora A, Kozera EK, Jepsen R, et al. Baseline clinical, hormonal and molecular markers associated with clinical response to IL-23 antagonism in hidradenitis suppurativa: A prospective cohort study. Exp Dermatol 2023;32:869–77.

65. Zagaria O, Ruggiero A, Fabbrocini G, et al. Wound care, adalimumab, and multidisciplinary approach in a patient affected by PASH syndrome. Int Wound J 2020;17:1528–31.

66. Garg A, Malviya N, Strunk A, et al. Comorbidity screening in hidradenitis suppurativa: Evidence-based recommendations from the US and Canadian Hidradenitis Suppurativa Foundations. J Am Acad Dermatol 2022;86:1092–101.

67. Cawen I, Navarrete J, Agorio C. PASH syndrome: a novel surgical approach. An Bras Dermatol 2022; 97:121–3.

68. Marzano AV, Trevisan V, Gattorno M, et al. Pyogenic arthritis, pyoderma gangrenosum, acne, and hidradenitis suppurativa (PAPASH): a new autoinflammatory syndrome associated with a novel mutation of the PSTPIP1 gene. JAMA Dermatol 2013;149:762–4.

69. Ursani MA, Appleyard J, Whiteru O, et al. Pyogenic Arthritis, Pyoderma Gangrenosum, Acne, Suppurative Hidradenitis (PA-PASH) Syndrome: An Atypical Presentation of a Rare Syndrome. Am J Case Rep 2016;17:587–91.

70. Kotzerke M, Mitri F, Marbach F, et al. A case of PA-PASH syndrome in a young man carrying a novel heterozygote missense variant in PSTPIP1. J Eur Acad Dermatol Venereol 2021;35:e439–40.

71. Kawanishi K, Nishiwaki H, Oshiro T, et al. A case of myeloperoxidase-antineutrophil cytoplasmic antibody and anticardiolipin antibody-positive pyogenic arthritis, pyoderma gangrenosum, acne and hidradenitis suppurativa (PAPASH) syndrome with colitis. Mod Rheumatol Case Rep 2021;5: 333–6.

72. Garzorz N, Papanagiotou V, Atenhan A, et al. Pyoderma gangrenosum, acne, psoriasis, arthritis and suppurative hidradenitis (PAPASH)-syndrome: a new entity within the spectrum of autoinflammatory syndromes? J Eur Acad Dermatol Venereol 2016; 30:141–3.

73. Monte Serrano J, de la Fuente Meira S, Cruañes Monferrer J, et al. PAPASH syndrome with MEFV gene mutation. Med Clin 2021;156:313.

74. Gottlieb J, Madrange M, Gardair C, et al. PAPASH, PsAPASH and PASS autoinflammatory syndromes:

phenotypic heterogeneity, common biological signature and response to immunosuppressive regimens. Br J Dermatol 2019;181:866–9.

75. Gillard M, Anuset D, Maillard H, et al. Comorbidities of pyoderma gangrenosum: a retrospective multicentric analysis of 126 patients. Br J Dermatol 2018;179:218–9.

76. Al Ghazal P, Herberger K, Schaller J, et al. Associated factors and comorbidities in patients with pyoderma gangrenosum in Germany: a retrospective multicentric analysis in 259 patients. Orphanet J Rare Dis 2013;8:136.

77. Binus AM, Qureshi AA, Li VW, et al. Pyoderma gangrenosum: a retrospective review of patient characteristics, comorbidities and therapy in 103 patients. Br J Dermatol 2011;165:1244–50.

78. Garg A, Hundal J, Strunk A. Overall and Subgroup Prevalence of Crohn Disease Among Patients With Hidradenitis Suppurativa: A Population-Based Analysis in the United States. JAMA Dermatol 2018;154:814–8.

79. Egeberg A, Jemec GBE, Kimball AB, et al. Prevalence and Risk of Inflammatory Bowel Disease in Patients with Hidradenitis Suppurativa. J Invest Dermatol 2017;137:1060–4.

80. Moschella SL. Is there a role for infliximab in the current therapy of hidradenitis suppurativa? A report of three treated cases. Int J Dermatol 2007;46:1287–91.

81. Lee JS, Tato CM, Joyce-Shaikh B, et al. Interleukin-23-Independent IL-17 Production Regulates Intestinal Epithelial Permeability. Immunity 2015;43: 727–38.

82. Maronese CA, Zelin E, Moltrasio C, et al. Genetic screening in new onset inflammatory bowel disease during anti-interleukin 17 therapy: unmet needs and call for action. Expert Opin Biol Ther 2021;21:1543–6.

83. Saternus R, Schwingel J, Müller CSL, et al. Ancient friends, revisited: Systematic review and case report of pyoderma gangrenosum-associated autoinflammatory syndromes. J Transl Autoimmun 2020;3:100071.

84. Saraceno R, Babino G, Chiricozzi A, et al. PsA-PASH: a new syndrome associated with hidradenitis suppurativa with response to tumor necrosis factor inhibition. J Am Acad Dermatol 2015;72: e42–4.

85. Nikolakis G, Kreibich K, Vaiopoulos A, et al. Case Report: PsAPSASH syndrome: an alternative phenotype of syndromic hidradenitis suppurativa treated with the IL-17A inhibitor secukinumab. F1000Res 2021;10:381.

86. Bruzzese V. Pyoderma gangrenosum, acne conglobata, suppurative hidradenitis, and axial spondyloarthritis: efficacy of anti-tumor necrosis factor α therapy. J Clin Rheumatol 2012;18:413–5.

87. Schwob E, Bessis D, Boursier G, et al. PASS: a rare syndrome within the autoinflammatory diseases that still lacks a genetic marker. J Eur Acad Dermatol Venereol 2020;34:e478–80.

88. Leuenberger M, Berner J, Di Lucca J, et al. PASS Syndrome: An IL-1-Driven Autoinflammatory Disease. Dermatology 2016;232:254–8.

89. Li M, Xiang H, Liang Y, et al. Secukinumab for PASS syndrome: A new choice for therapeutic challenge? Dermatol Ther 2022;35:e15507.

90. Tzanetakou V, Kanni T, Giatrakou S, et al. Safety and Efficacy of Anakinra in Severe Hidradenitis Suppurativa: A Randomized Clinical Trial. JAMA Dermatol 2016;152:52–9.

91. Niv D, Ramirez JA, Fivenson DP. Pyoderma gangrenosum, acne, and hidradenitis suppurativa (PASH) syndrome with recurrent vasculitis. JAAD Case Rep 2017;3:70–3.

92. Chen W, Ito T, Lin SH, et al. Does SAPHO syndrome exist in dermatology? J Eur Acad Dermatol Venereol 2022;36:1501–6.

93. Ozyemisci-Taskiran O, Bölükbasi N, Gögüs F. A hidradenitis suppurativa related SAPHO case associated with features resembling spondylarthropathy and proteinuria. Clin Rheumatol 2007;26:789–91.

94. Li C, Xu H, Wang B. Is SAPHO Syndrome Linked to PASH Syndrome and Hidradenitis Suppurativa by Nicastrin Mutation? A Case Report. J Rheumatol 2018;45:1605–7.

95. Genovese G, Caorsi R, Moltrasio C, et al. Successful treatment of co-existent SAPHO syndrome and hidradenitis suppurativa with adalimumab and methotrexate. J Eur Acad Dermatol Venereol 2019;33(Suppl 6):40–1.

96. Vekic DA, Woods J, Lin P, et al. SAPHO syndrome associated with hidradenitis suppurativa and pyoderma gangrenosum successfully treated with adalimumab and methotrexate: a case report and review of the literature. Int J Dermatol 2018;57:10–8.

97. De Souza A, Solomon GE, Strober BE. SAPHO syndrome associated with hidradenitis suppurativa successfully treated with infliximab and methotrexate. Bull NYU Hosp Jt Dis 2011;69:185–7.

98. Crowley EL, O'Toole A, Gooderham MJ. Hidradenitis suppurativa with SAPHO syndrome maintained effectively with adalimumab, methotrexate, and intralesional corticosteroid injections. SAGE Open Med Case Rep 2018;6. 2050313X18778723.

99. Richette P, Molto A, Viguier M, et al. Hidradenitis suppurativa associated with spondyloarthritis – results from a multicenter national prospective study. J Rheumatol 2014;41:490–4.

100. Hurtado-Nedelec M, Chollet-Martin S, Chapeton D, et al. Genetic susceptibility factors in a cohort of 38 patients with SAPHO syndrome: a study of PSTPIP2, NOD2, and LPIN2 genes. J Rheumatol 2010;37:401–9.

101. Guo C, Tian X, Han F, et al. Copy Number Variation of Multiple Genes in SAPHO Syndrome. J Rheumatol 2020;47:1323–9.

102. Klimiuk PA, Yang H, Goronzy JJ, et al. Production of cytokines and metalloproteinases in rheumatoid synovitis is T cell dependent. Clin Immunol 1999; 90:65–78.

103. Berthelot JM, Corvec S, Hayem G. SAPHO, autophagy, IL-1, FoxO1, and Propionibacterium (Cutibacterium) acnes. Joint Bone Spine 2018;85: 171–6.

104. Guo C, Li C, Han F, et al. Association analysis of interleukin-23 receptor SNPs and SAPHO syndrome in Chinese people. Int J Rheum Dis 2019;22: 2178–84.

105. Cai R, Dong Y, Fang M, et al. Genome-Wide Association Identifies Risk Pathways for SAPHO Syndrome. Front Cell Dev Biol 2021;9:643644.

106. Daoussis D, Konstantopoulou G, Kraniotis P, et al. Biologics in SAPHO syndrome: A systematic review. Semin Arthritis Rheum 2019;48:618–25.

107. Wang G, Zhuo N, Li J. Off-label Use of Secukinumab: A Potential Therapeutic Option for SAPHO Syndrome. J Rheumatol 2022;49:656.

108. Ji Q, Wang Q, Pan W, et al. Exceptional response of skin symptoms to secukinumab treatment in a patient with SAPHO syndrome: Case report and literature review. Medicine (Baltim) 2022;101: e30065.

109. Xia R, Diao Z, Zhang Z, et al. Successful treatment of synovitis, acne, pustulosis, hyperostosis and osteitis syndrome with ixekizumab. Clin Exp Dermatol 2022;47:978–80.

110. Licata G, Gambardella A, Calabrese G, et al. SAPHO syndrome successful treated with tildrakizumab. Dermatol Ther 2021;34:e14758.

111. Li C, Li Z, Cao Y, et al. Tofacitinib for the Treatment of Nail Lesions and Palmoplantar Pustulosis in Synovitis, Acne, Pustulosis, Hyperostosis, and Osteitis Syndrome. JAMA Dermatol 2021;157:74–8.

112.. Ma M, Lu S, Hou X, et al. Novel JAK-1 inhibitor upadacitinib as a possible treatment for refractory SAPHO syndrome: A case report. Int J Rheum Dis 2023;26(11):2335–7.

113. Luzzati M, Simonini G, Filippeschi C, et al. SAPHO syndrome: the supposed trigger by isotretinoin, the efficacy of adalimumab and the specter of depressive disorder: a case report. Ital J Pediatr 2020;46: 169.

114. Fania L, Moro F, Clemente A, et al. Successful treatment of Sapho syndrome and hidradenitis suppurativa: A therapeutic challenge. Dermatol Ther 2020;33:e13453.

115. Briede K, Valiukeviciene S, Kucinskiene V, et al. Biologic Therapy for Hidradenitis Suppurativa Plus Conglobate Acne Associated with SAPHO

Syndrome: A Case Report. Acta Derm Venereol 2020;100:adv00311.

116. Burgemeister LT, Baeten DL, Tas SW. Biologics for rare inflammatory diseases: TNF blockade in the SA PHO syndrome. Neth J Med 2012;70:444–9.

117. Correia CP, Martins A, Oliveira J, et al. Systemic Amyloidosis with Renal Failure: A Challenging Diagnosis of SAPHO Syndrome. Eur J Case Rep Intern Med 2019;6:001087.

118. Falahati V, Aronowitz PB. SAPHO Syndrome from Hidradenitis Suppurativa. J Gen Intern Med 2020; 35:1307–8.

119. Azevedo VF, Dal Pizzol VI, Lopes H, et al. Metotrexato no tratamento da síndrome SAPHO complicadas por quelóides [Methotrexate to treat SAPHO syndrome with keloidal scars]. Acta Reumatol Port 2011;36:167–70.

120. Louter L, van Kats MA, Huisman AM. Een vrouw met pijn, stijfheid en huidafwijkingen [A woman with pain, stiffness and skin abnormalities]. Ned Tijdschr Geneeskd 2014;158:A7857.

121. Flora A, Holland R, Smith A, et al. Rapid and sustained remission of synovitis, acne, pustulosis, hyperostosis, and osteitis (SAPHO) syndrome with IL-23p19 antagonist (risankizumab). JAAD Case Rep 2021;14:33–6.

122. Yuan F, Luo J, Yang Q. SAPHO Syndrome Complicated by Ankylosing Spondylitis Successfully Treated With Tofacitinib: A Case Report. Front Immunol 2022;13:911922.

123. Bechara FG, Podda M, Prens EP, et al. Efficacy and Safety of Adalimumab in Conjunction With Surgery in Moderate to Severe Hidradenitis Suppurativa: The SHARPS Randomized Clinical Trial. JAMA Surg 2021;156:1001–9.

124. Garg A, Neuren E, Cha D, et al. Evaluating patients' unmet needs in hidradenitis suppurativa: Results from the Global Survey Of Impact and Healthcare Needs (VOICE) Project. J Am Acad Dermatol 2020;82:366–76.

125. Moltrasio C, Tricarico PM, Moura R, et al. Clinical and molecular characterization of hidradenitis suppurativa: a practical framework for novel therapeutic targets. Dermatology 2023;239(5):836–9.

126. Maronese CA, Ingram JR, Marzano AV. Has the time come to assess small molecule/biologic drug combination for the management of moderate-to-severe hidradenitis suppurativa? Br J Dermatol 2023;189(4):467–8.

Pediatric Neutrophilic Dermatoses

Ester Moreno-Artero, MD[a], Antonio Torrelo, MD[b],*

KEYWORDS

- Pediatric neutrophilic dermatoses • Sweet syndrome • Pyoderma gangrenosum • Behçet disease

KEY POINTS

- Neutrophilic dermatoses are a heterogeneous group of diseases, not frequent in children, often associated with an underlying internal noninfectious disease.
- They share an overlapping histopathologic background characterized by perivascular and diffuse neutrophilic infiltrates in one or more layers of the skin, and extracutaneous neutrophilic infiltrates may be associated.
- In children, some neutrophilic dermatoses can be the presentation of rare genetic diseases, justifying a more extensive diagnostic workup in this age group.

INTRODUCTION

The term neutrophilic dermatoses (NDs) encompasses a heterogeneous group of diseases, often associated with an underlying internal noninfectious disease, with an overlapping histopathologic background characterized by perivascular and diffuse neutrophilic infiltrates in one or more layers of the skin; extracutaneous neutrophilic infiltrates may be associated with the ND.[1,2] NDs are not frequent in children and are even rarer in newborns and infants.[1–3] When an ND appears in this age group, it represents a diagnostic and therapeutic challenge. Besides the classic NDs such as pyoderma gangrenosum (PG), Sweet syndrome (SS), and Behçet disease (BD), an ND can be the presentation of rare genetic diseases of the innate immune system, such as autoinflammatory diseases (AIDs), justifying a more extensive diagnostic workup in this age group.[2] The link between ND and AIDs is being object of recent research.[1–3]

In this article, the authors review the most important NDs that can present in children (**Box 1**) and emphasize the peculiar aspects of NDs in children from a diagnostic and therapeutic perspective.

SWEET SYNDROME
Clinical Care Points

- Sweet syndrome is characterized by the abrupt development of tender erythematous papules and plaques, often accompanied by fever and leukocytosis in peripheral blood.
- A significant association with malignancy is seen in both adults and children over 3 years, notably hematologic malignancies.
- Widespread vesiculobullous or oral mucosal lesions as well as the presence of anemia and/or thrombocytopenia are more frequently seen if associated malignancy.
- Systemic steroids are the first choice of treatment. A commonly used dose in children is 1 to 2 mg/kg/day of prednisone until skin lesions have resolved, followed by tapering.

SS, also known as acute febrile ND, has been classified into three primary groups: the classical form, the drug-induced, and the malignancy-associated

[a] Department of Dermatology, Hospital de Galdácano-Usansolo, Vizcaya, Bilbao 48007, Spain; [b] Department of Dermatology, Hospital Infantil Universitario Niño Jesús, Menendez Pelayo 65, Madrid 28009, Spain
* Corresponding author.
E-mail address: atorrelo@aedv.es

Dermatol Clin 42 (2024) 267–283
https://doi.org/10.1016/j.det.2023.12.005

Box 1
Neutrophilic dermatoses in children

Sweet syndrome

Pyoderma gangrenosum

Behçet disease

Neutrophilic eccrine hidradenitis

Neutrophilic dermatosis as the presentation of autoinflammatory disease in children

- CANDLE/PRAAS
- DIRA, DITRA, pustular psoriasis, and related pustular skin diseases
- APLAID/PLAID syndrome
- PAAND
- CAPS and NLRP1-related disorders

Neutrophilic dermatosis and autoimmunity

SS.[1] The classical type of SS is the most frequent in childhood, and most of the children with classical SS have suffered an upper respiratory or gastrointestinal tract infection within the previous 1 to 3 weeks.[3] Neonates, infants, and children, with a mean age of 5 years, may be affected.[4–9] A female predilection has been reported in adults, but there is a male predominance under 3 years of age, and an equal sex distribution in older children.[5] **Table 1** summarizes the main differences between childhood and adult SS.

Cutaneous Features

SS is clinically characterized by the abrupt development of tender erythematous papules and plaques, often accompanied by fever and leukocytosis in peripheral blood (**Fig. 1**). Lesions may enlarge and coalesce to form plaques with a mamillated surface and are often dusky, with a targetoid or erythema multiforme-like appearance. They can develop a pseudovesicular or vesicular appearance with remarkable edema, and this vesiculobullous variant is more often associated with acute myelogenous leukemia.[1] Pustules may also occur. Lesions arise principally on the head, neck, and upper extremities, but in malignancy-associated cases, they often show a widespread distribution.[1] Oral mucosa is often spared and, when involved, malignancy should be investigated.[4,5]

Extracutaneous Features and Associations

Fever is present in most patients and typically precedes the cutaneous lesions by days to weeks. Because neutrophils can infiltrate other organs and systems, musculoskeletal involvement may occur, presenting as myalgias and, in 20%, bony disease (arthritis, arthralgia, tibial pain, or osteomyelitis). Ocular involvement, including episcleritis, scleritis, and limbal nodules, occurs in up to 70% of adults with classical SS, but is much less common in pediatric cases.[5–7] Other organ systems that may be rarely involved include the central nervous system (CNS), liver, gastrointestinal (GI) tract, pulmonary and cardiovascular systems, spleen, kidneys, and bone.[4]

A notable association with malignancy is seen in both adults and children older than 3 years. Approximately 15% to 30% of adult patients present with an internal malignancy (more frequent hematological than solid organ). In a literature review of 66 pediatric patients with SS, malignancy or premalignant disorders were seen in 24% of the cases, all malignancies were hematologic, and all cases were older than 3 years of age. In fact, when looking only at cases between 3 and 18 years, up to 44% of patients had an associated malignancy or a premalignant disorder.[5]

Certain drugs have been related with SS in children, such as trimethoprim, all-trans-retinoic acid, and granulocyte colony-stimulating factor.[10–12] Other associations described in children have

Table 1
Main differences between childhood and adult Sweet syndrome[3–7]

	Children Disease	Adult Disease
Sex predominance	- Male predominance <3 y - Equal sex distribution >3–18 y	- Female predominance
Extracutaneous features	- More common cardiac involvement	- Ocular involvement is more common
Associations	- Stronger association with primary and secondary immunodeficiency - Malignancy remains unreported <3 y	- Notable association with malignancy in adults and children >3 y - Most frequent are myeloid line hematologic disorders (especially acute myelogenous leukemia)

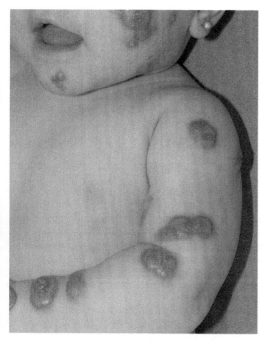

Fig. 1. Sweet syndrome in an infant.

been primary or secondary immune deficiency in 10%, nonmalignant hematologic disorders such as aplastic anemia, and other rare associations including alpha-1-antitrypsin deficiency, aseptic meningitis, autoimmune hepatitis, glycogen storage disease type 1b, systemic lupus erythematosus (SLE), and systemic inflammatory response syndrome.[5,10,11]

Malignancy must be searched for when the clinical history or the physical examination are suspicious, in the absence of an associated systemic disease, drug, or an infectious trigger, when clinical features are more related to the malignancy-associated type of SS, such as widespread, vesiculobullous or oral mucosal lesions, or in the presence of anemia and/or thrombocytopenia.[3]

Histopathology

SS in children, as in adults, is characterized the presence of a dense, perivascular or diffuse, neutrophilic infiltrate of the papillary and reticular dermis, with occasional eosinophils. In the subcutaneous variant, the neutrophilic infiltrate is seen in the subcutis. Edema of the papillary dermis and leukocytoclasia without frank vasculitis are additional features.[3]

Diagnosis

Criteria for diagnosis have been established (Box 2) and are equally operative for children.

Both major and 2 of 4 minor criteria are needed for the diagnosis. The presence of vasculitis does not exclude the diagnosis.

Prognosis and Outcome

SS heals without scarring, except for ulcerated lesions; post-inflammatory dyspigmentation is possible. Cardiovascular complications (sterile pericarditis, dilatation of the great vessels, valvular disease, and myocardial infarction) occur in 15% of pediatric cases, with a mortality of 40%, and are more common than in adults.[2,5]

Acquired cutis laxa secondary to SS, also known as Marshall's syndrome, manifests with post-inflammatory elastolysis of the heart and/or aorta, and may be fatal.[13–17] It has been reported that patients showing pathergy have a greater risk of Marshall's syndrome.[3] Thus, cardiovascular evaluation, including echocardiography, is mandatory when a cutis laxa phenotype develops.[3]

Most patients report rapid improvement after 1 to 3 days of corticosteroid therapy, and this is a cardinal feature of this disease. Recurrence occurs in approximately 20% to 30% of cases, or more frequently in case of hematologic disorders (50%),[1] with similar rates of recurrence in adults and children.[5,12,18–22]

Treatment

Although cutaneous lesions may resolve spontaneously within weeks or months, treatment is recommended (Table 2).

Table 2
Treatment of pediatric neutrophilic dermatoses

Condition	Therapy
Sweet syndrome[1,21]	Systemic steroids are the first choice: 1–2 mg/kg/day of prednisone until skin lesions have resolved, followed by tapering.[21] Other drugs used with variable success: colchicine, potassium iodine, cyclosporin, doxycycline, dapsone, clofazimine, IVIG, methotrexate, and indomethacin.[1]
Pyoderma gangrenosum[2,3,23–28]	Limited disease may be controlled with topical corticosteroids, but systemic corticosteroids are often needed (0.5–1 mg/kg/day prednisone, with potential use of higher doses up to 3 mg/kg and/or corticosteroid pulses). Second-line agents include dapsone, methotrexate, mycophenolate mofetil, and azathioprine.[3,24,25] TNF antagonists, such as infliximab and adalimumab, are used frequently with or without adjunctive systemic steroids, particularly when associated with IBD.[2,23,25] When PG appears in the context of autoinflammatory syndromes, IL-1 inhibitors such as anakinra are used.[23] In cases of severe, recalcitrant disease: • A trial of intravenous immune globulin or alkylating agents such as cyclophosphamide may be warranted. • IL-17 inhibitors, ixekizumab, brodalumab, and secukinumab, have also been used in refractory cases, and the latter has completed a phase I–II pilot study to evaluate the efficacy and safety in monotherapy for PG treatment.[26,27] However, there are several reports of paradoxic PG with secukinumab.[28] • IL-23 inhibitors, such as ustekinumab, tildrakizumab, guselkumab and risankizumab, have also been used in PG, as well as JAK inhibitors, including oral tofacitinib, oral ruxolitinib, and baricitinib.[27]
Behçet disease[29,30]	For mucocutaneous and articular phenotype (oral and genital ulcers, as well as musculoskeletal manifestations): colchicine in divided doses, alone or in combination with topical or intralesional corticosteroids, topical tacrolimus or pimecrolimus, topical lidocaine, or topical sucralfate have been recommended. For refractory cases, oral prednisolone 1 mg/kg/day, intravenous methylprednisolone 1 g/day for 3 d, methotrexate (0.2–0.4 mg/kg/week), or azathioprine (2.5 mg/kg/day) can be used. Apremilast has been approved for the treatment of BD in adults, and a clinical trial in children is ongoing. For extracutaneous manifestations and severe cases, the use of immunosuppressants, mainly azathioprine, and TNF-α inhibitors should be considered. Many clinical trials are expanding the therapeutic possibilities, including anti-IL-6 (tocilizumab), anti-IL-1 (anakinra and canakinumab), and anti-IL-17 agents (secukinumab), small molecules, and IFN-α.
Neutrophilic eccrine hidradenitis[31]	Treatment is not needed, as the condition has a self-resolving nature, but topical corticosteroids or oral analgesia can be used for pain control. If frequent recurrences, systemic treatment such as colchicine may be needed.
Neutrophilic dermatosis as the presentation of autoinflammatory disease in children[32–37]	CANDLE/PRAAS: • Oral corticosteroids and methotrexate provide only slight clinical benefit.[32] • Baricitinib, a Janus kinase 1/2 inhibitor, has demonstrated clinical and analytical improvement in patients with CANDLE syndrome.[32] DIRA: • Anakinra, the recombinant IL-1 receptor antagonist, and canakinumab have been used.[34]

(continued on next page)

Table 2 (*continued*)	
Condition	Therapy
	DITRA:
	• It has been treated with variable success with TNF-α, IL-12/23, and IL-17 inhibitors, whereas anti-IL-1 treatment has been showed less effective.[35]
	• Spesolimab is a monoclonal antibody targeting the IL-36 receptor and has been approved for the treatment of flares of pustular psoriasis and thus DITRA.[35]
	• Other antagonists of the IL-36 receptor, together with gevokizumab and canakinumab, two novels IL-1β inhibitors, are under preclinical and clinical trials in patients with autoinflammatory pustular psoriasis.[33]
	APLAID/PLAID syndrome:
	• Systemic corticosteroids may induce some clinical improvement and partial symptom control, but management is challenging.
	• Antihistamines, omalizumab, dapsone, and hydroxychloroquine may improve particular skin features.
	• Immunoglobulin replacement and prophylactic antibiotics may be administered for prevention of infectious diseases.
	• Anti-inflammatory therapy with anti-IL-1 and anti-TNF-α agents has induced heterogeneous responses.[37]
	For PAAND, CAPS, and NLRP1-related disorders, the anti-IL-1 treatment is highly effective.

Abbreviations: IVIG, intravenous immunoglobulin; TNF, tumor necrosis factor.

PYODERMA GANGRENOSUM
Clinical Care Points

- Pyoderma gangrenosum (PG) is a cutaneous ulcerative disease which usually manifests in adults as a single, painful ulcer on the lower extremities. In children, it is more frequently disseminated and shows no specific location, but head and neck are frequently involved.

- No underlying disease is identified in approximately half of the cases of PG in children; in the other half, inflammatory bowel disease is the most prevalent association. There is less frequent association with hematologic disorders than in adults.

- It may develop in the setting of the autoinflammatory disease spectrum of PAPA, PASH, and PAPASH.

- Limited disease may be controlled with topical corticosteroids, but systemic treatment is often needed. IL-1 inhibitors such as anakinra have been used in children when PG appears in the context of autoinflammatory syndromes.

PG is a cutaneous ulcerative disease frequently associated with systemic disease. PG may occur in all age groups but is more frequent between 20 and 50 years and only 4% of cases occur in children.[1] There is a female predominance in adults, but an equal sex distribution in children.[3] PG in infants is rare, with a few reports of PG before 1 year of age.[38]

An abnormal neutrophil trafficking, abnormal inflammation, and genetic factors with family cases of PG reported contribute to the pathogenesis of the disease. PG may develop in the setting of the AID spectrum of PAPA (pyogenic sterile arthritis, PG, and acne), PASH syndrome (PG, acne, hidradenitis suppurativa), and PAPASH (psoriatic arthritis, PG, acne, hidradenitis suppurativa). In a few cases of this spectrum, genetic variants in *NCSTN* and *PSTPIP1* have been identified, thus reinforcing the link between NDs and AIDs.[3,39–41] In addition, IL-18 and IL-16, a chemotactic agent increased in auto-inflammatory syndromes such as PAPA, play an important role in the induction of PG lesions.[23] Other potentially involved mediators are IL-1 and TNF-α.

Cutaneous Features

In adults, classical PG usually manifests as a single painful ulcer on the lower extremities, although it can occur anywhere (**Fig. 2**). In children, however, PG is more frequently disseminated and shows no specific location, but head and neck are frequently involved.[42] In infants, a particular distribution of perianal and genital lesions has been described.[38] Typically, PG begins as a tender

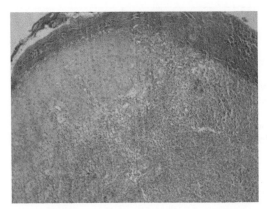

Fig. 2. Infantile pyoderma gangrenosum. Histology showing dense accumulation of neutrophils (H&E stain, original magnification 20X).

papule, pustule or bulla, nodule, or bulla with a surrounding erythematous or violaceus induration. This lesion undergoes necrosis, leading to a central ulcer with a purulent base and a gunmetal-colored border that usually extends centrifugally. The ulcer may expose tendons or muscles. Healing reepithelization starts in the ulcer borders and leaves atrophic, cribriform, pigmented scars.[1] Clinical variants of PG are presented in **Table 3**.

Associations

No underlying disease is identified in approximately half of the cases of PG in children; in the other half, inflammatory bowel disease (IBD) is the most prevalent association (Crohn's disease in 11% and ulcerative colitis in 10%), followed by hematologic disorders (8%), vasculitis (6%), immune deficiency (6%), and PAPA syndrome (4%).[23] As mentioned above, PG may be associated with specific genetic syndromes, including PAPA, PASH, and PAPASH.[23] Other associations reported in children are trauma-induced hyperzincemia and hypercalprotectinemia, isotretinoin-induced PG, Wilson's disease, type 1 diabetes, SLE, Sjogren's disease, and varicella.[23] PG may occur before, concurrent with, or after development of related systemic symptoms, with or without exacerbation of the underlying disease.[43–47]

In a review of pediatric PG, the association with hematologic malignancies and idiopathic cases tend to occur in pre-adolescent children, whereas IBD and PAPA are associated with PG in older children. **Table 4** summarizes the main differences between childhood and adult disease.

Histopathology

Histopathologic findings are not specific, but a biopsy is required to rule out alternative diagnoses,

mainly infections (see **Fig. 2**). Tissue from the ulcer edge should be sent for bacterial, mycobacterial, and fungal cultures, as well as for histopathologic study with routine and microbial stains.[3]

Diagnosis

Diagnostic criteria of PG are established and work well also in children (**Box 3**).

The major criteria and four minor criteria are needed for the diagnosis.

Treatment

Limited disease may be controlled with topical corticosteroids, but systemic treatment is often needed. It is summarized in **Table 2**.

BEHÇET DISEASE
Clinical Care Points

- Behçet disease (BD) is a chronic multisystem inflammatory disorder characterized by recurrent oral and genital ulcers with additional variable involvement of multiple organ systems.
- Ocular manifestations are the second most prevalent. Recurrent attacks of uveitis are reported in 70% of pediatric patients, with a reduction in visual acuity in 68% of pediatric cases, but 80% of the affected eyes improves after therapy
- The most severe manifestation of BD is central nervous system disease, which occurs in 5% to 25% of patients. Unlike adults, irreversible impairments are less frequent in children, with only definite sequelae in 17% of these.
- Treatment varies according to the many different presentations of BD in terms of severity and organ damage.

BD is a chronic multisystem inflammatory disorder characterized by recurrent oral and genital ulcers with additional variable involvement of multiple organ systems, including ocular, mucocutaneous, skeletal, vascular, GI, and nervous.[1,3] The pathogenesis of BD involves neutrophil-induced vascular injuries and autoimmunity.[1] BD affects people in their late 20s and early 30s, but children represent 4% to 26% of cases, including a transient variant seen in neonates whose mothers are diagnosed of BD. In a recent study including 230 children with BD, the mean age of the first symptom was 7.4 years, being oral ulcers the presenting sign in 87% to 98%.[48] The interval between the first and the second symptom was 2 years, which

Table 3
Clinical variants of pyoderma gangrenosum[1,3]

Variant	Clinical Aspect	Location	Particular Associations	Histology
Ulcerative (classic)	Inflammatory tender papule, pustule or bulla or nodule with a surrounding erythematous or violaceus induration that undergoes necrosis, leading to a central ulcer with a purulent base and a gunmetal border	Trunk and lower extremities		Neutrophilic abscess (center) and a lymphocytic angiocentric infiltrate (borders)
Bullous	Rapidly developing inflammatory bullae, which quickly evolve to superficial ulcers	Face and upper extremities	Hematologic diseases	Subepidermal bulla formation, intraepidermal vesicle formation, and neutrophilic dermal infiltrate
Pustular	Rapid development of multiple pustules with surrounding erythema		Fever and arthralgia. Inflammatory bowel disease	Subcorneal pustule, perifollicular neutrophilic infiltrate, dense dermal infiltrate with subepidermal edema
Vegetative/ superficial	Solitary nodule, plaque, or ulcer with more indolent presentation, verrucous surface and without undermined borders or purulent base.	Head and neck		Pseudoepitheliomatous hyperplasia, dermal neutrophilic abscesses, sinus tracts, and palisading granulomatous reaction

Table 4
Main differences between childhood and adult pyoderma gangrenosum[1,23,42]

	Children Disease	Adult Disease
Prevalence	• 4% of PG	• More frequent between 20 and 50 y
Sex distribution	• Equal sex distribution	• Female predominance
Location	• Disseminated, without a specific distribution pattern. • Head and neck more frequent locations than in adults • In infants, perianal, and genital ulcers	• Lower extremities and trunk
Clinical aspect	• Lesions are multiple more frequently than in adults	
Pathergy	• Frequently positive (62%)	• Rarely positive
Associations	• Idiopathic in about 50% of cases • IBD is most common both in children and adults • Less frequent association with hematologic disorders	• Between 50% and 70% have an underlying condition. • More frequent with hematologic disease (15%–25%)

Box 3
Diagnostic criteria of pyoderma gangrenosum[42]

Major

- Neutrophilic infiltrate on a biopsy of the ulcer edge

Minor

- Exclusion of infection on histologic stains and tissue cultures
- Pathergy
- History of inflammatory bowel disease or inflammatory arthritis
- Papule, vesicle, or pustule that rapidly ulcerates
- Peripheral erythema, undermined ulcer edge, and local tenderness
- Multiple ulcerations, with at least one on the anterior lower leg
- Cribriform scarring
- Improvement with 1 month of immunosuppressive therapy

Adapted from Schoch JJ, Tolkachjov SN, Cappel JA, Gibson LE, Davis DM. Pediatric Pyoderma gangrenosum: A retrospective review of clinical features, etiologic associations, and treatment. Pediatr Dermatol. 2017; 34: 39-45.

contributes to diagnostic delay.[48] In children, both males and females are equally affected, but clinical features are different; uveitis, vascular disease, and mortality are more common in boys, whereas genital aphthosis and erythema nodosum (EN) occur more frequently in girls. BD is more prevalent along the ancient Silk Road from eastern Asia to the Mediterranean coast, with highest prevalence in Turkey (420 per 100,000). HLA-B51/B5 has a strong association with BD, with a described prevalence of 57.2% in a large adult cohort, and a lower risk of gastrointestinal involvement. Familial cases are reported more frequently in children (10%–50% of cases). Genetic variants in the gene *TNFAIP3* gene, which causes haploinsufficiency of A20 (HA20), have been reported in a few children with BD clinical features as well as recurrent fever, severe gastrointestinal involvement, and absence of association with HLA-B51. Other gene loci have been involved in the pathogenesis of BD, such as *TLR4* and *MEFV*.[49]

Cutaneous Features

Clinically, BD is characterized by recurrent crops of oral ulcers that vary in size between several millimeters to more than 1 cm. The aphthae may be single or multiple, but mostly of the herpetiform type, with small foci of oral erythema developing into shallow, round to oval ulcerations, with regular and discrete borders, covered by a white, gray, or yellowish pseudomembrane.[1] Oral aphthae may arise on the mucous side of the lips, oral mucosa, tongue, or gingiva, whereas palate, tonsils, and pharynx are rarely involved. The ulcers tend to resolve without scarring in a few days, in the case of minor ulcers, but larger ulcers can take several weeks and result in scarring.[1,3] Genital ulcers are less frequent than oral ulcers, are less frequent in children (32%–82%) than in adults, and tend to be deeper and larger than oral ulcers; scarring is common. The perianal region may be also involved.[3] Other cutaneous manifestations are folliculitis, pustular and acneiform lesions on atypical sites, superficial thrombophlebitis, PG and EN-like lesions, palpable purpura, nailfold capillary abnormalities, and targetoid lesions. Pathergy is common, especially in endemic areas.[49]

Extracutaneous Features and Associations

Ocular manifestations are the second most prevalent (20%–50%) and include uveitis (more commonly anterior than posterior), hypopyon, necrotizing retinal vasculitis, posterior synechiae, cataracts, and cystoid macular edema or maculopathy. Recurrent attacks of uveitis are reported in 70% of pediatric patients, with a reduction in visual acuity in 68% of pediatric cases, but 80% of the affected eyes improves after therapy.[50] Gastrointestinal symptoms (abdominal pain, diarrhea, ulceration, bleeding and perforation) are not infrequent, affecting 4.8% to 56.5% of patients; they are related to the involvement of mainly terminal ileum or the ileocecal region.[51–53] Pediatric rate of vascular events ranges between 2% and 21%; vascular disease affects all sizes of vessels and deep vein thrombosis is the most frequent vascular event, as in adults. Arterial disease may present as aneurysm, pseudoaneurysm, thrombosis, and stenosis.[54] Musculoskeletal involvement occurs in 20% to 50%, with arthralgia or arthritis. The most severe manifestation of BD is CNS disease, which occurs in 5% to 25% of patients. CNS involvement may be "parenchymal" (transverse myelitis, brainstem, cerebral and multifocal disease manifesting as chronic headaches, hemiplegia, cranial nerve palsy, seizures, psychosis or cognitive dysfunctions, recurrent aseptic meningitis, meningoencephalitis, and optic neuropathy) and "non-parenchymal" disease (cerebral venous thrombosis, pseudotumor cerebri, and stroke). In contrast to adults, most of the children present with non-parenchymal disease and cerebral venous thrombosis is the most common manifestation. Unlike adults, irreversible impairments are less frequent in children, with only definite sequelae in 17% of these. Oral aphthae precede neurologic manifestations by years in children, whereas only one-third of adults have oral aphthae as the presenting symptom.[51–53] The clinical differences between pediatric and adult BD are summarized in **Table 5**.

Histopathology

Biopsy is not always useful, as inflammatory changes are not specific. Mucocutaneous lesions are due to a neutrophilic vascular reaction characterized by an obliterative/angiocentric lymphocytic infiltration of vessels of all sizes. Leukocytoclastic vasculitis, endothelial cell swelling, erythrocyte extravasation, fibrinoid necrosis, or vascular thrombosis can be seen. In later stages, an angiocentric lymphocytic infiltrate predominates.[1,3,5]

Regarding pustular or acneiform lesions, a neutrophilic vascular reaction is usually seen, but suppurative or mixed suppurative and granulomatous folliculitis also occurs.[1,3,5] BD-associated EN demonstrates septal panniculitis with medium vessel vasculitis, which differs from EN.[1–3]

Diagnosis

Diagnostic criteria have been redefined on several occasions. Criteria for childhood BD have been recently reviewed, and three of the following six criteria are required for a diagnosis of BD. The pathergy test is not included:[55]

1. Recurrent oral aphthosis (at least three flares per year)
2. Genital ulceration, typically with scar
3. Skin involvement: necrotic folliculitis, acneiform lesions, and erythema nodosum
4. Ocular involvement: anterior and posterior uveitis and retinal vasculitis
5. Neurologic signs, excluding isolated headaches
6. Vascular signs: venous thrombosis, arterial thrombosis, and arterial aneurysm

Treatment

Treatment varies according to the many different presentations of BD, in terms of severity and organ damage (see **Table 2**).[29]

NEUTROPHILIC ECCRINE HIDRADENITIS
Clinical Care Points

- Neutrophilic eccrine hidradenitis is characterized by crops of asymptomatic or painful erythematous papules, nodules, and plaques at different anatomic areas, especially palms and soles.

- In adults, it is mandatory to rule out an associated malignancy, while in children, it is often idiopathic with a self-resolving course, although some cases in association with acute myeloid leukemia and synovial sarcoma have been reported.

- In children, differential diagnosis may be established with the hot-foot syndrome, due to a *Pseudomonas aeruginosa* superficial infection of eccrine glands.

- Treatment is not needed, as the condition has a self-resolving nature, but topical corticosteroids or oral analgesia can be used for pain control.

Neutrophilic eccrine hidradenitis (NEH) is a benign ND due to a neutrophilic infiltration of the eccrine

---

Table 5
Main differences between pediatric and adult Behçet disease[49,50]

	Children	Adults
Familial aggregation	• High (10%–50%)	• Low (2.2%)
Mucocutaneous lesions (oral ulcers)	• Most patients present with recurrent oral ulcers (87%–98%) • Genital ulcers less frequent	• Only one-third of adults at initial presentation. • Genital ulcers more common than in children
Systemic manifestations	• More gastrointestinal symptoms, CNS involvement and arthralgia, and more acute exacerbations of uveitis (but visual prognosis is similar)	
Prognosis	• Better, lower BD severity scores and activity index	

glands and secretory coils, leading to their necrosis.[56] NEH is more frequent in adults, males, with a 2:1 male-to-female ratio, and often occurs associated with malignancy, especially in the context of using antineoplastic drugs, but this is uncommon in children.[31]

Cutaneous Features

NEH is characterized by crops of asymptomatic or painful erythematous papules, nodules, and plaques at different anatomic areas.[56]

Associations

First cases of NEH were described in adults diagnosed of acute myeloid leukemia and treated with chemotherapy, mostly cytarabine and daunorubicin. Lesions resolved when chemotherapy was finished, but reappeared in subsequent chemotherapy cycles when the same drug was used.[57] Later on, new etiologic factors have been implied, such as trauma or vigorous activity before the onset of symptoms or viral agents (HIV, hepatitis C, and COVID-19).[31,58]

In a recent cohort of 33 patients, 15 of 21 adults (71%) had an associated malignancy, most commonly acute myeloid leukemia. In this series, cutaneous lesions in the adult group not associated with tumors were localized to palms and soles, as in children. In children, NEH is more uncommon, but probably underreported, occurs specially during summer, is localized to palms and soles, and is often idiopathic with a self-resolving course (Table 6). Median age is 8.5 years.[31]

In the literature, there are cases of NEH in children associated with malignancy (acute myeloid leukemia, synovial sarcoma), although this is infrequent. In these cases, lesions are not localized to palms and soles, but arise in trunk and extremities.[31]

Diagnosis

Diagnosis is mainly clinic, although on histology there is a neutrophilic or mixed lymphocytic–neutrophilic infiltrate around eccrine glands and the secretory coils, but the hallmark of this disease is eccrine gland necrosis. Other possible features are eccrine intraductal abscesses, syringometaplasia, mild epidermal spongiosis, basal cell vacuolization with keratinocyte necrosis, or focal to superficial panniculitis.[31]

In children, differential diagnosis may be established with the hot-foot syndrome due to a *P aeruginosa* superficial infection of eccrine glands. Hot-foot syndrome develops after exposure to pool water containing high concentrations of *P aeruginosa* and has a benign self-limited course. Other conditions to rule out are EN, insect bites, or traumatic-pressure urticaria.[58,59]

Prognosis and Outcome

Prognosis is generally good. However, malignancy-associated cases have less recurrences than idiopathic ones, which more often need systemic treatment such as colchicine. Thus, in children, the recurrence rate has been described of 33%, higher than in adults, probably due to the more frequent idiopathic cases.[31]

Treatment

Treatment is summarized in **Table 2**.

NEUTROPHILIC DERMATOSIS AS THE PRESENTATION OF AUTOINFLAMMATORY DISEASE IN CHILDREN
Clinical Care Points

- Several infantile-onset autoinflammatory diseases (AIDs) can present with prominent skin manifestations with neutrophilic infiltration.

- Chronic atypical neutrophilic dermatosis (ND) with lipodystrophy and elevated temperature is an autoinflammatory type I interferonopathy which is included within the group of NDs because histologic features are very characteristic, with dense skin neutrophilic infiltrates.

- The deficiency of interleukin-36 receptor antagonist and deficiency of interleukin-1 receptor antagonist are autoinflammatory syndromes characterized by recurrent episodes of generalized pustular psoriasis since childhood.

- In *PLCG2*-associated antibody deficiency and immune dysregulation or autoinflammation and *PLCG2*-associated antibody deficiency and immune dysregulation, alterations in PLCG2 lead to an abnormal activation of neutrophils and monocytes triggered by cold.

- Pyrin-associated autoinflammation with ND is a monogenic AID presenting with different NDs such as acne, hidradenitis suppurativa (HS), pyoderma gangrenosum, neutrophilic small vessel vasculitis, and sterile skin abscesses.

- Cryopyrin-associated periodic syndrome is a group of hereditary autoinflammatory syndromes encompassing familial cold autoinflammatory syndrome as the mildest form, Muckle–Wells syndrome as the intermediate variant, and neonatal-onset multisystem inflammatory disease as the most severe phenotype; histopathology is characterized by a neutrophil-rich dermal infiltrate.

Table 6
Main differences between childhood and adult neutrophilic eccrine hidradenitis[31]

	Children	Adults
Associations	Idiopathic > malignancy-associated	Malignancy, most commonly hematologic, and chemotherapy
Preferred anatomic location	Palmoplantar	Axillae, face, trunk, extremities
Prognostic	More recurrences	Less recurrences

As it has been mentioned above, several infantile-onset AIDs can present with prominent skin manifestations with neutrophilic infiltration, thus considered within the spectrum of ND. As these autoinflammatory disorders have a different etiopathogenic basis, the therapeutic targets are different and are summarized in **Table 2**.

Chronic Atypical Neutrophilic Dermatosis Neutrophilic Dermatosis with Lipodystrophy and Elevated Temperature Syndrome

Chronic atypical ND with lipodystrophy and elevated temperature (CANDLE), also named proteasome-associated autoinflammatory syndrome (PRAAS), is a prototypic autoinflammatory type I interferonopathy.[60–62]

Clinical Features

Patients with type I interferonopathies present early in life, even within the first week, but late-onset cases during the second decade have been described. Among skin manifestations, patients may present with acral perniotic lesions, not always triggered by cold exposure, and mostly located on the nose, ears, fingers, or toes. These lesions are more prominent in newborns and infants, and less frequent since childhood, and may overlap with those of other interferonopathies, such as stimulator of interferon genes (STING)-associated vasculopathy with onset in infancy (SAVI), and Aicardi–Goutieres syndrome (AGS). Certain cutaneous findings are characteristic of CANDLE, such as periorbital and, less commonly, perioral edema, violaceous annular plaques with raised border and a flat purpuric center, and neutrophilic panniculitis that leads to progressive lipodystrophy (**Fig. 3**). Although there is some degree of continuous skin involvement, common triggers of exacerbations are cold and viral infections.[62,63]

Patients present with almost daily recurrent fever or elevated temperature, growth delay, and progressive loss of fat. There is also chronic and/or episodic systemic inflammation in other organs, such as CNS, joints, or cartilages, among others.[63]

Diagnosis

Histologic features are very characteristic, with a perivascular and interstitial infiltrate extending to the subcutaneous fat, as a lobar neutrophilic panniculitis. The presence in the infiltrate of immature myeloid, mononuclear cells, as well as neutrophils and karyorrhexis is most indicative of CANDLE syndrome (see **Fig. 3**).[57] Immunohistochemistry shows positivity for myeloperoxidase and CD68 in the infiltrate; CD123 positivity in clusters is also characteristic.[61]

The presence of a chronically elevated peripheral blood interferon (IFN) signature is also a common finding in patients with the type I interferonopathies CANDLE, SAVI, and AGS.[62]

Genetic diagnosis is recommended.[53] Biallelic PSMB8 variants are the most common cause of CANDLE, but digenic heterozygous variants in other genes encoding proteasome or immunoproteasome subunits have also been reported.[62,63]

Deficiency of Interleukin-1 Receptor Antagonist, Deficiency of Interleukin-36 Receptor Antagonist, Pustular Psoriasis, and Related Pustular Skin Diseases

Several genetic variants in six genes have been implicated in pustular psoriasis: the interleukin-36 receptor antagonist (IL36RN), the caspase recruitment domain-containing protein 14 (CARD14), adaptor protein complex 1 subunit sigma 3 (AP1S3), TNFAIP3-interacting protein 1 (TNIP1), serine protease inhibitor gene serpin family A member 3 (SERPINA3), and the IL-1 receptor antagonist (IL-1RA) gene (IL1RN). Mutations in these genes lead to an absence of opposition to the pro-inflammatory activity of cytokines IL-1α and IL-1β, and NF-κB activation.[33] The deficiency of interleukin-36 receptor antagonist (DITRA) and deficiency of interleukin-1 receptor antagonist (DIRA) are autoinflammatory syndromes characterized by recurrent episodes of generalized pustular psoriasis since childhood.[64]

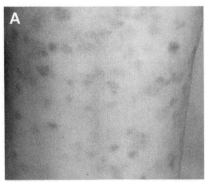
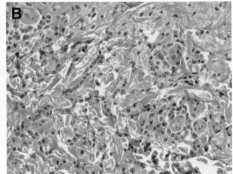

Fig. 3. CANDLE syndrome. (*A*) Purpuric, round, and annular lesions. (*B*) Histology showing interstitial infiltrate of mononuclear cells with atypical nuclei (H&E stain, original magnification 100X).

Cutaneous Features

Skin lesions are innumerable, generalized, sterile pustules that may have an acute, subacute, or, occasionally, chronic presentation (**Fig. 4**).[33]

Extracutaneous Features

DIRA may present with severe systemic complications such as respiratory insufficiency and thrombotic events, and mortality secondary to multiorgan failure has been described, though rarely. Bone changes, including epiphyseal ballooning of long bones, anterior rib-end widening, periosteal elevation of long bones and multifocal osteolytic lesions, have been also described. CNS involvement secondary to vasculitis may be rarely seen in DIRA.[64,65]

DITRA begins early in childhood and skin lesions are accompanied by high fever, asthenia and elevation of inflammatory laboratory markers, with less systemic involvement in comparison with DIRA.[64,66]

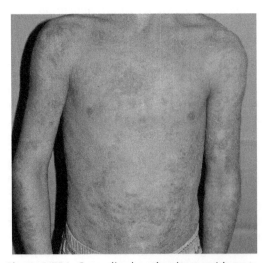

Fig. 4. DITRA. Generalized erythroderma with pustular lesions.

Treatment

Anakinra, the recombinant IL-1 receptor antagonist, and canakinumab have been used to treat patients with DIRA.[34] DITRA has been treated with variable success with TNF-α, IL-12/23, and IL-17 inhibitors, whereas anti-IL-1 treatment has been showed less effective.[64] Spesolimab is a monoclonal antibody blocking IL-36 signature and has been approved for the treatment of flares of pustular psoriasis and thus DITRA.[36] Other antagonists of the IL-36 receptor and gevokizumab, an experimental IL-1β inhibitor, are under preclinical and clinical trials in patients with autoinflammatory pustular psoriasis.[33]

PLCG2-Associated Antibody Deficiency and Immune Dysregulation and Autoinflammation and PLCG2-Associated Antibody Deficiency and Immune Dysregulation Syndromes

Gain-of-function variants in the *phospholipase C gamma 2 (PLCG2)* gene can cause *PLCG2*-associated antibody deficiency and immune dysregulation (PLAID) or autoinflammation and *PLCG2*-associated antibody deficiency and immune dysregulation (APLAID) syndrome.[67] In PLAID and APLAID, alterations in PLCG2 lead to an abnormal activation of neutrophils and monocytes at subphysiologic temperature, which may be enhanced in colder temperatures. This results in macrophage activation and granuloma formation, predominantly on cold skin surfaces, sparing intertriginous warmer areas.[67]

Cutaneous Features

Cutaneous features in PLAID and APLAID syndromes are triggered by cold or arise in colder body areas.

In PLAID, spontaneous ulceration of the nasal tip developing on the early neonatal period is characteristic, with a hemorrhagic crusted appearance that undergoes spontaneous resolution within several weeks or continues until tissue destruction and erosion of the nasal cartilage.[67] Patients with PLAID may also develop granulomas which spare warmer skin folds, areas of friction, or the skin overlying the vertebral column, and have the aspect of erythematous plaques or nodules on the face, sparing the scalp, the nasolabial folds, and the periorbital regions, which evolve into scaly red-brown or yellowish plaques with telangiectasias as well as hypertrichosis.[68] Cold urticaria in PLAID develops within the first year of life and often resolves with antihistamines, cold avoidance, or rapid rewarming.[68]

The most characteristic cutaneous manifestation of APLAID is the so-called "perforating neutrophilic and granulomatous dermatitis of the newborn," which appears very early in the neonatal period as an extensive pustular eruption (Fig. 5). Later, new lesions in the form of erythematous papules and plaques that later become hemorrhagic, pustular, and crusted, to eventually leave cribriform scarring. Histopathology shows a combination of interstitial granulomatous inflammation, sometimes with palisading, and accumulation of neutrophils in the upper dermis. The granulomatous material is extruded through transepidermal elimination.[69,70] Patients with APLAID lack cold-induced urticaria, but there are cases of overlapping PLAID/APLAID syndromes.[37]

Extracutaneous Features

As PLCG2 is expressed in lymphoid and myeloid cells except T cells, patients with PLAID have an impaired B-cell and NK cell activation. Thus, two-thirds of patients present with a high frequency of positive antinuclear antibodies, autoimmunity, and immunosuppression.[37]

Patients with APLAID present with symptoms of autoinflammation, such as uveitis, colitis, lung inflammation, and recurrent bacterial and viral sinopulmonary infections due to inappropriate production of antibodies. Unlike PLAID, APLAID patients do not have substantial autoantibody formation and inflammatory markers are normal.[71]

Treatment

Management is challenging. Systemic corticosteroids may induce some clinical improvement and partial symptom control. Antihistamines, omalizumab, dapsone, and hydroxychloroquine may improve some skin features. Immunoglobulin replacement and prophylactic antibiotics may be administered for prevention of infectious diseases. Anti-inflammatory therapy with anti-IL-1 and anti-TNF-α agents has induced heterogeneous responses.[37]

Pyrin-Associated Autoinflammation with Neutrophilic Dermatosis and Cryopyrin-Associated Periodic Syndrome

Pyrin-associated autoinflammation with ND (PAAND) is a monogenic AID caused by the p.S242 R MEFV variant.[72] Although MEFV is also mutated in patients with familial Mediterranean fever (FMF), and there is a high degree of overlap between PAAND and FMF, patients with PAAND present with different NDs such as acne, HS, PG, neutrophilic small vessel vasculitis, and sterile skin abscesses, evidencing also a high degree of overlap between PAPA and PAAND syndromes.[72,73] PAAND may rarely be complicated by amyloidosis.[74]

Cryopyrin-associated periodic syndrome (CAPS) is a group of hereditary autoinflammatory syndromes encompassing familial cold autoinflammatory syndrome (FCAS) as the mildest form, Muckle–Wells syndrome (MWS) as the intermediate variant, and neonatal-onset multisystem inflammatory disease (NOMID) as the most severe phenotype (Table 7).[75]

CAPS is due to 200 different underlying heterozygous gain-of-function variants within the nucleotide-binding domain like receptor protein 3 (NLRP3) gene, a protein necessary to the assembly of the NLRP3 inflammasome. CAPS presents with cutaneous atypical, rarely-itching, urticarial lesions or a maculo-papular rash, which is often symmetrically distributed on the trunk and/or extremities. Skin lesions may cause burning sensations and pain, occur daily, last for up to 24 h and aggravate during the course of the day, with a peak in the evening. In the case of FCAS and MWS, they are triggered and exacerbated by cold air or evaporative cooling of the skin, whereas direct cold exposure does not induce the skin lesions. Histopathology is characterized by a neutrophil-rich dermal infiltrate. Skin lesions

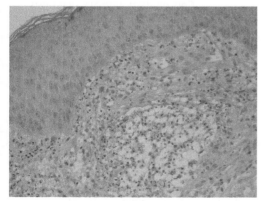

Fig. 5. APLAID. Subepidermal accumulation of neutrophils with some histiocytes (H&E stain, original magnification 40X).

Table 7
Cryopyrin-associated periodic syndromes[72]

	FCAS	MWS	NOMID
Duration of episodes	12–24 h	1–3 d	Chronic, with flares each 1–3 d
Triggers of skin lesions	Cold air-induced urticarial rash	Cold air-induced urticarial rash	Urticarial rash
Musculoskeletal	Arthralgias, myalgias	Arthralgias, myalgias, arthritis	Arthralgias, myalgias, arthritis, femur overgrowth
Ocular	Conjunctivitis, keratitis	Conjunctivitis, keratitis, uveitis	Conjunctivitis, keratitis, uveitis, papillitis
CNS symptoms	Headache	Headache, sensorineural hearing loss	Sensorineural hearing loss, sterile meningitis, elevated intracranial pressure, developmental delay
Amyloidosis	Rare	Possible	Possible

Adapted from Moghaddas F, Llamas R, De Nardo D, et al. A novel Pyrin-Associated Autoinflammation with Neutrophilic Dermatosis mutation further defines 14-3-3 binding of pyrin and distinction to Familial Mediterranean Fever. Ann Rheum Dis. 2017 Dec; 76(12): 2085-2094.

are accompanied by recurrent fever episodes and elevated levels of inflammatory markers.[75] The anti-IL-1 treatment is highly effective.

NEUTROPHILIC DERMATOSIS AS THE PRESENTATION OF SYSTEMIC LUPUS ERYTHEMATOSUS IN CHILDREN
Clinical Care Points

- Neutrophilic infiltrates in patients with systemic lupus erythematosus are well-described, such as neutrophilic urticarial dermatosis and Sweet-like neutrophilic dermatosis.

- They may be the initial symptom in one-third of cases and have also been reported within neonatal lupus erythematosus.

Neutrophilic infiltrates in patients with SLE are rare and transient, but well-described, and may appear as bullous SLE, leukocytoclastic vasculitis, SS, PG, palisaded neutrophilic granulomatous dermatitis, amicrobial pustulosis of the folds, neutrophilic

Table 8
Main differences within neutrophilic urticarial dermatosis and Sweet-like neutrophilic dermatosis [76]

	NUD	SLND
Associations	Schnitzler syndrome, adult-onset Still's disease, SLE, and cutaneous LE	Malignancy, most commonly hematologic, and chemotherapy
Diagnosis	Often after SLE diagnosis	Concomitant with SLE diagnosis in 60%
Skin lesions	Asymptomatic, or slightly pruritic, erythematous flat macules or patches or minimally raised papules	Pruritic or asymptomatic erythematous-edematous plaques or nodules
Anatomic location	Face, trunk, and extremities	Never appears on the trunk
Photodistributed	Never	Always
Systemic symptoms	Fever and arthralgias	Systemic signs of SLE
Flares of SLE	Rarely coincident	Coincident in 80% of cases
Histology	Perivascular or interstitial neutrophilic infiltration	Higher density of neutrophilic infiltration
Differential diagnosis	Adult-onset Still's disease (NUD lacks leukocytosis, lymphadenopathy, hepatosplenomegaly, and elevation of serum ferritin and shows positivity for serum antinuclear antibodies)	SS (SLND is photodistributed and shows less intense neutrophilic infiltrate)

urticarial dermatosis (NUD), and Sweet-like ND (SLND) (**Table 8**).

These nonbullous or nonvasculitic NDs in patients with LE have also named as autoimmunity-related ND. They may be the initial symptom of SLE patients in one-third of cases and have also been reported within neonatal lupus erythematosus.[76,77]

DISCLOSURE

The authors declare that they have no conflicts of interest.

REFERENCES

1. Davis MD, Moschella SL. Neutrophilic dermatosis. In: Bologna JL, Jorizzo JL, Schaffer JM, editors. *Dermatology*. 4th edition. Philadelphia: Elsevier-Saunders; 2018. p. 453–71.
2. Bucchia M, Barbarot S, Reumaux H, et al. Groupe de recherche de la Société Française de Dermatologie Pédiatrique; Société Francophone pour la rhumatologie et les Maladies Inflammatoires en Pédiatrie (SOFREMIP). Age-specific characteristics of neutrophilic dermatoses and neutrophilic diseases in children. J Eur Acad Dermatol Venereol 2019;33:2179–87.
3. Levy R, Lara-Corrales I. Neutrophilic and eosinophilic diseases. In: Torrelo A. Schachner & Hansen pediatric Dermatology. New Delhi: Jaypee Brothers; 2023. p. 759–82.
4. Cohen PR. Sweet's syndrome - a comprehensive review of an acute febrile neutrophilic dermatosis. Orphanet J Rare Dis 2007;2:34.
5. Halpern J, Salim A. Pediatric sweet syndrome: case report and literature review. Pediatr Dermatol 2009; 26:452–7.
6. Cohen PR, Kurzrock R. Sweet's syndrome and cancer. Clin Dermatol 1993;11:149–57.
7. Davies R. Limbal nodules in Sweet's syndrome. Aust N Z J Ophthalmol 1992;20:263–5.
8. Gray PE, Bock V, Ziegler DS, et al. Neonatal Sweet syndrome: a potential marker of serious systemic illness. Pediatrics 2012;129:e1353–9.
9. Parsapour K, Reep MD, Gohar K, et al. Familial Sweet's syndrome in 2 brothers, both seen in the first 2 weeks of life. J Am Acad Dermatol 2003;49:132–8.
10. Al-Saad K, KhananiMF, Naqvi A, et al. Sweet syndrome developing during treatment with all-trans retinoic acid in a child with acute myelogenous leukaemia. J Pediatr Hematol Oncol 2004;26:197–9.
11. Shimizu T, Yoshida I, Eguchi H, et al. Sweet syndrome in a child with aplastic anemia receiving recombinant granulocyte colony stimulating factor. J Pediatr Hematol Oncol 1996;18:282–4.
12. Uihlein LC, Brandling-Bennett HA, Lio PA, et al. Sweet syndrome in children. Pediatr Dermatol 2012;29:38–44.
13. Christensen CC, Gonzalez-Crussi F. Postinflammatory elastolysis and cutis laxa: report of a case with aortitis. Pediatr Pathol 1983;1:199–210.
14. Muster AJ, Bharati S, Herman JJ, et al. Fatal cardiovascular disease and cutis laxa following acute febrile neutrophilic dermatosis. J Pediatr 1983;102:243–8.
15. Guia JM, Frias J, Castro FJ, et al. Cardiovascular involvement in a boy with Sweet's syndrome. Pediatr Cardiol 1999;20:295–7.
16. Guhamajumdar M, Agarwala B. Sweet syndrome, cutis laxa, and fatal cardiac manifestations in a 2-year-old girl. Texas Heart Institute J 2011;38:285–7.
17. Hwang ST, Williams ML, McCalmont TH, et al. Sweet's syndrome leading to acquired cutis laxa (Marshall's syndrome) in an infant with alpha 1-antitrypsin deficiency. Arch Dermatol 1995;131:1175–7.
18. Cohen PR, Kurzrock R. Sweet's syndrome: A neutrophilic dermatosis classically associated with acute onset and fever. Clin Dermatol 2000;18:265–82.
19. Fitzgerald RL, McBurney EI, Nesbitt LT Jr. Sweet's syndrome. Int J Dermatol 1996;35:9–15.
20. Fett DL, Gibson LE, Su WP. Sweet's syndrome: systemic signs and symptoms and associated disorders. Mayo Clin Proc 1995;70:234–40.
21. Boatman BW, Taylor RC, Klein LE, et al. Sweet's syndrome in children. South Med J 1994;87:193–6.
22. Cohen PR, Talpaz M, Kurzrock R. Malignancy-associated Sweet's syndrome: a review of the world literature. J Clin Oncol 1988;6:1887–97.
23. Kechichian E, Haber R, Mourad N, et al. Pediatric pyoderma gangrenosum: a systematic review and update. Int J Dermatol 2017;56:486–95.
24. Wollina U. Pyoderma gangrenosum-a review. Orphanet J Rare Dis 2007;2:19.
25. Alavi A, French LE, Davis MD, et al. Pyoderma Gangrenosum: An Update on Pathophysiology, Diagnosis and Treatment. Am J Clin Dermatol 2017;18:355–72.
26. Tantcheva-Poor I, Broekaert IJ. Infliximab is an appropriate second-line therapy in infants with steroid refractory pyoderma gangrenosum. J Eur Acad Dermatol Venereol 2022;36:e376–8.
27. Maronese CA, Pimentel MA, Li MM, et al. Pyoderma Gangrenosum: An Updated Literature Review on Established and Emerging Pharmacological Treatments. Am J Clin Dermatol 2022;23:615–34.
28. Avcı C, Akın G, Akarsu S, et al. Pyoderma gangrenosum and Behçet's-like disease induced by secukinumab: a paradoxical drug reaction. J Dermatolog Treat 2023;34:2235040.
29. Bettiol A, Hatemi G, Vannozzi L, et al. Treating the Different Phenotypes of Behçet's Syndrome. Front Immunol 2019;10:2830.
30. Giani T, Luppino AF, Ferrara G. Treatment Options in Pediatric Behçet's Disease. Paediatr Drugs 2023; 25(2):165–91.

31. Isaq NA, Anand N, Camilleri MJ, et al. Neutrophilic eccrine hidradenitis: a retrospective study. Int J Dermatol 2023;62(9):1142–6.

32. Kanazawa N, Ishii T, Takita Y, et al. Efficacy and safety of baricitinib in Japanese patients with autoinflammatory type I interferonopathies (NNS/CANDLE, SAVI, And AGS). Pediatr Rheumatol Online J 2023; 21(1):38.

33. Uppala R, Tsoi LC, Harms PW, et al. "Autoinflammatory psoriasis"-genetics and biology of pustular psoriasis. Cell Mol Immunol 2021;18(2):307–17.

34. Romano M, Arici ZS, Piskin D, et al. The 2021 EULAR/American College of Rheumatology points to consider for diagnosis, management and monitoring of the interleukin-1 mediated autoinflammatory diseases: cryopyrin-associated periodic syndromes, tumour necrosis factor receptor-associated periodic syndrome, mevalonate kinase deficiency, and deficiency of the interleukin-1 receptor antagonist. Ann Rheum Dis 2022;81(7):907–21.

35. Hospach T, Glowatzki F, Blankenburg F, et al. Scoping review of biological treatment of deficiency of interleukin-36 receptor antagonist (DITRA) in children and adolescents. Pediatr Rheumatol Online J 2019;17(1):37.

36. Blair HA. Spesolimab: First Approval. Drugs 2022; 82(17):1681–6.

37. Welzel T, Oefelein L, Holzer U, et al. Variant in the PLCG2 Gene May Cause a Phenotypic Overlap of APLAID/PLAID: Case Series and Literature Review. J Clin Med 2022;11(15):4369.

38. Graham JA, Hansen KK, Rabinowitz LG, et al. Pyoderma gangrenosum in infants and children. Pediatr Dermatol 1994;11(1):10–7.

39. Demidowich AP, Freeman AF, Kuhns DB, et al. Brief report: genotype, phenotype, and clinical course in five patients with PAPA syndrome (pyogenic sterile arthritis, pyoderma gangrenosum, and acne). Arthritis Rheum 2012;64:2022–7.

40. Marzano AV, Trevisan V, Gattorno M, et al. Pyogenic arthritis, pyoderma gangrenosum, acne, and hidradenitis suppurativa (PAPASH): a new autoinflammatory syndrome associated with a novel mutation of the PSTPIP1 gene. JAMA Dermatol 2013;149:762–4.

41. Duchatelet S, Miskinyte S, Join-Lambert O, et al. First nicastrin mutation in PASH (pyoderma gangrenosum, acne and suppurative hidradenitis) syndrome. Br J Dermatol 2015;173:610–2.

42. Schoch JJ, Tolkachjov SN, Cappel JA, et al. Pediatric Pyoderma gangrenosum: A retrospective review of clinical features, etiologic associations, and treatment. Pediatr Dermatol 2017;34:39–45.

43. Powell FC, Perry HO. Pyoderma gangrenosum in childhood. Arch Dermatology 1984;120:757–61.

44. Powell FC, Schroeter AL, Su WP, et al. Pyoderma gangrenosum: a review of 86 patients. Quarterly J Med 1985;55:173–86.

45. Farhi D, Cosnes J, Zizi N, et al. Significance of erythema nodosum and pyoderma gangrenosum in inflammatory bowel diseases: A cohort study of 2402 patients. Medicine 2008;87:281–93.

46. Blitz NM, Rudikoff D. Pyoderma gangrenosum. Mt Sinai. J Med 2001;68:287–97.

47. Katz SK, Gordon KB, Roenigk HH. The cutaneous manifestations of gastrointestinal disease. PrimaryCare 1996;23:455–76.

48. Lesmeister LM, Peitz J, von Kleist-Retzow JC, et al. Consensus classification criteria for paediatric Behçet's disease from a prospective observational cohort: PEDBD. Ann Rheum Dis 2016;75(6):958–64.

49. Burns E, Cooper E, Peterson R, et al. Pediatric Behçet disease: Update in diagnosis and management. Pediatr Dermatol 2022;39(2):173–81.

50. Kramer M, Amer R, Mukamel M, et al. Uveitis in juvenile Behçet's disease: clinical course and visual outcome compared with adult patients. Eye (Lond). 2009;23(11):2034–41.

51. Karincaoglu Y, Borlu M, Toker SC, et al. Demographic and clinical properties of juvenile-onset Behçet's disease: a controlled multicenter study. J Am Acad Dermatol 2008;58:579–84.

52. Nanthapisal S, Klein NJ, Ambrose N, et al. Paediatric Behçet's disease: a UK tertiary centre experience. Clin Rheumatol 2016;35:2509–16.

53. Gallizzi R, Pidone C, Cantarini L, et al. A national cohort study on pediatric Behçet's disease: crosssectional data from an Italian registry. Pediatr Rheumatol Online J 2017;15:84.

54. Yıldız M, Köker O, Adrovic A, et al. Pediatric Behçet's disease - clinical aspects and current concepts. Eur J Rheumatol 2019;7(Suppl 1):1–10.

55. Batu ED. Diagnostic/classification criteria in pediatric Behçet's disease. Rheumatol Int 2019;39(1):37–46.

56. Nelson CA, Stephen S, Ashchyan HJ, et al. Neutrophilic dermatoses: pathogenesis, Sweet syndrome, neutrophilic eccrine hidradenitis, and Behcet disease. J Am Acad Dermatol 2018;79:987–1006.

57. Harrist TJ, Fine JD, Berman RS, et al. Neutrophilic eccrine hidradenitis. A distinctive type of neutrophilic dermatosis associated with myelogenous leukemia and chemotherapy. Arch Dermatol 1982;118:263–6.

58. Ben-Amitai D, Hodak E, Landau M, et al. Idiopathic palmoplantar eccrine hidradenitis in children. Eur J Pediatr 2001;160:189–91.

59. Fiorillo L, Zucker M, Sawyer D, et al. The pseudomonas hot-foot syndrome. N Engl J Med 2001; 345(5):335–8.

60. Torrelo A, Patel S, Colmenero I, et al. Chronic atypical neutrophilic dermatosis with lipodystrophy and elevated temperature (CANDLE) syndrome. J Am Acad Dermatol 2010;62(3):489–95.

61. Torrelo A, Colmenero I, Requena L, et al. Histologic and Immunohistochemical Features of the Skin

Lesions in CANDLE Syndrome. Am J Dermatopathol 2015;37(7):517–22.

62. Cetin Gedik K, Lamot L, Romano M, et al. The 2021 European Alliance of Associations for Rheumatology/American College of Rheumatology points to consider for diagnosis and management of autoinflammatory type I interferonopathies: CANDLE/PRAAS, SAVI and AGS. Ann Rheum Dis 2022; 81(5):601–13.

63. Torrelo A. CANDLE Syndrome As a Paradigm of Proteasome-Related Autoinflammation. Front Immunol 2017;8:927.

64. Marzano AV, Damiani G, Genovese G, et al. A dermatologic perspective on autoinflammatory diseases. Clin Exp Rheumatol 2018;36(Suppl 110):32–8.

65. Aksentijevich I, Masters SI, Ferguson PJ, et al. An autoinflammatory disease with deficiency of the interleukin-1-receptor antagonist. N Engl J Med 2009;360:2426–37.

66. Marrakchi S, Guigue P, Renshaw BR, et al. Interleukin-36-receptor antagonist deficiency and generalized pustular psoriasis. N Engl J Med 2011;365:620–8.

67. Aderibigbe OM, Priel DL, Lee CC, et al. Distinct Cutaneous Manifestations and Cold-Induced Leukocyte Activation Associated With PLCG2 Mutations. JAMA Dermatol 2015;151(6):627–34.

68. Milner JD. PLAID: a Syndrome of Complex Patterns of Disease and Unique Phenotypes. J Clin Immunol 2015;35(6):527–30.

69. Morán-Villaseñor E, Sáez-de-Ocariz M, Torrelo A, et al. Expanding the clinical features of autoinflammation and phospholipase Cγ2-associated antibody deficiency and immune dysregulation by description of a novel patient. J Eur Acad Dermatol Venereol 2019;33(12):2334–9.

70. Torrelo A, Vera A, Portugués M, et al. Perforating neutrophilic and granulomatous dermatitis of the newborn-a clue to immunodeficiency. Pediatr Dermatol 2007;24(3):211–5.

71. Zhou Q, Lee GS, Brady J, et al. A hypermorphic missense mutation in PLCG2, encoding phospholipase Cγ2, causes a dominantly inherited autoinflammatory disease with immunodeficiency. Am J Hum Genet 2012;91(4):713–20.

72. Moghaddas F, Llamas R, De Nardo D, et al. A novel Pyrin-Associated Autoinflammation with Neutrophilic Dermatosis mutation further defines 14-3-3 binding of pyrin and distinction to Familial Mediterranean Fever. Ann Rheum Dis 2017;76(12):2085–94.

73. Vahidnezhad H, Youssefian L, Saeidian AH, et al. Homozygous MEFV Gene Variant and Pyrin-Associated Autoinflammation With Neutrophilic Dermatosis: A Family With a Novel Autosomal Recessive Mode of Inheritance. JAMA Dermatol 2021;157(12):1 466–1471.

74. Kiyota M, Oya M, Ayano M, et al. First case of pyrin-associated autoinflammation with neutrophilic dermatosis complicated by amyloidosis. Rheumatology 2020;59(9):e41–3.

75. Booshehri LM, Hoffman HM. CAPS and NLRP3. J Clin Immunol 2019;39(3):277–86.

76. Lee WJ, Kang HJ, Shin HJ, et al. Neutrophilic urticarial dermatosis and Sweet-like neutrophilic dermatosis: under-recognized neutrophilic dermatoses in lupus erythematosus. Lupus 2018;27(4):628–36.

77. Satter EK, High WA. Non-bullous neutrophilic dermatosis within neonatal lupus erythematosus. J Cutan Pathol 2007;34(12):958–60.

Neutrophilic Panniculitides

Ganesh B. Maniam, MD, MBA*, Anne Coakley, MD, Giang Huong Nguyen, MD, DPhil,
Afsaneh Alavi, MD, Mark D.P. Davis, MD

KEYWORDS

- Neutrophilic dermatoses • Neutrophilic panniculitis • Pancreatic panniculitis
- Alpha-1 antitrypsin deficiency • Pfeifer-Weber-Christian disease • Sweet syndrome
- subcutaneous sweet syndrome • Drug-induced panniculitis

KEY POINTS

- Panniculitides are a clinically and histopathologically diverse group of conditions for which the unifying feature is prominent inflammation of subcutaneous fat under histopathological examination.
- Vacuoles, E1 enzyme, X-linked, Autoinflammatory, Somatic syndrome is an example of a newly described autoinflammatory disorder with spectrum of cutaneous manifestations including neutrophilic dermatoses and panniculitides.
- Treatments for most panniculitides are based on case reports and case series, which indicate a need for larger studies through multi-institutional collaboration.

INTRODUCTION

Neutrophilic panniculitis is characterized by neutrophilic inflammation involving the subcutaneous fat tissue. As panniculitides are a wide spectrum of inflammatory conditions affecting the subcutis, there are several conditions that could cause panniculitis.[1] Despite the diverse clinical etiologies of neutrophilic panniculitis, there are monotonous morphologic findings, and thus, biopsy is usually required for definitive diagnosis. Although recently proposed clinical algorithms split panniculitides into commonly ulcerative or nonulcerative processes (**Fig. 1**), most rely on histopathological characteristics to split panniculitides into septal versus lobular inflammation followed by the presence or absence of vasculitis. There are a large number of panniculitides that fall into the overlap of septal and lobar panniculitis with a mixed inflammatory infiltrate. The predominant cell type of the inflammatory infiltrate is often helpful in narrowing down the underlying etiology of panniculitis, in addition to other histopathological clues such as granuloma formation or fat necrosis.[2,3]

When the inflammatory infiltrate of panniculitis is predominantly composed of neutrophilic granulocytes, there are several conditions that lead to the differential diagnosis (**Box 1**). This review focuses on the clinicopathological characteristics of the most common causes of neutrophilic panniculitis.

NEUTROPHILIC PANNICULITIDES THAT ARE COMMONLY ULCERATIVE
Pancreatic Panniculitis

Pancreatic panniculitis is a rare complication of various pancreatic diseases but is mostly associated with alcoholic pancreatitis. Also known as pancreatic fat necrosis or enzymatic panniculitis, this condition has also been associated with pancreatic malignancy (including hepatic malignancy with pancreatic involvement) and pancreatic pseudocyst. The underlying mechanism is thought to be pancreatic inflammation leading to the release of pancreatic enzymes into circulation.[4] This subsequently increases vascular permeability, causes endothelial damage, and triggers fat hydrolysis. A combination of these

Mayo Clinic Department of Dermatology, 200 First Street Southwest, Rochester, MN 55905, USA
* Corresponding author.
E-mail address: maniam.ganesh@mayo.edu

Dermatol Clin 42 (2024) 285–295
https://doi.org/10.1016/j.det.2023.08.005

derm.theclinics.com

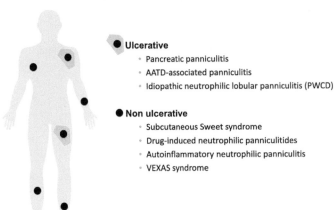

Neutrophilic Panniculitis

Ulcerative
- Pancreatic panniculitis
- AATD-associated panniculitis
- Idiopathic neutrophilic lobular panniculitis (PWCD)

Non ulcerative
- Subcutaneous Sweet syndrome
- Drug-induced neutrophilic panniculitides
- Autoinflammatory neutrophilic panniculitis
- VEXAS syndrome

Fig. 1. Overview of neutrophilic panniculitis divided into ulcerative and non-ulcerative clinical classifications. (*From* Anand NC, Takaichi M, Johnson EF, Wetter DA, Davis MDP, Alavi A. Suggestions for a new clinical classification approach to panniculitis based on a Mayo Clinic experience of 207 Cases. Am J Clin Dermatol 2022;23(5):739-746.)

effects leads to the characteristic fat necrosis with neutrophilic inflammation of pancreatic panniculitis.[1,4] Other proposed mechanisms include immune complex deposition and the release of adipokines or other cytokines.[4]

This type of panniculitis most commonly affects men or persons with an alcohol use disorder.[4] Pancreatic panniculitis may precede the diagnosis of pancreatic disease, in which case abdominal pain or serositis can be important clinical clues and makes the role of dermatologists in early diagnosis very important.[1] The lesions are tender erythematous to violaceus subcutaneous nodules and are most often disseminated on the extremities[4] (**Fig. 2**). Pancreatic panniculitis is commonly ulcerated with an oily brown discharge secondary to the enzymatic fat necrosis.[3,4] A rare clinical association is joint involvement via intraosseous fat necrosis, leading to "pancreatitis, panniculitis, and polyarthritis" syndrome.[4]

Diagnosis of pancreatic panniculitis is through clinicopathological correlation of underlying pancreatic disease with biopsy demonstrating characteristic histopathological findings. Pancreatic disease is best assessed through either laboratory studies demonstrating elevated levels of pancreatic enzymes or imaging findings consistent with a pancreatic disorder.[4] Histopathological examination reveals a neutrophilic infiltration which may be septal in early lesions but is characteristically lobular. This inflammation surrounds the fat liquefaction and saponification that leads to the necrotic, enucleated remnants known as "ghost cells." There may be dystrophic fat calcification, lipophages, or homogenous deposits of basophilic material; there is notably an absence of vasculitis.[1,2,4]

Management of pancreatic panniculitis is through medical or surgical treatment of the underlying pancreatic disease. Supportive treatment is important through fluid resuscitation and pain management, whereas cases of lower extremity involvement may benefit from compression or elevation of the affected limb.[1,2,4] There has been experimental use of octreotide in cases of pancreatic panniculitis, as this medication inhibits pancreatic enzyme production through its effects as a synthetic somatostatin biosimilar.[4]

Alpha-1 Antitrypsin Deficiency Panniculitis

Panniculitis may occur in the setting of alpha-1 antitrypsin deficiency (AATD), a rare genetic disorder most common in European populations, which is characterized by a deficiency of the serine protease inhibitor alpha-1 antitrypsin (AAT) due to mutations in the *SERPINA1* gene.[1,5] This deficiency is due to dysfunctional hepatic synthesis of AAT causing protein misfolding and polymerization before hepatic sequestration and accumulation; this causes the characteristic liver disease of AATD. If there is a clinically significant decrease in the circulatory levels of AAT, the resulting protease/antiprotease imbalance impairs the inhibition of neutrophil elastase in the lungs, causing elastic degradation and early-onset obstructive lung disease.

There is an unclear pathophysiological mechanism driving the subcutaneous inflammation in AATD panniculitis. The inhibition of interleukin (IL)-1β by AAT enzymes or chemoattraction of neutrophils to polymerized AAT proteins may play a role in pathogenesis.[1,4,5] Although the significance is unknown, another important pathophysiological

Box 1
Neutrophilic panniculitides

Neutrophilic panniculitides that are commonly ulcerative

Pancreatic panniculitis

AATD-associated panniculitis

Idiopathic neutrophilic lobular panniculitis (PWCD)

Neutrophilic panniculitides that are commonly non-ulcerated

Subcutaneous Sweet syndrome

Drug-induced neutrophilic panniculitides

Autoinflammatory neutrophilic panniculitis

- Rheumatoid arthritis (RA)-associated panniculitis
- Inflammatory bowel disease (IBD)-associated panniculitis
- Subcutaneous involvement of bowel bypass dermatitis
- Subcutaneous involvement of Behcet syndrome
- VEXAS syndrome

Late stages of certain panniculitides (early stages are less neutrophilic)

- Late stages of erythema induratum
- Late stages of traumatic panniculitis

Neutrophilic variants of other panniculitides

- Neutrophilic variant of lupus panniculitis
- Neutrophilic variant of subcutaneous fat necrosis of the newborn

Abbreviations: AATD, alpha-1 antitrypsin deficiency; IBD, inflammatory bowel disease; PWCD, Pfeifer-Weber-Christian disease; RA, rheumatoid arthritis; VEXAS syndrome, Vacuoles, E1 enzyme, X-linked, Autoinflammatory, Somatic syndrome.

consideration is the presence of polymerized AAT proteins in the skin biopsies and lung specimens of those with this AATD panniculitis and pulmonary disease, respectively.[5]

Although a diagnosis of AATD is made in the setting of characteristic hepatopulmonary disease, the presentation AATD-related panniculitis often precedes symptomatic liver or lung involvement.[5] This condition typically presents in women aged 30 to 60 years with severe AATD. It is also known to affect the pediatric population and, despite the relative rarity of its underlying disease, is the most common neutrophilic panniculitis affecting children.[1] Often triggered by trauma or iatrogenic interventions, this panniculitis clinically presents as tender subcutaneous nodules that are often ulcerated with an oily yellow discharge.[2,5] These lesions are erythematous to violaceous in coloration, distributed more commonly on the extremities and lower trunk (**Fig. 3**), and often heal as atrophic scars.[1,2,5] The diagnosis of AATD-related panniculitis requires both adequate histopathological evidence and, if not previously obtained, confirmatory genetic studies. Biopsies demonstrate a lobular pattern without vasculitis, though early lesions may have a septal pattern. Although there are some histiocytes, the infiltrate is predominantly neutrophilic with inflammation that is classically described as "splaying" between collagen bundles in the early stages.[5] There is also significant fat necrosis which may have skip areas or, in later stages, "floating fat."[2,5]

The rarity of this AATD panniculitis has limited research into the management of this condition.[5] Depending on the relevant family history, genetic screening of close relatives may be warranted. In regard to treatment, intravenous infusions of AAT proteins can correct the underlying enzymatic deficiency by reaching serum levels above 57 mg/dL.[1,5] Dapsone has also been found to be a successful treatment option, as it decreases neutrophil

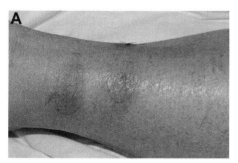
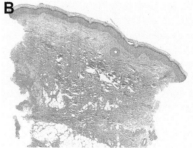

Fig. 2. A 76-year-old woman with history of multiple myeloma presenting with eight subcutaneous nodules (*A*) that are tender to touch and are predominantly found around the ankles but also in her thighs, as well as jaundice, with skin biopsy (*B*) consistent with pancreatic panniculitis.

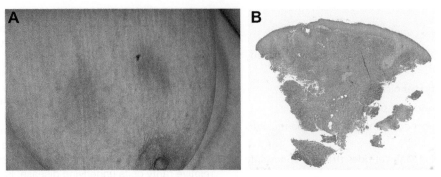

Fig. 3. A 66-year-old woman with multiple bounds of fat necrosis (*A*) with further biopsy (*B*) and clinical testing suggesting of alpha-1 antitrypsin deficiency with associated panniculitis and bullous emphysema.

adhesion and migration via CD11b inhibition and is currently considered the first line of therapy.[1] Other treatment options include plasma exchange and liver transplantation.[5] Corticosteroids, tetracyclines, and immunosuppressants have been trialed in the past with limited utility.[5] Promoting IL-1 receptor antagonism through anakinra administration is also an emerging therapy that mimics the anti-inflammatory effects of AAT.[1] There are novel therapies are being investigated for AATD in several clinical trials (**Table 1**).[6–9]

Idiopathic Neutrophilic Lobular Panniculitis (Pfeifer-Weber-Christian Disease)

Idiopathic neutrophilic lobular panniculitis is also known as Pfeifer-Weber-Christian disease (PWCD) and is a rare disease characterized by lobular panniculitis of adipose tissue with systemic symptoms and multiorgan involvement. It is a rare disease of unknown etiology with predominance in women.[10] Clinically, it is characterized by relapsing fever, fatigue, polyarthralgia, and tender subcutaneous nodules.[10] Other systemic symptoms due to visceral involvement may occur. Hepatomegaly and splenomegaly have also been documented in the case literature.[10] Other visceral organ involvement including the lungs, heart, kidneys, and adrenal glands are documented in case series but are uncommon in PWCD.

This diagnosis is confirmed via biopsy with histopathology of lobular panniculitis. Of note, the existence of PWCD as a separate entity from other panniculitides is debated. Many cases of PWCD have been reclassified as other forms of panniculitis including lipodermatosclerosis, AATD, lupus panniculitis, and traumatic panniculitis.[11]

Infective Panniculitis

Microbial infiltration of adipose tissue can cause panniculitis, and certain infectious can have a predominantly neutrophilic inflammation in certain cases. Immunocompromise is a major risk factor for the development of any infection, including infective panniculitis. In general, the most common location of infection-induced panniculitis is the lower extremity. This occurs most commonly through direct inoculation into the subcutaneous tissue (such as a penetrating injury), which causes a nodular wound surrounded by infection and inflammation. Hematogenous dissemination of an infectious microorganism, such as fungemia or bacterial sepsis, can also cause panniculitis which presents as multiple nodules. The direct extension of an underlying infection can also reach the adipose layer to cause panniculitis.[12] However, it is important to note that the clinical presentation of infective panniculitis depends on the immune status of the host.[13] The etiologies of infective panniculitis can be generally subdivided into bacterial, mycobacterial, and fungal etiologies given that viral etiologies are exceedingly rare (**Table 2**).[12,13]

PANNICULITIDES THAT ARE COMMONLY NON-ULCERATIVE
Subcutaneous Sweet Syndrome

The most common cause of neutrophilic panniculitis is the subcutaneous variant Sweet syndrome (SS).[3] Although neutrophilic dermatoses are associated with hematological malignancies, this association among neutrophilic panniculitides primarily relates to subcutaneous SS.[14] SS (acute febrile neutrophilic dermatosis) can be idiopathic, drug-induced, or related to malignancy. It is an uncommon disease that primarily affects adults aged 30 to 60 years old. The exact pathogenesis of SS is unknown. One hypothesis is that SS is a hypersensitivity reaction given its association with medications and underlying malignancies.[15,16] Granulocyte colony-stimulating factors (G-CSF), all-trans retinoic acid (ATRA), and FMS-like tyrosine kinase-3 inhibitors have also been hypothesized to play a central role

Table 1
Recent clinical trials for alpha-1 antitrypsin deficiency

Study	Intervention	Population/Study Design	Status
NCT04722887[6]	A multicenter, single-dose and repeat-dose over 8 weeks, sequential cohort study to evaluate safety and tolerability as well as pharmacokinetics of two different doses of alpha1-proteinase inhibitor subcutaneous (human) 15% administered subcutaneously in subjects with alpha1-antitrypsin deficiency	16 participants/non-randomized, sequential assignment, open label	Recruiting
NCT02363946[7]	A double-blind, placebo-controlled, dose-escalating, phase 1 study to determine the safety, tolerability, pharmacokinetics and effect of circulating alpha-1 antitrypsin levels of ARC-AAT in healthy volunteer subjects and in patients with alpha-1 antitrypsin deficiency (AATD)	65 participants/Randomized, parallel assignment, triple masking	Terminated
NCT04204252[8]	A prospective phase III multicenter, placebo-controlled, double-blind study to evaluate the efficacy and safety of "Kamada-AAT for Inhalation" 80 mg per day in adult patients with congenital alpha-1 antitrypsin deficiency with moderate and severe airflow limitation ($40\% \leq FEV1 \leq 80\%$ of predicted; $FEV1/SVC \leq 70\%$)	220 participants/randomized, parallel assignment, quadruple masking	Recruiting
NCT03815396[9]	An open-label, multicenter, phase 1 study to assess the safety, pharmacokinetics, and pharmacodynamics of single and multiple ascending intravenous doses of inhibrx rhAAT-Fc (INBRX-101) in adults with alpha-1 antitrypsin deficiency (AATD)	31 participants/non-randomized, sequential assignment, open label	Completed

Abbreviations: AATD, alpha-1 antitrypsin deficiency; FEV1, forced expiratory volume in 1 second; SVC, slow vital capacity.

in the pathogenesis of subcutaneous SS.[17] High levels of G-CSF in the blood of patients with underlying autoimmunity or malignancy have been associated with SS. Similarly, exogenous G-CSF has also been associated with SS supporting this hypothesis of elevated G-CSF leading to a maladaptive innate immune response.[17] Many medications have been implicated with drug-induced SS (**Table 3**).[17] The most common medication associated with SS is GM-CSF.[15]

Clinically, these lesions present as tender erythematous nodules or indurations. These lesions are typically on the extremities, especially the posterior lower extremities, but may be generalized.[2] The lesions are frequently tender and can form vesicles or bullae secondary to the underlying edema. Associated systemic symptoms include fever, headache, malaise, arthralgias, and myalgias.[16] Diagnosis is through utilization of major and minor criteria for SS (**Box 2**) and drug-induced SS (**Box 3**)—and both require histopathological confirmation.[14] Histopathology for subcutaneous SS reveals lobular neutrophilic panniculitis, which may have associated vasculitis; early lesions may have a septal inflammatory pattern.[5]

The treatment of choice for SS is systemic glucocorticoids. Other first-line agents include colchicine and potassium iodide. For drug-induced SS, cessation of the offending medication is important for the resolution of cutaneous manifestations.

Table 2
Etiologies of infective panniculitis

Pathogens	Diagnosis	Management
Bacterial agents *Streptococcus* species, *Staphylococcus aureus*, *Pseudomonas* species, *Actinomycosis* species, *Nocardia* species, *Klebsiella* species, *Brucella* species	Histology in a lobular or mixed pattern. Diagnostic confirmation via tissue cultures and staining (PAS, Gram stain)	Identification of the infectious agent guides treatment, though broad spectrum antibiotics should be initiated in cases of sepsis.
Mycobacterial agents *Mycobacterium tuberculosis* Nontuberculous mycobacterial agents: *M chelonae, M fortuitum, Mycobacterium avium intracellulare complex, M marinum, M ulcerans*, and other atypical mycobacterial species	Histology with granulomas and neutrophilic abscesses. Diagnostic confirmation via PCR as well as IHC (Ziehl-Nielsen, anti-BCG, and so forth) Tissue cultures have low sensitivities	A workup for a systemic infection should be initiated. Surgical debridement may be considered. Identification of the infectious agent guides treatment. Other than rifampin/rifabutin and ethambutol, other commonly used antibiotics include macrolides, fluoroquinolones, tetracyclines, and aminoglycosides.
Fungal agents causing subcutaneous mycosis: sporotrichosis (*Sporothrix schenckii*), chromoblastomycosis (pigmented fungi including: *Phialophora verrucosa, Fonsecaea pedrosoi, Fonsecaea compacta,* and *Cladophialophora carrionii*), and mycetomas (most commonly *Madurella mycetomatis*) *Systemic fungal diseases*: *Blastomycosis dermatitidis, Candida* species, *Aspergillus* species, *Fusarium, Histoplasma* *Rarer fungal etiologies of panniculitis*: Phaeohyphomycosis (several possible pigmented fungal agents), lobomycosis (*Lacazia loboi*), rhinosporidiosis (*Rhinosporidium seeberi*), and mucormycosis (*Rhizopus, Mucor*)	Histology with suppurative granulomas. Diagnostic confirmation via fungal tissue cultures or special staining	Identification of the infectious agent guides treatment. Systemic fungal infection is a life-threatening condition and requires prompt intervention. Systemic antifungals should be initiated in cases of systemic fungal infection, such as includes itraconazole or amphotericin B. Other fungal etiologies can be treated based on their specific presentation. For example, sporotrichosis could be treated with oral saturated solution of potassium iodide, itraconazole, or terbinafine. Surgical interventions may be needed, such as patients with eumycetoma who should have surgical excision as well as initiation of oral ketoconazole or itraconazole.

Abbreviations: BCG, bacillus calmette-guérin; PAS, periodic acid-Schiff; PCR, polymerase chain reaction; IHC, immunohistochemistry.

Second-line agents include clofazimine, cyclosporin, indomethacin, and dapsone.[15,17] IL-1 and tumor necrosis factor (TNF)-alpha inhibitors are also shown to be effective in treating SS. Other treatments still under investigation include granulocyte and monocyte adsorption apheresis.[17]

Drug-Induced Neutrophilic Panniculitides

Drug-induced panniculitis, also known as iatrogenic panniculitis, is a rare complication of medical therapies and can present as different form of panniculitides including granulomatous panniculitis, subcutaneous sweet or neutrophilic panniculitis.

Table 3 Medications associated with drug-induced Sweet syndrome	
Antibiotics	Clindamycin, Tetracyclines, Ofloxacin, Norfloxacin Nitrofurantoin, Piperacillin, and Tazobactam, TMP-SMX, Quinupristin, and Dalfopristin
Antiepileptics	Carbamazepine, diazepam
Antifungal	Fluconazole, ketoconazole
Antihypertensives	Hydralazine, furosemide
Anti-inflammatory	NSAIDs, sulfasalazine, mesalamine
Antineoplastic	ATRA, azacitidine, bortezomib, imatinib, ipilimumab, lenalidomide, mitoxantrone, ruxolitinib, topotecan, vemurafenib, vorinostat
Antiplatelets	Ticagrelor
Antipsychotics	Clozapine
Antithyroid	Propylthiouracil
Antivirals	Abacavir
Bone marrow stimulating agents	G-CSF or GM-CSF
Immunomodulators	Adalimumab, infliximab, interferon-beta, IL-2 therapy
Hormonal agents	Oral contraceptives, hormonal IUD
Other	Isotretinoin, PPIs, vaccination

Abbreviations: TMP-SMX, trimethoprim/sulfamethoxazole; NSAIDs, nonsteroidal anti-inflammatory drugs; ATRA, all-trans retinoic acid; G-CSF, granulocyte colony-stimulating factor; GM-CSF, granulocyte-macrophage colony stimulating factor; IL, interleukin; IUD, intrauterine device; PPIs, proton-pump inhibitors.

Clinical presentation varies based on the underlying etiology, and some have been associated with fever or arthralgias.[15] The histologic patterns vary from lobular to septal to mixed, but vasculitis is mostly absent. There are several drugs that have been implicated in this form of panniculitis (**Box 4**).[1,15] Drug discontinuation is dependent on the severity of skin disease and the medical necessity of continued drug administration.

Autoinflammatory-Related Panniculitis

There are several autoinflammatory or autoimmune diseases that have been associated with neutrophilic panniculitis (**Table 4**). Subcutaneous involvement of other autoinflammatory neutrophilic dermatoses, such as bowel bypass dermatitis and Behcet syndrome, are not included;

Box 2
Major and minor criteria for Sweet syndrome must meet both major criteria and at least two minor criteria

Major criteria:

Abrupt onset of painful cutaneous plaques or nodules

Histopathologic evidence of a neutrophilic dermatosis or panniculitis

Minor criteria:

Fever greater than 38°C

Preceded by an upper respiratory or gastrointestinal infection or vaccination.

Three of the following four laboratory abnormalities on presentation: ESR greater than 20, positive CRP, WBC greater than 8000/mL with greater than 70% neutrophils

Skin improvement with treatment with systemic corticosteroids or potassium iodide

C = Celsius, ESR = erythrocyte sedimentation rate, CRP = C-reactive protein, WBC = white blood count

---

Box 3
Diagnostic criteria for drug-induced Sweet syndrome must meet all criteria

Abrupt onset of painful cutaneous plaques or nodules

Fever greater than 38°C

Histopathologic evidence of a neutrophilic dermatosis or panniculitis

Temporal association between initiation of the drug and cutaneous manifestations

Skin improvement with drug cessation or treatment with systemic corticosteroids

C = Celsius

newborn, are outside the scope of this review. VEXAS syndrome is another autoinflammatory disorder which can present with neutrophilic panniculitis, and this is covered in more detail below. A prior study has linked neutrophilic autoinflammation with increased levels of TNF-α, IL-1β, IL-17, and IL-8. Of particular importance, IL-8 is known to play a significant role in the chemotaxis of neutrophil chemotaxis. This same study found that this autoinflammation is associated with increased metalloproteinases which caused neutrophil-mediated tissue damage.[18–20] The specific pathophysiological mechanisms are not yet fully understood.

these entities are covered elsewhere, and other than subcutaneous involvement, there are not typically other unique features.[1] Neutrophilic variants of other panniculitides, such as lupus panniculitis and subcutaneous fat necrosis of the

Vacuoles, E1 enzyme, X-linked, Autoinflammatory, Somatic Syndrome

VEXAS syndrome (Vacuoles, E1 enzyme, X-linked, Autoinflammatory, Somatic) is a severe inflammatory disease due to a mutation in the X-linked

Table 4
Selected autoinflammatory-related neutrophilic panniculitides

Entity	Clinical Presentation	Histopathology
Rheumatoid arthritis	Examination reveals subcutaneous nodules, especially on lower extremities, typically presents in middle-aged females with history of RA and elevated serum RF[1,19]	Lobular neutrophilic pattern as well as histiocytes in the inflammatory infiltrate; fat necrosis and vascular involvement may also be seen, whereas true LCV is a rare finding[1]
CANDLE syndrome	This is a genetic disorder caused by *PSMB8* gene mutations.[1] The condition may be triggered by cold temperature, infections, or other stressors in the neonatal period. This presents with erythematous and edematous maculopapular lesions which may be pruritic. This initially affects the face, especially the lips and eyelids, before caudal progression. Other findings include fever and lipodystrophy.[20]	Neutrophilic panniculitis with mononuclear cells and atypical myeloid cells (demonstrated by IHC); there may also be eosinophils. Dermal involvement is both perivascular and interstitial.[20] IHC: positive staining for STAT1, MPO, CD 163, and CD 123[1]
Recurrent lipoatrophic panniculitis of children	Presents in pediatric population as tender subcutaneous nodules with fever, malaise, abdominal pain, arthralgias, and/or recurrent lipoatrophy; laboratory evaluation reveals elevated acute phase reactants[1]	Lobular neutrophilic panniculitis (especially early stages) with associated fat necrosis; notably without vasculitis. IHC: positive staining for STAT1[1]

Abbreviations: RA, rheumatoid arthritis; RF, rheumatoid factor; LCV, leukocytoclastic vasculitis; CANDLE, chronic atypical neutrophilic dermatosis with lipodystrophy and elevated temperature; IHC, immunohistochemistry; STAT, signal transducer and activator of transcription; MPO, myeloperoxidase; CD, cluster of differentiation.

gene, ubiquitin-activating enzyme 1 (UBA1).[21] Inactivating somatic mutations in UBA1 leads to disruption of the ubiquitination protein degradation pathway. The regulation of UBA1b translation has been shown to be fundamental in both the pathogenesis and prognosis of VEXAS syndrome.[22] This disorder most commonly affects men in the fifth decade of life or later.[23] The overall incidence of VEXAS is estimated to be 1 in 13,591 unrelated individuals, 1 in 4269 men older than 50 years, and 1 in 26,238 women older than 50 years.[21]

Clinically, VEXAS syndrome presents with treatment-resistant inflammatory diseases with concurrent hematologic abnormalities. Patients with VEXAS often have overlying features of many inflammatory disorders including SS, relapsing polychondritis, polyarteritis nodosa, and giant cell arteritis.[21] Other systemic symptoms commonly include fever, skin lesions (**Fig. 4**), chondritis, and sterile neutrophilic pulmonary infiltrates.[23] Associated hematologic disorders include macrocytic anemia, thrombocytopenia, thromboembolic disease, and bone marrow failure which can subsequently evolve into hematologic malignancies. Thromboembolic disease is a significant contributor to disease morbidity and mortality.[23] These hematologic abnormalities are also thought to account for the higher rates of myelodysplastic syndromes in VEXAS patients than in patients with clonal hematopoietic disease. In addition to myelodysplastic syndromes, VEXAS patients also have a greater risk of developing multiple myeloma (**Table 5**).[24,25]

VEXAS syndrome is diagnosed with genetic testing using peripheral blood to assess for mutations in the UBA-1 gene.[23] Hematologic disorders commonly seen in VEXAS syndrome include

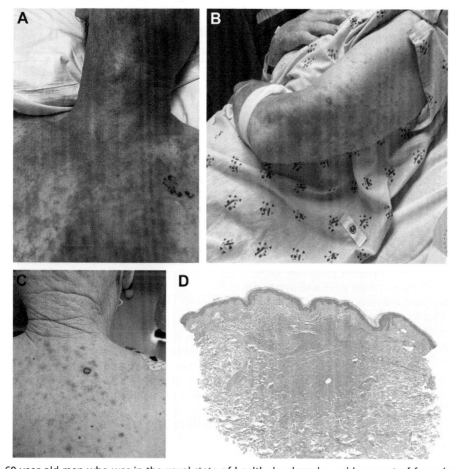

Fig. 4. A 60-year-old man who was in the usual state of health developed a sudden onset of fever, leukopenia, spontaneous pneumothorax, phlebitis, and diffuse hemorrhagic rash (*A-C*) with essential negative workup for connective tissue disorder but bone marrow biopsy showing vacuolization and on further genetic testing consistent with VEXAS. Biopsy of a skin lesion (*D*) is consistent with neutrophilic urticarial dermatosis as a reactive phenomenon.

Table 5
Systemic manifestations of Vacuoles, E1 enzyme, X-linked, Autoinflammatory, Somatic syndrome

Systemic	Fever
Eyes	Inflammatory eye disease, periorbital edema
Ears	Ear chondritis, sensorineural hearing loss
Nose	Nose chondritis
Lungs	Pleural effusion, neutrophilic alveolitis
Heart	Myocarditis
Bone	Myelodysplastic syndrome, multiple myelomas, cytopenias, vacuoles in myeloid and erythroid cells
Abdomen	Hepatosplenomegaly, colitis
Musculoskeletal	Inflammatory arthritis
Pelvic	Orchitis, epididymitis
Lower extremities	DVT
Cutaneous	Neutrophilic dermatoses, medium vessel vasculitis, leukocytoclastic vasculitis

Abbreviations: VEXAS syndrome, Vacuoles; E1 enzyme, X-linked; Autoinflammatory, Somatic syndrome; DVT, deep venous thrombosis.

macrocytic anemia, lymphopenia, and monocytopenia.[23] Other characteristic laboratory findings include elevated inflammatory markers including erythrocyte sedimentation rate and C-reactive protein. The bone marrow of VEXAS patients reveals characteristic abundant cytoplasmic vacuoles in myeloid and erythroid precursor cells.[25] The contents of the vacuoles in VEXAS syndrome remain unclear and are a source of ongoing study. The differential for cytoplasmic vacuoles in bone marrow precursor cells includes alcohol intoxication, copper deficiency, zinc toxicity, and myeloid neoplasms. The cytoplasmic vacuoles of VEXAS can be distinguished from other causes in this differential by the presence of autoinflammatory disorders and/or other hematologic abnormalities.[25]

VEXAS syndrome has a high morbidity and mortality rate, and treatment options are currently limited. A recent study of 80 VEXAS patients found overall survival at 10 years was 60%.[26] Poor clinical outcomes were associated with moderate thrombocytopenia, transfusion-dependent anemia, and typical clonal hematopoiesis mutations.[26] For treatment, glucocorticoids are helpful in

controlling the inflammatory component of this disease but have high toxicity associated with long-term use.[23] There are currently no steroid-sparing agents that exist for the treatment of VEXAS syndrome. One future therapeutic consideration is autologous and allogenic bone marrow transplants, which eliminates the clonal stem cell populations.[23] Small molecule inhibitors that target the ubiquitin protease pathway developed in cancer therapies could also have potential in the treatment of VEXAS syndrome.[27]

SUMMARY

Panniculitides are a diverse group of disorders with similar morphology. Neutrophilic panniculitides are an important subgroup with a link to systemic and sometimes life-threatening disorders. This article provides a review of panniculitis affecting adults highlighting the neutrophilic panniculitis and their association.

CLINICS CARE POINTS

- Pancreatic panniculitis may precede pancreatic disease, thus early diagnosis by a dermatologist can be impactful.
- Treat subcutaneous Sweet's syndrome with systemic glucocorticoids as the first-line therapy, along with other options such as calcimine and potassium iodide.
- Drug-induced neutrophilic panniculitides may require discontinuation of the offending medication depending on both the severity of skin disease and the necessity of continued drug administration.

DISCLOSURE

No financial conflicts of interest nor funding sources to disclose for all authors except A Alavi is an investigator for BI and Processa Pharmaceuticals, serves as a board member of the Hidradenitis Suppurativa Foundation, and is a consultant for AbbVie, BI, InflaRx, Novartis, and UCB.

REFERENCES

1. Llamas-Velasco M, Fraga J, Sanchez-Schmidt, et al. Neutrophilic infiltrates in panniculitis: comprehensive review and diagnostic algorithm proposal. Am J Dermatopathol 2020;42(10):717–30.
2. Shavit E, Marzano AV, Alavi A. Ulcerative versus non-ulcerative panniculitis: is it time for a novel

clinical approach to panniculitis? Int J Dermatol 2021;60(4):407–17.

3. Anand NC, Takaichi M, Johnson EF, et al. Suggestions for a new clinical classification approach to panniculitis based on a Mayo Clinic experience of 207 Cases. Am J Clin Dermatol 2022;23(5):739–46.

4. Miulescu R, Balaban DV, Sandru F, et al. Cutaneous manifestations in pancreatic diseases - a review. J Clin Med 2020;9(8):2611.

5. Franciosi AN, Ralph J, O'Farrell NJ, et al. Alpha-1 antitrypsin deficiency–associated panniculitis. J Am Acad Dermatol 2022;87(4):825–32.

6. A study to evaluate safety, tolerability and pharmacokinetics of two different doses of alpha1-proteinase inhibitor subcutaneous (human) 15% in participants with alpha1-antitrypsin deficiency. ClinicalTrials.gov identifier: NCT04722887. Updated February 27, 2023 https://clinicaltrials.gov/ct2/show/NCT04722887. Accessed June 14, 2023.

7. A study of ARC-AAT in healthy volunteer subjects and patients with alpha-1 antitrypsin deficiency (AATD). ClinicalTrials.gov identifier: NCT02363946. Updated August 3, 2018 https://clinicaltrials.gov/ct2/show/NCT02363946. Accessed June 14, 2023.

8. Evaluate efficacy and safety of "Kamada-AAT for inhalation" in patients with AATD (InnovAATe). ClinicalTrials.gov identifier: NCT04204252. Updated May 3, 2023 https://clinicaltrials.gov/ct2/show/NCT04204252. Accessed June 14, 2023.

9. Phase 1 study to assess the safety, PK, and PD of INBRX-101 in adults with alpha-1 antitrypsin deficiency (rhAAT-Fc). ClinicalTrials.gov identifier: NCT03815396. Updated September 13, 2022 https://clinicaltrials.gov/ct2/show/NCT03815396. Accessed June 14, 2023.

10. Rotondo C, Corrado A, Mansueto N, et al. Pfeifer-Weber-Christian disease: A case report and review of literature on visceral involvements and treatment choices. Clin Med Insights Case Rep 2020;13. https://doi.org/10.1177/1179547620917958. 1179547620917958.

11. Khan GA, Lewis FI. Recognizing Weber-Christian disease. Tenn Med 1996;89(12):447–9.

12. Morrison LK, Rapini R, Willison CB, et al. Infection and panniculitis. Dermatolog Ther 2010;23:328–40.

13. Delgado-Jiminez Y, Fraga J, Garcia-Diez A. Infective panniculitis. Dermatol Clin 2008;26(4):471–80.

14. Chan MP, Duncan LM, Nazarian RM. Subcutaneous Sweet syndrome in the setting of myeloid disorders: A case series and review of the literature. J Am Acad Dermatol 2013;68(6):1006–15.

15. Coromilas AJ, Gallitano SM. Neutrophilic drug reactions. Clin Dermatol 2020;38:648–59.

16. Moschella SL. Review of so-called aseptic neutrophilic dermatoses. Australas J Dermatol 1983;24(2):55–62.

17. Heath MS, Ortega-Loayza AG. Insights into the pathogenesis of Sweet's syndrome. Front Immunol. 2019; 10. Available at: https://doi.org/10.3389/fimmu.2019.00414. Accessed June 15, 2023.

18. Marzano AV, Damiani G. Neutrophilic panniculitis and autoinflammation: what's the link? [letter to the editor]. Br J Dermatol 2016;175:646–7.

19. Tran TA, DuPree M, Carlson JA. Neutrophilic lobular (pustular) panniculitis associated with rheumatoid arthritis: a case report and review of the literature. Am J Dermatopathol 1999;21(3):247–52.

20. Symmank D, Borst C, Drach M, et al. Dermatologic manifestations of noninflammasome-mediated autoinflammatory diseases. JID Innovations 2023;3(2):100176.

21. Beck DB, Ferrada MA, Sikora KA, et al. Somatic mutations in UBA1 and severe adult-onset autoinflammatory disease. N Engl J Med 2020;383(27):2628–38.

22. Ferrada MA, Savic S, Cardona DO, et al. Translation of cytoplasmic UBA1 contributes to VEXAS syndrome pathogenesis. Blood 2022;140(13):1496–506.

23. Patel B, Ferrada MA, Grayson PC, et al. VEXAS syndrome: an inflammatory and hematologic disease. Semin Hematol 2021;58:201–2023.

24. Ferrada M. VEXAS syndrome. NIH National Institute of Arthritis and Musculoskeletal and Skin Diseases. Updated April 2023. Available at: https://www.niams.nih.gov/labs/grayson-lab/vexas. Accessed June 15, 2023.

25. Grayson PC, Patel BA, Young NS. VEXAS syndrome. Blood 2021;137(26):3591–4.

26. Gutierrez-Rodrigues F, Kusne Y, Fernandez J, et al. Spectrum of clonal hematopoiesis in VEXAS syndrome. Blood. 2023. Available at: https://doi.org/10.1182/blood.2022018774. Accessed June 15, 2023.

27. Hyer M, Milhollen M, Ciavarri J, et al. A small-molecule inhibitor of the ubiquitin activating enzyme for cancer treatment. Nat Med 2018;24:186–93.

Palisaded Neutrophilic Granulomatous Dermatitis, Bowel-Associated Dermatosis–Arthritis Syndrome, and Rheumatoid Neutrophilic Dermatitis

Mika Yamanaka-Takaichi, MD, PhD, Afsaneh Alavi, MD*

KEYWORDS

- Neutrophilic disorder • Palisaded neutrophilic granulomatous dermatitis
- Bowel-associated dermatosis–arthritis syndrome • Rheumatoid neutrophilic dermatitis
- Reactive granulomatous disorder

KEY POINTS

- Palisaded neutrophilic granulomatous dermatitis (PNGD), bowel-associated dermatosis–arthritis syndrome, and rheumatoid neutrophilic dermatitis are rare inflammatory skin disorders that can be associated with underlying systemic diseases such as autoimmune disorders, malignancies, inflammatory bowel disease, and rheumatoid arthritis.
- As treating underlying disorders is the mainstay of therapy, patients with these neutrophilic inflammatory conditions should be screened for systemic disease.
- Because PNGD, interstitial granulomatous dermatitis, and interstitial granulomatous drug reaction share some clinical and histologic features, the authors recommend using the term "reactive granulomatous dermatitis" in dermatologic practice to avoid confusion.

INTRODUCTION

Neutrophilic dermatosis is a heterogeneous group of inflammatory skin diseases characterized by the presence of a sterile neutrophilic infiltrate on histopathology.[1] The classification of neutrophilic dermatoses is based on the recognition of clinical and pathologic features and identification of associated disorders. The pathogenesis of neutrophilic dermatoses is not well understood. Recent studies demonstrated the occurrence of neutrophilic dermatosis in autoinflammatory diseases and the similarities in clinical and histologic features, cytokine profiles, and therapeutic approaches between neutrophilic dermatosis and autoinflammatory diseases, suggesting that autoinflammation may be a cause of neutrophilic dermatoses.[2] Three specific types of neutrophilic dermatoses are reviewed in this article, including palisaded neutrophilic granulomatous dermatitis (PNGD), bowel-associated dermatosis–arthritis syndrome (BADAS), and rheumatoid neutrophilic dermatitis (RND). PNGD is typically associated with underlying disease states, including autoimmune connective tissue disease, lymphoproliferative disorders, and inflammatory arthritis.[3] RND is a rare cutaneous manifestation of rheumatoid arthritis (RA).[4] BADAS is another uncommon syndrome characterized by the triad

Department of Dermatology, Mayo Clinic, Rochester, MN, USA
* Corresponding author. Department of Dermatology, Gonda 16, Mayo Clinic, 200 First Avenue, Rochester, MN 55905.
E-mail address: alavi.afsaneh@mayo.edu

Dermatol Clin 42 (2024) 297–305
https://doi.org/10.1016/j.det.2023.08.008
0733-8635/24/© 2023 Elsevier Inc. All rights reserved.

of gastrointestinal symptoms, arthritis, and skin eruption.[1] Although these conditions share some similarities, they have distinct clinical features and underlying causes. Here, the authors have reviewed the literature and described the clinical and histopathologic features, etiology of the disease, and its relationship to various systemic diseases.

ETIOPATHOGENESIS
Palisaded Neutrophilic Granulomatous Dermatitis

PNGD is a rare inflammatory neutrophilic cutaneous disorder with varied clinical presentations (**Fig. 1**).[4] The cause and pathogenesis of PNGD is not well understood. Abnormal activation of neutrophils, deposition of circulating immune complexes, delayed hypersensitivity-type reactions, and low-grade small vessel vasculitis have been proposed as etiologies.[3] PNGD often occurs in patients with immunoreactive systemic diseases, especially autoimmune diseases, with the formation of immune complexes in dermal vessels proposed as the initiating event. After this, the activated neutrophils and complement damage the dermal collagen, leading to a granulomatous response.[5]

In addition, cases of PNGD induced after the use of etanercept for RA, Sjögren's syndrome,

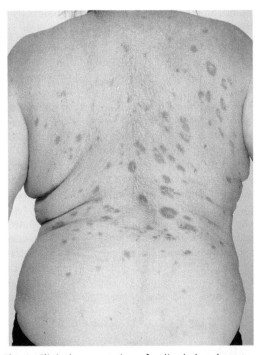

Fig. 1. Clinical presentation of palisaded and neutrophilic granulomatous dermatitis. Symmetric distributed erythematous papules with umbilication and central crusting.

and juvenile idiopathic arthritis have been reported.[6,7] Unlike other tumor necrosis factor (TNF)-α inhibitors, etanercept does not strongly suppress the activation of TNF-α, which may allow TNF-α-induced granuloma formation and may also modulate cytokines other than TNF that other TNF inhibitors do not, which may have contributed to PNGD induction.[6]

Bowel-Associated Dermatosis–Arthritis Syndrome

BADAS, also known as bowel bypass syndrome and blind loop syndrome, is most common in patients who have undergone bowel bypass surgery or other gastrointestinal surgery with blind loop, and in patients with a history of inflammatory bowel disease (IBD).[8] BADAS is a noninfectious neutrophilic dermatosis prominently characterized by skin eruptions and joint pain. In 1981, 7 of 105 patients who underwent a jejunal-ileal bypass for morbid obesity were reported to have developed an episodic illness featuring inflammatory skin lesions, usually associated with a nondestructive polyarthritis, as well as tenosynovitis, myalgia, and fever.[9] Dicken and Seehafer named this condition "bowel bypass syndrome",[10] and the term "bowel-associated dermatosis-arthritis syndrome" was coined by Jorizzo and colleagues.[11] The syndrome is usually more common in adults, and few pediatric cases with IBD and short bowel syndrome have also been reported.[12–14] Although the pathogenesis of BADAS is unclear, the prevailing hypothesis is that abnormalities in the intestinal tract in IBD or abnormal immune responses in the remaining intestine after intestinal survey cause bacterial overgrowth resulting in the formation of immune complexes, which circulate and deposit in tissues and organs.[15] Xhao and colleagues described a patient with BADAS induced by small intestinal bacterial overgrowth with no history of gastrointestinal surgery and IBD.[15] Ely and colleagues showed that skin testing with *Streptococcus pyogenes* antigen causes an exacerbation of BADAS or may provoke the entire syndrome de novo. They proposed the mechanism that a bacterial allergy is generated to the high concentration of altered gut flora in the patients with BADAS. Based on the fact that bacterial peptidoglycans, especially those of *group A streptococci*, produced similar arthritis and skin lesions in animal models, they indicated that peptidoglycans from numerous intestinal bacteria share common structural and antigenic features with *S pyogenes* peptidoglycan and could be causative of the toxic and immunologic features of the syndrome (**Fig. 2**).[16]

Rheumatoid Neutrophilic Dermatitis

RND is a rare neutrophilic skin condition that has been associated with RA, which was first described by Ackerman.[1] RND is a specific cutaneous manifestation of RA, which can also be observed in the patients with seronegative arthritis.[1,4] The activity of RND often parallels that of RA.[17,18] RND in a patient with RA taking tocilizumab has been reported, and it has been speculated that a paradoxic reaction may be triggered by a cytokine imbalance that increased IL-6.[17] The disease is more common in women, with a male-to-female ratio of 1:2.[4] The etiology is unknown, but it has been suggested that it is an immune complex-mediated disease (Fig. 3).[19]

CLINICAL AND HISTOLOGIC PRESENTATION
Palisaded Neutrophilic Granulomatous Dermatitis or Reactive Granulomatous Dermatitis

PNGD presents with a variety of clinical manifestations. Typical clinical presentations include erythematous papules with crusting, perforation, or umbilication and symmetrically distributed on extensor surfaces of the upper extremities, most commonly the elbows and hands.[1,20] Other clinical manifestations can include patches, nodules, linear cords, and plaques.[1] PNGD is often asymptomatic but can be accompanied by pruritus or tenderness.[21] PNGD was first described in 1994 as a papular eruption on the extremities in several patients with systemic lupus erythematosus, RA, or uncharacterized collagen vascular disease.[22] Many cases of PNGD have been described by several names, including linear subcutaneous bands, interstitial granulomatous dermatitis (IGD) with cutaneous cords and arthritis, rheumatoid papules, Churg–Strauss granuloma, eosinophilic granulomatosis with polyangiitis, cutaneous extravascular necrotizing granuloma, and Winkelmann granuloma.[23,24] In addition, the clinical and histopathologic features of PNGD overlap with IGD and interstitial granulomatous drug reaction (IGDR), with few strictly distinguishing features between them. Therefore, Rosenbach and English coined the simplified unifying term "reactive granulomatous dermatitis (RGD)" as an umbrella term for these diseases.[3]

Histopathologic findings of PNGD may vary depending on the stage of the disease. Early lesions show leukocytoclastic vasculitis with diffuse pan-dermal infiltrates composed of neutrophils, nuclear debris, and strands of amorphous basophilic material, whereas late lesions usually lack leukocytoclasia and are characterized by palisaded granulomas and degenerated collagen.[1]

Retrospective multicenter study of 52 patients with IGD and PNGD showed that neutrophilic infiltrates, karyorrhexis, and skin lesions with limited clinical course were mainly associated with

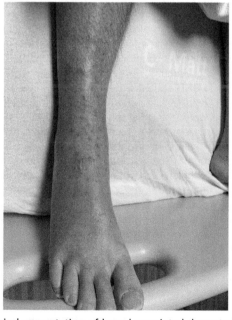
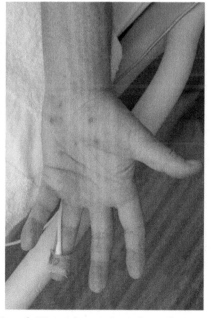

Fig. 2. Clinical presentation of bowel-associated dermatosis–arthritis syndrome. Central papule or pustule with an erythematous basis on the extremities.

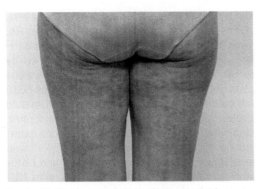

Fig. 3. Clinical presentation of rheumatoid neutrophilic dermatitis. Small erythematous plaques on the trunk.

PNGD.[25] The presence of vasculitis has been reported to be useful in differentiating PNGD from IGD.[3] However, a recent retrospective study of the clinical and histopathologic features of patients with RGD including IGD, PNGD, and IGDR found no significant association between histopathologic features of RGD and underlying disease and suggested that RGD is a clinically relevant umbrella term that should be routinely used in dermatologic practice.[26] Although there is still controversy over whether to classify these conditions as a single disease on the spectrum or as separate diseases, we suggest that when a patient is ultimately diagnosed with RGD by clinicopathologic findings, the clinician should consider screening for underlying systemic disease, regardless of whether the histopathologic diagnosis was IGD, PNGD, or IGDR.

Bowel-Associated Dermatosis–Arthritis Syndrome

Patients with BADAS present with a serum sickness-like syndrome characterized by fever, arthritis, and myalgia, which frequently precede the inflammatory skin eruption. Arthritis is an asymmetric, nondestructive, episodic polyarthritis, involves predominantly peripheral joints, and can be accompanied by tendinitis.[1] Diarrhea and malabsorption are other significant features of BADAS.[27] The most characteristic skin lesions are small erythematous macules with a central papule or pustule, often located on the upper extremities or trunk, but may also present with skin manifestations including erythema nodosum, panniculitis, ecchymosis, and pustular vasculitis.[1,27] In most patients, cutaneous symptoms seem after flu-like symptoms such as fever, malaise, and arthralgia.[12] Skin symptoms typically resolve spontaneously in about a week, with the potential for ongoing flares every 4 to 6 weeks over a period of years.[12,28] Symptoms of BADAS typically

develop 3 months to 5 years after gastrointestinal surgery,[8] although a case of BADAS 10 years after bariatric surgery and 18 years after jejunoileal bypass has been reported.[27,29]

In histopathology, early lesions show papillary edema and subepidermal vesiculation. Late lesions show a dense infiltration of neutrophils in the dermis and perivascular infiltrates and typically do not show the vasculitis changes of fibrinoid necrosis.[28] However, one case demonstrated a large subcorneal pustule without a significant dermal neutrophilic infiltrate, which suggests that the histology in BADAS may not necessarily be identical to Sweet syndrome, and the clinical picture alone plays an important role in diagnosis.[30]

One case of PET scan performed on BADAS was reported as being useful in eliminating other diagnoses, characterizing skin lesions, and potentially helping in the choice of lesion for the skin biopsy.[31]

Rheumatoid Neutrophilic Dermatitis

Cutaneous manifestation of RND includes nontender and resemble urticaria or appears crusted, annular, erythematous, subcutaneous papules, plaques, and nodules.[18,32] The skin lesions are typically symmetric and favor the trunk, shoulders, neck, and extremities, particularly the hands and forearms.[1,32] The duration of individual lesions varies from 1 to 3 weeks.[32] Resolution occurs spontaneously or with improvement of the underlying RA. Lesions tend to heal without scarring, but temporary hyperpigmentation may result.[32]

Histopathologic features of RND include dense neutrophilic infiltration of the dermis (particularly the upper to middle dermis) without the presence of vasculitis.[1,32] Leukocytoclasia can been seen in RND and infiltrate can involve in the panniculus. Cellulitis is distinguished by conspicuous dermal edema and lymphatic dilatation.[32] Spongiotic intraepidermal blisters, subepidermal bullae, or papillary neutrophilic micro-abscesses may be seen.[33] The histopathological differential is Sweet syndrome and dermatitis herpetiformis. Dermatitis herpetiformis can be distinguished by performing immunofluorescence, which reveals granular immunoglobulin A (IgA) deposits localized to the dermal papillae.[32] Sweet syndrome could be the most difficult differential consideration as the diseases seem similar histopathologically. The differentiation between these two conditions should be based on a comprehensive set of clinical findings, yet the presence of plasma cells may be helpful in distinguishing RND from Sweet's disease histopathologically.[1]

ASSOCIATIONS

Palisaded Neutrophilic Granulomatous Dermatitis

PNGD has been reported to be associated with systemic diseases, especially autoimmune diseases. Common underlying diseases in PNGD include connective tissue diseases (especially systemic lupus erythematosus), inflammatory arthritis, and blood diseases, with rare cases induced by infection or drugs being reported.[3] Table 1 shows the underlying diseases in PNGD reported to date (see **Table 1**).

Reactive granulomatous skin findings, including PNGD, are also seen in some cases associated with myeloproliferative disorders such as myelodysplastic syndrome, leukemia, lymphoma, and paraproteinemia.[1]

Bowel-Associated Dermatosis–Arthritis Syndrome

BADAS may occur in up to 20% of patients undergoing jejunal bypass surgery and has been reported in patients with several other gastrointestinal conditions, including bariatric surgery, peptic ulcers, diverticulitis, appendicitis, IBD, and cystic fibrosis.[11,12,34] The potential risk of developing BADAS is much lower with conventional bariatric interventions. However, there are sporadic reports of BADAS after modern bariatric procedures, including Roux-en-Y jejunostomy, ileoanal pouch anastomosis, biliopancreatic diversion, Billroth II, and most recently laparoscopic gastric bypass.[28,35–38]

Rheumatoid Neutrophilic Dermatitis

Of the cutaneous manifestation of RA, rheumatoid nodules are the most common and occur in 20% of affected persons.[39] RA-related skin diseases include Sweet's syndrome, pyoderma gangrenosum (PG), PNGD, Raynaud's phenomenon, livedo racemosa IGD with arthritis (IGDA), and erythema elevatum diutinum (EED), which may occur in association with other diseases.[4,40] The prevalence of RND in all RA patients was reported to be 0.9% to 1.8%, which can also be seen in the patients with seronegative arthritis.[1,4]

Table 1
Underlying systemic disease in palisaded neutrophilic granulomatous dermatitis[3,6,7,20,23,42,48–52]

Connective Tissue Disease	Arthritis
Lupus erythematous (SLE and DLE)	Rheumatoid arthritis
Limited systemic sclerosis	Ankylosing spondylitis
Undifferentiated connective tissue disease	Juvenile idiopathic arthritis
ANCA-associated vasculitis	
Granulomatosis with polyangiitis	
Erythema elevatum diutinum	
Sjögren's syndrome	
Mixed cryoglobulinemia	
Takayasu's arteritis	
Lymphoproliferative disease	*Infections*
Acute myeloid leukemia	Subcutaneous bacterial endocarditis
Chronic myelomonocytic leukemia	Hepatitis
Multiple myeloma	Streptococcal infection
Lymphoma (MF, CTCL, Hodgkin lymphoma and non-Hodgkin's lymphoma)	AIDS
	Borrelia
Monoclonal gammopathy	Lyme disease
Medications	*Others*
TNF inhibitors (adalimumab, etanercept)	Sarcoidosis
IL-6 inhibitors (tocilizumab)	Ulcerative colitis
Allopurinol	Celiac disease and type I diabetes
Ledipasvir/sofosbuvir	Behcet's disease
	Multiple sclerosis
	Breast cancer
	Still's disease

Abbreviations: AIDS, acquired immunodeficiency syndrome; ANCA, antineutrophilic cytoplasmic antibody; CTCL, cutaneous T-cell lymphoma; DLE, discoid lupus erythematosus; IL-6, interleukin-6; MF, mycosis fungoides; SLE, systemic lupus erythematosus; TNF, tumor necrosis factor.

EVALUATION AND MANAGEMENT
Palisaded Neutrophilic Granulomatous Dermatitis

The diagnosis of PNGD is based on correlation of clinical and histologic findings. Although there are cases without detectable systemic disease, patients with cutaneous and histologic features of PNGD and lacking a diagnosis of associated underlying disease should be evaluated for systemic disease.[1] In addition to a systematic physical examination and history, chest radiographs and blood tests (antinuclear antibodies, antineutrophil cytoplasmic antibody, rheumatoid factor, cyclic citrullinated peptide antibodies, and a complete blood count with differential) should be considered.

The differential diagnosis of PNGD includes leukocytoclastic vasculitis, urticaria, and granuloma annulare.[41] Skin biopsy is highly recommended to differentiate PNGD from other cutaneous granulomatous diseases with overlapping clinical features (granuloma annulare, granulomatous dermatitis interstitial, and granulomatous drug reaction interstitial).

PNGD often resolves spontaneously or during treatment of systemic diseases. By controlling the underlying disease, existing lesions can be resolved and recurrence prevented.[42] PNGD can be treated with topical, intralesional, or systemic steroids, with other reports of disease improvement with dapsone, hydroxychloroquine, disease-modifying antirheumatic drugs, and biologics.[3,42]

Bowel-Associated Dermatosis–Arthritis Syndrome

BADAS is difficult to diagnose due to the lack of characteristic laboratory findings. The deferential diagnosis of BADAS included other neutrophil-mediated skin disorders such as PG, Sweet's syndrome, pustular vasculitis of the hands, leukocytoclastic vasculitis, septic vasculitis, Behçet's syndrome, rheumatoid neutrophilic dermatosis, acute generalized exanthematous pustulosis, erythema nodosum, and Henoch–Schönlein purpura.[43]

The diagnosis should be determined comprehensively by the history, physical examination, and pathology findings.

Treatment options for BADAS are the surgical reduction of the blind loops of bowel, systemic corticosteroids, dapsone, and antibiotics. The long-term antibiotics, such as tetracyclines, metronidazole, and erythromycin, are used to decrease bacterial loads in the affected gut.[16,28] Dapsone was reported to be effective in suppressing the skin and joint symptoms when metronidazole and tetracycline had failed.[9] Topical or oral corticosteroids

(10–20 mg/day) are also an alternative treatment option.[9,16] Immunosuppressants such as cyclosporine and mycophenolate mofetil can be used to reduce steroid dose or as a treatment of IBD.[44]

Ustekinumab has been reported to completely resolve skin lesions and improve gastrointestinal symptoms in patients with BADAS secondary to Crohn's proctitis.[45]

A case report showed that ruxolitinib and a Janus kinase inhibitor were used to treat the pediatric patient with BADAS who had severe very early-onset IBD.[12]

Rheumatoid Neutrophilic Dermatitis

The differential diagnosis for RND includes Sweet syndrome, PG, cellulitis, EED, neutrophilic urticaria, and dermatitis herpetiformis.[32] Other possible diagnoses include BADAS, sporotrichosis, cutaneous lymphoma, and reaction to a foreign body, and other neutrophilic dermatoses.[4,46] It is particularly challenging histopathologically to distinguish RND from Sweet's disease. The main differentiators from Sweet syndrome are the presentation, symptoms, disease course, and associated diseases.[32]

Although PNGD is sometimes described as a variant of RND, it should be considered as a separate entity given the lack of granuloma on histopathologic findings.[1]

RND usually resolves spontaneously or ameliorates with treatment of RA.[32] Treatment of RND includes topical or systemic corticosteroids or dapsone (50–100 mg/day). Antimalarials such as hydroxychloroquine and cyclophosphamide (200 mg twice daily) have been reported to be effective in some cases.[39,47–52]

SUMMARY

The three neutrophilic dermatoses highlighted here, PNGD, BADAS, and RND, are rare dermatologic conditions that can be challenging to diagnose due to their wide range of clinical features, histopathologic findings, and association with various systemic diseases. A multidisciplinary approach is necessary for the diagnosis and management of these rare conditions. Further research is needed to better understand the pathogenesis of these conditions and their association with systemic diseases. These diseases highlight an important aspect of dermatology that cutaneous eruptions can serve as a sign of systemic disease, and patients with these suspected conditions should promptly undergo workup for underlying systemic disease. The correct diagnosis prevents a myriad of laboratory tests and allows for more effective symptom management.

CLINICS CARE POINTS

- RND is a specific cutaneous manifestation of RA with a parallel activity with the underlying RA disease, which can also be observed in the patients with seronegative arthritis.
- Patients with reactive granulomatous dermatitis including PNGD, IGD, IGDR should be screened for underlying systemic disease.
- Treatment of BADAS includes surgical reduction of the blind loops of bowel in adition to systemic medical therapies.

FUNDING

None.

ETHICS APPROVAL

Not applicable.

CONSENT TO PARTICIPATE/PUBLISH

Not applicable.

AVAILABILITY OF DATA AND MATERIAL

Not applicable.

CONFLICTS OF INTERESTS/COMPETING INTERESTS

M. Yamanaka-Takaichi: no conflicts of interest to disclose. A. Alavi is a consultant for Abbvie, BI, Incyte , InflaRx, Novartis and UCB and investigator for BI, Processa.

REFERENCES

1. Alavi A, Sajic D, Cerci FB, et al. Neutrophilic dermatoses: an update. Am J Clin Dermatol 2014;15:413–23.
2. Satoh TK, Mellett M, Contassot E, et al. Are neutrophilic dermatoses autoinflammatory disorders? Br J Dermatol 2018;178:603–13.
3. Rosenbach M, English JC 3rd. Reactive Granulomatous Dermatitis: A Review of Palisaded Neutrophilic and Granulomatous Dermatitis, Interstitial Granulomatous Dermatitis, Interstitial Granulomatous Drug Reaction, and a Proposed Reclassification. Dermatol Clin 2015;33:373–87.
4. Żuk G, Jaworecka K, Samotij D, et al. Rheumatoid neutrophilic dermatitis. Reumatologia 2019;57:350–3.
5. Deen J, Banney L, Perry-Keene J. Palisading neutrophilic and granulomatous dermatitis as a presentation of Hodgkin lymphoma: A case and review. J Cutan Pathol 2018;45:167–70.
6. Ishikawa M, Yamamoto T. Etanercept-induced palisaded neutrophilic granulomatous dermatitis. An Bras Dermatol 2021;96:117–9.
7. Nguyen TA, Celano NJ, Matiz C. Palisaded Neutrophilic Granulomatous Dermatitis in a Child with Juvenile Idiopathic Arthritis on Etanercept. Pediatr Dermatol 2016;33:e156–7.
8. Richarz NA, Bielsa I, Morillas V, et al. Bowel-associated dermatosis–arthritis syndrome (BADAS). Australas J Dermatol 2020;62:241–2.
9. Kennedy C. The spectrum of inflammatory skin disease following jejuno-ileal bypass for morbid obesity. Br J Dermatol 1981;105:425–35.
10. Dicken CH, Seehafer JR. Bowel bypass syndrome. Arch Dermatol 1979;115(7):837–9.
11. Jorizzo JL, Apisarnthanarax P, Subrt P, et al. Bowel-bypass syndrome without bowel bypass. Bowel-associated dermatosis-arthritis syndrome. Arch Intern Med 1983;143:457–61.
12. Havele SA, Clark AK, Oboite M, et al. Bowel-associated dermatosis-arthritis syndrome in a child with very early onset inflammatory bowel disease. Pediatr Dermatol 2021;38:697–8.
13. Oldfield CW, Heffernan-Stroud LA, Buehler-Bota TS, et al. Bowel-associated dermatosis-arthritis syndrome (BADAS) in a pediatric patient. JAAD case reports 2016;2:272–4.
14. Pereira E, Estanqueiro P, Almeida S, et al. Bowel-associated dermatosis-arthritis syndrome in an adolescent with short bowel syndrome. J Clin Rheumatol : practical reports on rheumatic & musculoskeletal diseases 2014;20:322–4.
15. Zhao H, Zhao L, Shi W, et al. Is it bowel-associated dermatosis-arthritis syndrome induced by small intestinal bacteria overgrowth? SpringerPlus 2016;5:1551.
16. Ely PH. The bowel bypass syndrome: a response to bacterial peptidoglycans. J Am Acad Dermatol 1980;2:473–87.
17. Kubota N, Ito M, Sakauchi M, et al. Rheumatoid neutrophilic dermatitis in a patient taking tocilizumab for treatment of rheumatoid arthritis. J Dermatol 2017;44:e180–1.
18. Brown TS, Fearneyhough PK, Burruss JB, et al. Rheumatoid neutrophilic dermatitis in a woman with seronegative rheumatoid arthritis. J Am Acad Dermatol 2001;45:596–600.
19. Hirota TK, Keough GC, David-Bajar K, et al. Rheumatoid neutrophilic dermatitis. Cutis 1997;60:203–5.
20. Shenk MER, Ken KM, Braudis K, et al. Palisaded neutrophilic and granulomatous dermatitis associated with ledipasvir/sofosbuvir. JAAD case reports 2018;4:808–10.
21. Bremner R, Simpson E, White CR, et al. Palisaded neutrophilic and granulomatous dermatitis: an unusual cutaneous manifestation of immune-mediated disorders. Semin Arthritis Rheum 2004;34:610–6.

22. Chu P, Connolly MK, LeBoit PE. The histopathologic spectrum of palisaded neutrophilic and granulomatous dermatitis in patients with collagen vascular disease. Arch Dermatol 1994;130:1278–83.

23. Zabihi-Pour D, Bahrani B, Assaad D, et al. Palisaded neutrophilic and granulomatous dermatitis following a long-standing monoclonal gammopathy: A case report. SAGE open medical case reports 2021;9. 2050313X97956.

24. Sangueza OP, Caudell MD, Mengesha YM, et al. Palisaded neutrophilic granulomatous dermatitis in rheumatoid arthritis. J Am Acad Dermatol 2002;47: 251–7.

25. Rodríguez-Garijo N, Bielsa I, Mascaró JM, et al. Reactive granulomatous dermatitis as a histological pattern including manifestations of interstitial granulomatous dermatitis and palisaded neutrophilic and granulomatous dermatitis: a study of 52 patients. J Eur Acad Dermatol Venereol 2021;35:988–94.

26. Bangalore Kumar A, Lehman JS, Johnson EF, et al. Reactive granulomatous dermatitis as a clinically relevant and unifying term: a retrospective review of clinical features, associated systemic diseases, histopathology and treatment for a series of 65 patients at Mayo Clinic. J Eur Acad Dermatol Venereol 2022;36:2443–50.

27. Ashchyan HJ, Nelson CA, Stephen S, et al. Neutrophilic dermatoses: Pyoderma gangrenosum and other bowel- and arthritis-associated neutrophilic dermatoses. J Am Acad Dermatol 2018;79:1009–22.

28. Thrash B, Patel M, Shah KR, et al. Cutaneous manifestations of gastrointestinal disease: part II. J Am Acad Dermatol 2013;68. 211.e1-33; quiz 44-6.

29. Fisch C, Schiller P, Harr T, et al. First presentation of intestinal bypass syndrome 18 yr after initial surgery. Rheumatology 2001;40:351–3.

30. Patton T, Jukic D, Juhas E. Atypical histopathology in bowel-associated dermatosis-arthritis syndrome: A case report. Dermatol Online J 2009;15:3.

31. Hassold N, Jelin G, Palazzo E, et al. Bowel-associated dermatosis arthritis syndrome: A case report with first positron emission tomography analysis. JAAD case reports 2019;5:140–3.

32. Mashek HA. Rheumatoid Neutrophilic Dermatitis. Arch Dermatol 1997;133:757.

33. Lowe L, Kornfeld B, Clayman J, et al. Rheumatoid neutrophilic dermatitis. J Cutan Pathol 1992;19: 48–53.

34. Prpić-Massari L, Kastelan M, Brajac I, et al. Bowel-associated dermatosis-arthritis syndrome in a patient with appendicitis. Med Sci Mon Int Med J Exp Clin Res 2007;13:Cs97–100.

35. Dicken CH. Bowel-associated dermatosis-arthritis syndrome: bowel bypass syndrome without bowel bypass. J Am Acad Dermatol 1986;14:792–6.

36. Gómez-Diez S, Mas Vidal A, Soler T, et al. [Vitamin A deficiency and bowel-associated dermatosis-arthritis syndrome secondary to biliopancreatic diversion for obesity]. Actas Dermo-Sifiliográficas 2010;101:900–2.

37. Slater GH, Kerlin P, Georghiou PR, et al. Bowel-associated dermatosis-arthritis syndrome after biliopancreatic diversion. Obes Surg 2004;14: 133–5.

38. Tu J, Chan JJ, Yu LL. Bowel bypass syndrome/ bowel-associated dermatosis arthritis syndrome post laparoscopic gastric bypass surgery. Australas J Dermatol 2011;52:e5–7.

39. Sánchez JL, Cruz A. Rheumatoid neutrophilic dermatitis. J Am Acad Dermatol 1990;22:922–5.

40. Cugno M, Gualtierotti R, Meroni PL, et al. Inflammatory Joint Disorders and Neutrophilic Dermatoses: a Comprehensive Review. Clin Rev Allergy Immunol 2018;54:269–81.

41. Almutawa YM, Alherz W, Alali MO, et al. Palisaded neutrophilic and granulomatous dermatitis in a patient with Churg-strauss syndrome: a case report and literature review. Cureus 2022;14(10):e30085. https://doi.org/10.7759/cureus.

42. Yang C, Tang S, Li S, et al. Underlying systemic diseases in interstitial granulomatous dermatitis and palisaded neutrophilic granulomatous dermatitis: a systematic review. Dermatology (Basel, Switzerland) 2022;1–12.

43. Zakko L, Finch J, Rothe MJ, et al. Bowel-associated dermatosis–arthritis syndrome. New York: Springer; 2013. p. 55–7.

44. Cox NH, Palmer JG. Bowel-associated dermatitis-arthritis syndrome associated with ileo-anal pouch anastomosis, and treatment with mycophenolate mofetil. Br J Dermatol 2003;149:1296–7.

45. Heard M, Zhang M, Jorizzo JL. A case of bowel-associated dermatosis-arthritis syndrome treated with ustekinumab: The importance of targeting underlying gastrointestinal disease. JAAD case reports 2020;6:506–8.

46. Bevin AA, Steger J, Mannino S. Rheumatoid neutrophilic dermatitis. Cutis 2006;78:133–6.

47. Gerbing EK, Metze D, Luger TA, et al. [Interstitial granulomatous dermatitis without arthritis: successful therapy with hydroxychloroquine]. Journal der Deutschen Dermatologischen Gesellschaft = Journal of the German Society of Dermatology : JDDG 2003;1:137–41.

48. Enescu CD, Patel A, Friedman BJ. Unique Recognizable Histopathologic Variant of Palisaded Neutrophilic and Granulomatous Dermatitis that Is Associated With SRSF2-Mutated Chronic Myelomonocytic Leukemia: Case Report and Review of the Literature. Am J Dermatopathol 2022;44: e33–6.

49. Moreno C, Kutzner H, Palmedo G, et al. Interstitial granulomatous dermatitis with histiocytic pseudorosettes: a new histopathologic pattern in cutaneous

borreliosis. Detection of Borrelia burgdorferi DNA sequences by a highly sensitive PCR-ELISA. J Am Acad Dermatol 2003;48:376–84.

50. Fujimoto R, Fujiwara S, Takata M, et al. Palisaded neutrophilic granulomatous dermatitis as a paradoxical adverse reaction following tocilizumab use. Int J Dermatol 2023;62:103–5.

51. Akagawa M, Hattori Y, Mizutani Y, et al. Palisaded Neutrophilic and Granulomatous Dermatitis in a Patient with Granulomatosis with Polyangiitis. Case Rep Dermatol 2020;12:52–6.

52. Gill D, Mann K, Kaur S, et al. Palisaded Neutrophilic Granulomatous Dermatitis Associated with Adult Onset Still's Disease. Arch Med 2017;09.

Superficial and Bullous Neutrophilic Dermatoses

Sneddon–Wilkinson, IgA Pemphigus, and Bullous Lupus

Priya Manjaly, BA[a,b,1], Katherine Sanchez, BS[a,1], Samantha Gregoire, BS[a], Sophia Ly, BA[a], Kanika Kamal, BA[a], Arash Mostaghimi, MD, MPH, MPA[a,*]

KEYWORDS

• Neutrophilic dermatoses • Sneddon–Wilkinson • IgA pemphigus • Bullous lupus

KEY POINTS

- Sneddon–Wilkinson disease, IgA pemphigus, and bullous systemic lupus erythematosus are blistering skin disorders characterized by sterile neutrophilic infiltrate.
- Sneddon–Wilkinson disease and IgA pemphigus both present with grouped flaccid pustules in an annular pattern and have epidermal neutrophilic infiltrate on histology.
- IgA pemphigus is distinguished from Sneddon–Wilkinson disease with direct immunofluorescence showing intercellular IgA deposition.
- Bullous systemic lupus erythematosus presents with tense bullae, neutrophilic infiltrate in the dermis, and direct immunofluorescence showing linear IgG deposition along the dermal–epidermal junction.

INTRODUCTION

Neutrophilic dermatoses are a heterogenous group of inflammatory skin disorders characterized by neutrophilic skin infiltrate in the absence of infection, allergy, or autoimmunity.[1–3] It is postulated that the underlying pathophysiology of neutrophilic dermatoses is autoinflammation, which is distinguished from autoimmunity by the absence of auto-reactive lymphocytes or autoantibodies.[4] In these cases, normal mature neutrophils aberrantly react to autologous self-tissues despite the lack of an identifiable pathologic trigger.[4] There is also evidence for the involvement of cytokines interleukin (IL)-1B, IL-17, and tumor necrosis factor (TNF)-α due to their role in promoting neutrophil chemotaxis.[1–3,5]

The various neutrophilic dermatoses each present with distinct histopathological skin involvement, with neutrophilic infiltrate occupying either the epidermis, dermis, or hypodermis.[1,3] This results in location-specific cutaneous manifestations, including pustules and bullae, plaques and papules, or nodules and ulcers, respectively.[1,3] However, some experts have postulated that neutrophilic dermatoses exist as a spectrum of diseases due to their many overlapping features and pathophysiology.[1,2]

This review focuses on three neutrophilic dermatoses: Sneddon–Wilkinson disease (SWD), immunoglobulin A (IgA) pemphigus, and bullous systemic lupus erythematosus (BSLE). SWD and IgA pemphigus are classified as superficial neutrophilic dermatoses, whereas BSLE is considered a

[a] Department of Dermatology, Brigham and Women's Hospital, Boston, MA 02115, USA; [b] Boston University School of Medicine, Boston, MA 02118, USA
[1] Co-first authors.
* Corresponding author. Department of Dermatology, Brigham and Women's Hospital, 221 Longwood Avenue, Boston, MA 02115.
E-mail address: amostaghimi@bwh.harvard.edu

Dermatol Clin 42 (2024) 307–315
https://doi.org/10.1016/j.det.2023.08.010

bullous neutrophilic dermatosis due to its subepidermal involvement and characteristic tense bullae.[1,6] Owing to their many clinical and histopathological similarities, it is unclear if IgA pemphigus and SWD exist on a continuum or if they are truly distinct pathophysiological entities.[1] In this review, the authors present SWD and IgA pemphigus as two separate diseases. Given their many overlapping features and unique differences, this review aims to further elucidate the epidemiology, pathophysiology, and clinical features of SWD, IgA pemphigus, and BSLE.

DISCUSSION
Sneddon–Wilkinson Disease

Key features

- Most commonly presents in women aged 50 to 70 years.
- Presents as grouped, sterile superficial pustular eruptions with a relapsing and remitting course.
- Lesions typically localize to the trunk, intertriginous surfaces, and proximal extremities.
- Dapsone is the first-line treatment.

Epidemiology

SWD, also referred to as classic subcorneal pustular dermatosis, is a rare, benign, bullous neutrophilic dermatosis that was first described by Sneddon and Wilkinson.[7] The exact incidence and prevalence of SWD are unknown, and there are no known racial or geographic predispositions.[8] SWD predominantly affects middle-aged and elderly women between 50 and 70 years, with women affected at a rate four times greater than men.[8] Cases in children and young adults are rare and often present with unusual characteristics, such as an atypical distribution of lesions.[8–11] Only one case has been reported in a nonagenarian patient.[12]

Pathophysiology

The exact pathogenesis of SWD has not been fully elucidated. On histology, SWD consistently presents with sterile subcorneal blisters filled with polymorphonuclear leukocytes.[7] The infiltrate is predominantly neutrophilic, although rare cases of SWD have shown a small amount of subcorneal eosinophilic infiltrate as well.[13] The predominance of neutrophilic infiltrate in the subcorneal blisters has prompted the investigation of multiple chemotactic factors, including TNF-α, C5a, interleukin-8.[10,14] Prior in vivo investigations suggesting that TNF-α may play a crucial role in neutrophil recruitment in SWD are supported by excessive TNF-α levels found in serum and blister samples of

patients and the treatment response of patients on TNF-α inhibitors.[14,15]

Aside from subcorneal blisters, histologic specimen from patients with SWD typically lacks accompanying dermal or epidermal changes, including spongiosis or acantholysis.[7,9] The presence of epidermal acantholysis is suggestive of older lesions that have undergone secondary change.[16] Direct and indirect immunofluorescence is typically negative in cases of classic SWD.[16]

Clinical features

SWD has a chronic course with recurrent pustular eruptions with frequent flares.[17] The primary lesions of SWD characteristically present as spontaneous isolated or grouped, superficial, flaccid pustules that quickly progress to form an annular, circinate, or serpiginous configuration (**Fig. 1**).[15,18] The lesions most commonly involve the trunk, proximal extremities, and intertriginous regions while typically sparing the face, mucous membranes, palmar/plantar surfaces, and nails.[18] Localized symptoms including pain, pruritis, irritation, and underlying skin erythema may accompany lesions; however, systemic symptoms secondary to the SWD lesions are uncommon.[8]

Disease associations

The classic form of SWD is typically considered to be a benign disease without any systemic involvement.[16] However, SWD has been associated with numerous comorbid disease states, including hematologic and solid tumor malignancies such as IgA paraproteinemia and multiple myeloma, and other less commonly associated disease states such as pyoderma gangrenosum, thyroid disorders, thymoma, rheumatoid arthritis, systemic lupus erythematosus (SLE), Sjogren's syndrome, multiple sclerosis, inflammatory bowel disease, and synovitis, acne, pustulosis, hyperostosis, osteitis (SAPHO) syndrome.[16] Rare cases of drug and infection-induced SWD have also been reported.[19,20]

Diagnosis

Owing to its rare nature, there are no established diagnostic criteria for SWD.[16] The differential diagnosis of SWD includes other vesiculopustular and blistering diseases including pustular psoriasis, subcorneal IgA pemphigus, pemphigus foliaceus, dermatitis herpetiformis (DH), and acute generalized exanthematous pustulosis.[16] Diagnosis is typically made from a consistent clinical picture, hallmark findings on histology, and through exclusion of the remaining clinical differential.[16] The key diagnostic procedure is skin biopsy, but further workup to exclude underlying malignancy (ie, IgA paraproteinemia) or associated disease states (ie, connective tissue diseases, thyroid disorders)

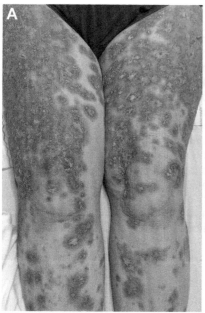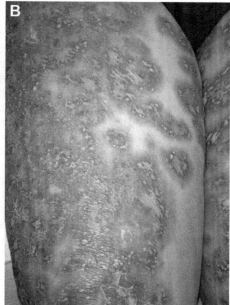

Fig. 1. Sneddon–Wilkinson disease presenting with grouped superficial flaccid pustules in an annular pattern on the extremities. (*A*) anterior bilateral legs, (*B*) close-up anterior leg. (*Courtesy of* Ryan Trowbridge, MD.)

include a complete blood count, urine and serum protein electrophoresis and immunofixation, antinuclear antibodies, and thyroid-stimulating hormone.[21]

Treatment

SWD is a chronic condition with a relapsing and remitting nature; however, treatment can help induce and maintain prolonged remission in some patients. Oral dapsone (50–200 mg daily) is the first-line treatment of SWD, with lesions typically resolving within a month of treatment initiation.[8] Dapsone can also be used in combination with topical or oral steroids, although it remains unclear if the addition of a steroid leads to faster clearance of lesions. Cessation of dapsone treatment is associated with recurrence of lesions; thus, maintenance therapy at a lower dose is recommended.[8] In patients who cannot tolerate dapsone or have developed dapsone resistance, successful treatments with retinoids (etretinate, acitretin), TNF inhibitors (etanercept, infliximab), light therapy (psoralen ultraviolet light [PUVA], ultraviolet B [UVB]) have also been documented.[8] For patients with underlying systemic disease, treatment of the underlying condition may help improve the associated SWD.

IgA Pemphigus

Key features

- Most commonly presents in individuals aged 40 to 60 years.

- Presents as vesicles, pustules, erosions, or erythematous plaques with a subacute course.
- Lesions typically localize to trunk, proximal extremities, intertriginous, and cephalic surfaces.
- Direct immunofluorescence shows intracellular deposition of IgA.
- The combination of corticosteroids and dapsone is the most effective treatment.

Epidemiology

IgA pemphigus, also referred to as intracellular IgA dermatosis, is a rare, benign, bullous neutrophilic dermatosis that was first described as a separate entity from SWD by Wallach and colleagues.[22,23] The exact incidence and prevalence of IgA pemphigus are unknown, and there are no known ethnic predispositions.[23] Similar to other pemphigus diseases, IgA pemphigus predominantly affects individuals between 40 and 60 years, with women affected at a slightly greater rate than men.[24] Cases in children and young adults are rare.[24]

Pathophysiology

IgA pemphigus can be classified into two subtypes: (1) subcorneal pustular dermatosis type (SPD type) or (2) intraepidermal neutrophilic IgA dermatosis (IEN type).[23] The pathogenesis of the SPD-type IgA pemphigus is due to the presence of human desmocollin-1, an autoantigen target for the IgA anti-keratinocyte cell surface autoantibodies.[25] In contrast, the exact pathogenesis of the IEN-type IgA pemphigus has not been fully elucidated.[24] Although the target antigens in the IEN type are unknown, previous studies have revealed the existence of a wide range of IgA antibodies directed against desmoglein 1 and 3, desmocollin 1 to 3, and non-desmosomal cell surface proteins.[26]

On histology, IgA pemphigus consistently presents with sterile intraepidermal clefts and pustules filled with polymorphonuclear leukocytes.[27] The infiltrate is predominantly neutrophilic in a majority of patients, although mixed neutrophilic and eosinophilic infiltrates are present in approximately 30% of patients.[23] Lymphocytic and eosinophilic dermal infiltrates have also been seen in a minority of patients.[23] In SPD-type IgA pemphigus, clefts and pustules localize to the subcorneal region.[27] In contrast, clefts and pustules present in the entire, mid, or lower epidermis in IEN-type IgA pemphigus.[26,27]

Histology typically reveals accompanying epidermal changes, including intraepidermal clefting and acantholysis, whereas dermal changes are typically absent.[23,28] In IgA pemphigus, direct immunofluorescence characteristically shows intercellular deposition of IgA.[23,28] IgA deposition can be isolated or concurrent with deposition of IgG, C3, and/or IgM.[23,28] Indirect immunofluorescence shows circulating IgA intercellular autoantibodies in a majority of cases.[23,28] It is important to note that the findings on direct and indirect immunofluorescence are the primary distinguishing features between IgA pemphigus and SWD (Table 1).

Clinical features

IgA pemphigus has a subacute onset.[27] The primary lesions of IgA pemphigus characteristically present as isolated or grouped, tense bullae that progress into translucent fluid-filled blisters (Fig. 2). The blisters can progress into vesicles, pustules, erosions, or erythematous plaques with central crusting in an annular or circinate configuration.[23,26,27] IgA pemphigus lesions most commonly involve the trunk, proximal extremities, intertriginous, and cephalic regions, and more rarely can affect the palmar/plantar surfaces and mucosal surfaces.[23,24] Widespread lesions and involvement of the face and/or scalp favor a diagnosis of IgA pemphigus rather than SWD.[29] Lesions typically have accompanying pain and pruritis.[23,30] Systemic symptoms secondary to the IgA pemphigus lesions are uncommon.[30]

Disease associations

IgA pemphigus is typically considered to be a benign disease.[31] However, IgA pemphigus has been shown to coexist with numerous disease states that potentially modify patients' overall life expectancies.[23] IgA pemphigus has been associated with underlying hematologic, lymphoproliferative, and solid tumor malignancies including IgA monoclonal gammopathy and multiple myeloma.[23] In addition, IgA pemphigus has been less commonly associated with other disease states, including ulcerative colitis, Sjögren syndrome, Crohn's disease, myasthenia gravis, rheumatoid arthritis, HIV infection, Wilson disease, and

---

Table 1
Comparison chart of Sneddon–Wilkinson disease, IgA pemphigus, and bullous systemic lupus erythematosus

	Sneddon–Wilkinson	IgA Pemphigus	BSLE
Neutrophilic Dermatoses			
Pathology	Chronic disease with neutrophilic infiltrate in subcorneal blisters	Subacute disease characteristic deposition of intracellular IgA	*Acute disease presenting with autoantibodies to type VII collagen*
Epidemiology	Most common in females from 50 to 70 y of age	Patients generally 40–60 y of age	Most common in females of African descent from 20–40 y of age
Clinical appearance	Recurrent, grouped, sterile, pustular eruptions	Vesicles, pustules, erosions, or erythematous plaques	Small vesicles to large, tense blisters
Treatment	Dapsone is first line and requires maintenance therapy to avoid recurrence	Corticosteroids in combination with dapsone show best results	Dapsone is first line. If not, steroids, or biologics

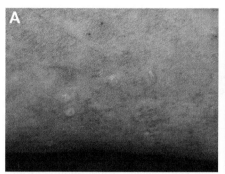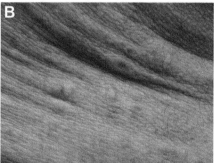

Fig. 2. IgA pemphigus disease presenting as small grouped vesicles. (*A*) extremities, (*B*) body folds. (*Courtesy of Ryan Trowbridge, MD.*)

alpha-1 antitrypsin deficiency.[23] Interestingly, an overlap of clinicopathologic and immunoserologic features between IgA pemphigus and pyostomatitis/pyodermatitis vegetans, another neutrophilic dermatosis, has been reported in the oral mucosa.[32,33]

Diagnosis

Owing to its rare nature, there are no established diagnostic criteria for IgA pemphigus. The differential diagnosis of IgA pemphigus includes SWD, pemphigus foliaceus, pemphigus herpetiformis, linear IgA bullous dermatosis, and bacterial skin infections.[30,32,33] Diagnosis is typically made from a consistent clinical picture, hallmark findings on histology, immunoserologic findings, and exclusion of the remaining clinical differential.[23] Diagnostic procedures include skin biopsy, direct immunofluorescence, and indirect immunofluorescence.[30] Further workup to exclude underlying malignancy and other systemic disease should be considered.

Treatment

IgA pemphigus is a milder and more limited disease compared with classic pemphigus, and treatment can induce remission of lesions without scarring.[30] The primary treatment for IgA pemphigus is topical or oral corticosteroids (eg, oral prednisone 0.5–1.5 mg/kg/day) or combination therapy with oral dapsone, which is more effective in treating IgA pemphigus than either drug alone.[23,30,34] Abrupt cessation of corticosteroids is associated with recurrence of lesions; thus, a gradual dosage reduction is recommended for cessation.[30] Other successful treatment options include vitamin A derivatives and immunosuppressants (cyclophosphamide, mycophenolate mofetil, azathioprine).[23] Refractory cases of IgA pemphigus have been managed with infliximab, adalimumab, intravenous immunoglobulin, and plasmapheresis.[23]

Bullous Systemic Lupus Erythematous

Key features

- Most commonly presents in females of African descent aged 20 to 40 years.
- Vesiculobullous lesions vary from small, clustered vesicles to large, tense blisters.
- Lesions localize most commonly to the head, neck, and extremities.
- Coexists with SLE.

Epidemiology

BSLE is a cutaneous manifestation of SLE.[6,35] It can be diagnosed in patients with preexisting SLE or it can present as the initial manifestation of SLE and be diagnosed concurrently.[35] BSLE was first described in a case report by Sunthonpalin and colleagues; however, diagnostic criteria were first formally established by Camisa and Sharma in 1983.[35–37] The prevalence of BSLE is unknown at this time due to its rarity.[35] Less than 1% of SLE patients develop BSLE.[38] Its estimated incidence is about 2% of all bullous cutaneous autoimmune disorders.[6] BSLE predominantly affects females of African descent between 20 and 40 years, although it may affect patients of all races, males, and those outside of that age range.[6] Cases in children are rare, and often present without extra-cutaneous symptoms.[39,40]

Pathophysiology

BSLE immunologic presentation depends on the subtype, of which there are three (**Table 2**). The most common is type I BSLE, involving the characteristic type VII collagen autoantibodies most frequently encountered in BSLE lesions.[41,42] The detection of antitype VII collagen autoantibodies can precede the physical signs and symptoms of BSLE; however, it is unknown how soon before disease manifestation these are detectable in the blood.[43] BSLE may also involve autoantibodies targeting non-collagenous domains 1 and 2 of type VII

Table 2
Bullous systemic lupus erythematosus subtypes

Type I	Type II	Type III
Autoantibodies to type VII collagen at the dermoepidermal junction	Type VII collagen autoantibodies absent	Autoantibodies to epidermal or simultaneous dermal and epidermal epitopes on the basement membrane

collagen at the dermoepidermal junction, which are detected by enzyme-linked immunoassay.[35,44]

Direct immunofluorescence reveals linear immunoglobulin G (IgG) deposits at the dermoepidermal junction along the basement membrane zone; IgA, IgM, and C3 deposits have also been reported in BSLE.[38,41,44,45] Indirect immunofluorescence typically reveals circulating autoantibodies against the basement membrane and a dermal pattern of IgG circulation.[41,42]

Histologically, BSLE is characterized by a dermal infiltrate of polynuclear neutrophils attaching to the basement membrane zone.[45] Subepidermal detachment and leukocytoclasis are also seen.[45] Mucin deposits in the absence of eosinophils are commonly seen on histology from skin biopsy.[41,46]

Clinical features

BSLE has a benign and acute course characterized by full remission in most cases within a year of diagnosis.[35,47] The primary lesions of BSLE are subepidermal vesicles and bullae that can vary in appearance from tense, large, fluid-filled blisters to small vesicular clusters (**Fig. 3**).[35,38,42] The development of these lesions is known to be fast, widespread, and often favoring sun-exposed areas, although BSLE presentation is not exclusively limited to any areas and involvement of non-sun-exposed areas is part of the diagnostic criteria.[38,46]

The lesions most commonly involve the head, neck, and extremities.[42] Other commonly affected sites include the trunk and mucosal surfaces, typically the buccal or genital mucosae.[42] Cases involving blistering of the tongue have also been documented.[42,48] Associated symptoms include pain, pruritis, crusting, bloody blisters, and concurrent edematous erythematous plaques.[42] In association with SLE, patients with BSLE frequently have or develop extra-cutaneous symptoms, especially renal disease, hemocytopenia, alopecia, serositis, arthritis, and urticaria.[35,42,45]

Disease associations

BSLE can lead to substantial morbidity, dyspigmentation, and scarring. It is also associated with a predisposition to systemic involvement, from which it is unknown if it is attributed to BSLE or to underlying SLE activity.[35,42,45] BSLE often results in higher SLE activity and can also be used as a prognosticator of SLE disease progression.[35,49] BSLE is also associated with leukocytoclastic vasculitis and a higher incidence of herpes zoster.[50,51]

Diagnosis

The diagnosis of BSLE is based on five main criteria (**Box 1**), the first being meeting the American College of Rheumatology (ACR) benchmarks for SLE[52] and the rest specifying clinical and histopathologic

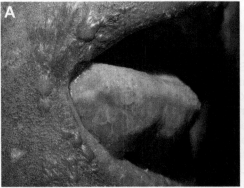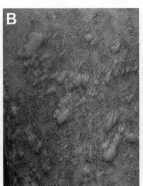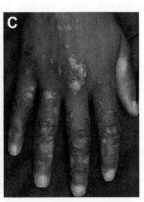

Fig. 3. BSLE presenting with tense, fluid-filled blisters, and vesicles on the mouth, trunk, and extremities. (*A*) face, (*B*) extremities, (*C*) posterior hand. (*Courtesy of* Ryan Trowbridge, MD.)

<table>
<tr><td>

Box 1
Bullous systemic lupus erythematosus diagnostic criteria

1. Satisfaction of ACR criteria for SLE diagnosis
2. Vesiculobullous presentation regardless of sun exposure
3. Histopathology shared with DH and leukocytoclastic vasculitis
4. Positive or negative indirect immunofluorescence of basement membrane antibodies
5. Positive direct immunofluorescence findings at basement membrane

</td></tr>
</table>

requirements.[38,53] The differential diagnosis of BSLE includes SLE with specific bullous lesions, DH, epidermolysis bullosa acquisita (EBA), IgA pemphigus, and bullous pemphigoid.[41] Diagnostic procedures include laboratory workups consisting of blister fluid biopsy, histologic confirmation, antinuclear antibody testing, and immunology panels.[35] A histologic confirmation of mucin deposits in the reticular dermis is critical for diagnosis of BSLE to distinguish it from SLE with specific bullous lesions as well as from DH.[35,54] In addition, antitype VII collagen autoantibodies are also found in EBA, so diagnosis of BSLE may also require IgG subtype variation testing, which is a fairly new practice.

Treatment

First-line treatment for BSLE is oral dapsone, starting at 50 mg daily and up to a maximum of 75 mg twice daily, which has shown up to 90% efficacy in providing full remission, cessation of new lesion formation in as little as 1 to 2 days, and disappearance of existing lesions within a matter of days.[35,38] Children should start with only 1.5 mg/kg/day and not exceed 2 mg/kg/day.[35] Additional treatments for BSLE include topical or systemic corticosteroid therapy, which are generally reserved for cases that cannot tolerate or are unresponsive to dapsone.[35,38,42] Systemic corticosteroids, as monotherapy or in combination with oral dapsone, can be used if there is systemic involvement.[35,38,42] Patients with refractory BSLE may benefit from treatment with immunomodulating biologics, such as rituximab and tofacitinib.[35,38,44,55]

SUMMARY

SWD, IgA pemphigus, and BSLE are rare diseases with overlapping clinical and pathophysiological features, highlighting the spectral nature of neutrophilic dermatoses and making diagnosis difficult. Diagnostic workup involves close attention to clinical presentation, histopathology, immune serology,

and evaluation of direct and indirect immunofluorescence. A careful history and workup aid in evaluating underlying disease states and comorbidities. The first-line treatment of all three diseases includes a combination of dapsone with corticosteroids or other immunosuppressive agents.

CLINICS CARE POINTS

- Diagnosis for Sneddon–Wilkinson disease (SWD), IgA pemphigus, and bullous systemic lupus erythematosus (BSLE) is based on clinical and histologic findings, with exclusion of other vesiculobullous diseases.
- On histology, SWD and IgA pemphigus are characterized by epidermal neutrophilic infiltrate, whereas BSLE demonstrates dermal neutrophilic infiltrate in the basement membrane zone.
- Positive direct and indirect immunofluorescence differentiates IgA pemphigus from SWD.
- In BSLE, direct immunofluorescence will show linear IgG deposition at the dermal–epidermal junction.
- Workup for underlying disease states and associated comorbidities is indicated.
- The first-line treatment for all three diseases is dapsone with corticosteroids or other immunosuppressive agents.

DISCLOSURE

A. Mostaghimi discloses consulting fees from Pfizer, Concert, Boehringer Ingelheim, Lilly, LEO, AbbVie, Equillium, Digital Diagnostics, hims and hers, ACOM, and Zest Dermatology outside of the scope of this work.

REFERENCES

1. Filosa A, Filosa G. Neutrophilic dermatoses: a broad spectrum of disease. Italian Journal of Dermatology and Venereology 2018;153(2).
2. Satoh TK, Mellett M, Contassot E, et al. Are neutrophilic dermatoses autoinflammatory disorders? Br J Dermatol 2018;178(3):603–13.
3. Marzano Av, Borghi A, Wallach D, et al. A Comprehensive Review of Neutrophilic Diseases. Clin Rev Allergy Immunol 2018;54(1):114–30.
4. Nelson CA, Stephen S, Ashchyan HJ, et al. Neutrophilic dermatoses. J Am Acad Dermatol 2018; 79(6):987–1006.

5. Griffin GK, Newton G, Tarrio ML, et al. IL-17 and TNF-α Sustain Neutrophil Recruitment during Inflammation through Synergistic Effects on Endothelial Activation. J Immunol 2012;188(12):6287–99.

6. Odonwodo A, Vashisht P. Bullous Systemic Lupus Erythematosus. [Updated 2023 May 22]. In: StatPearls [Internet]. Treasure Island (FL): StatPearls Publishing; 2023. Available at: https://www.ncbi.nlm.nih.gov/books/NBK557445/.

7. Sneddon IB, Wilkinson DS, Subcorneal Pustular Dermatosis. Br J Dermatol 1956;68(12):385–94.

8. Watts PJ, Khachemoune A. Subcorneal Pustular Dermatosis: A Review of 30 Years of Progress. Am J Clin Dermatol 2016;17(6):653–71.

9. Kretschmer L, Maul JT, Hofer T, et al. Interruption of Sneddon-Wilkinson Subcorneal Pustulation with Infliximab. Case Rep Dermatol 2017;9(1):140–4.

10. Alhafi MA, Janahi MI, Almossalli ZN. Subcorneal Pustular Dermatosis in Paediatrics: A Case Report and Review of the Literature. Cureus 2021. https://doi.org/10.7759/cureus.20221.

11. Scalvenzi M, Palmisano F, Annunziata MC, et al. Subcorneal Pustular Dermatosis in Childhood: A Case Report and Review of the Literature. Case Rep Dermatol Med 2013;2013:1–5.

12. Ranieri P, Bianchetti A, Trabucchi M. Sneddon-Wilkinson Disease: A Case Report of a Rare Disease in a Nonagenarian. J Am Geriatr Soc 2009;57(7):1322–3.

13. Bordignon M, Zattra E, Montesco MC, et al. Subcorneal Pustular Dermatosis (Sneddon-Wilkinson Disease) with Absence of Desmoglein 1 and 3 Antibodies. Am J Clin Dermatol 2008;9(1):51–5.

14. Grob JJ, Mege JL, Capo C, et al. Role of tumor necrosis factor-α in Sneddon-Wilkinson subcorneal pustular dermatosis. J Am Acad Dermatol 1991;25(5):944–7.

15. Romagnuolo M, Muratori S, Cattaneo A, et al. Successful treatment of refractory <scp>Sneddon-Wilkinson</scp> disease (subcorneal pustular dermatosis) with infliximab. Dermatol Ther 2022;35(7).

16. Cheng S, Edmonds E, Ben-Gashir M, et al. Subcorneal pustular dermatosis: 50 years on. Clin Exp Dermatol 2008;33(3):229–33.

17. Berk DR, Hurt MA, Mann C, et al. Sneddon-Wilkinson disease treated with etanercept: report of two cases. Clin Exp Dermatol 2009;34(3):347–51.

18. Mayba JN, Hawkins CN. First presentation of Sneddon-Wilkinson disease with unexpected immunoglobulin A gammopathy: A case report and review of the literature. SAGE Open Med Case Rep 2019;7. 2050313X1982643.

19. Tajiri K, Nakajima T, Kawai K, et al. Sneddon-Wilkinson Disease Induced by Sorafenib in a Patient with Advanced Hepatocellular Carcinoma. Intern Med 2015;54(6):597–600.

20. Bohelay G, Duong TA, Ortonne N, et al. Subcorneal pustular dermatosis triggered by Mycoplasma pneumoniae infection: a rare clinical association. J Eur Acad Dermatol Venereol 2015;29(5):1022–5.

21. Delaleu J, Lepelletier C, Calugareanu A, et al. Neutrophilic dermatoses. Rev Med Interne 2022;43(12):727–38.

22. Sluzevich JC, Mutasim D. IgA Pemphigus. In: XPharm: the comprehensive pharmacology reference. Elsevier; 2007. p. 1–6.

23. Kridin K, Patel PM, Jones VA, et al. IgA pemphigus: A systematic review. J Am Acad Dermatol 2020;82(6):1386–92.

24. Kridin K. Pemphigus group: overview, epidemiology, mortality, and comorbidities. Immunol Res 2018;66(2):255–70.

25. Hashimoto T, Kiyokawa C, Mori O, et al. Human Desmocollin 1 (Dsc1) Is an Autoantigen for the Subcorneal Pustular Dermatosis Type of IgA Pemphigus. J Invest Dermatol 1997;109(2):127–31.

26. Geller S, Gat A, Zeeli T, et al. The expanding spectrum of <scp>I</scp> g <scp>A</scp> pemphigus: a case report and review of the literature. Br J Dermatol 2014;171(3):650–6.

27. Tsuruta D, Ishii N, Hamada T, et al. IgA pemphigus. Clin Dermatol 2011;29(4):437–42.

28. Toosi S, Collins JW, Lohse CM, et al. Clinicopathologic features of IgG/IgA pemphigus in comparison with classic (IgG) and IgA pemphigus. Int J Dermatol 2016;55(4):e184–90.

29. Niimi Y, Kawana S, Kusunoki T. IgA pemphigus: A case report and its characteristic clinical features compared with subcorneal pustular dermatosis. J Am Acad Dermatol 2000;43(3):546–9.

30. Aslanova M, Yarrarapu SNS, Zito PM. IgA Pemphigus. [Updated 2023 Jul 24]. In: StatPearls [Internet]. Treasure Island (FL): StatPearls Publishing; 2023. Available at: https://www.ncbi.nlm.nih.gov/books/NBK519063/.

31. Porro AM, Caetano L de VN, Maehara L de SN, et al. Non-classical forms of pemphigus: pemphigus herpetiformis, IgA pemphigus, paraneoplastic pemphigus and IgG/IgA pemphigus. An Bras Dermatol 2014;89(1):96–106.

32. Wolz MM, Camilleri MJ, McEvoy MT, et al. Pemphigus vegetans variant of IgA pemphigus, a variant of IgA pemphigus and other autoimmune blistering disorders. Am J Dermatopathol 2013;35(3):e53–6.

33. Clark LG, Tolkachjov SN, Bridges AG, et al. Pyostomatitis vegetans (PSV)-pyodermatitis vegetans (PDV): A clinicopathologic study of 7 cases at a tertiary referral center. J Am Acad Dermatol 2016;75(3):578–84.

34. Moreno ACL, Santi CG, Gabbi TVB, et al. IgA pemphigus: Case series with emphasis on therapeutic response. J Am Acad Dermatol 2014;70(1):200–1.

35. Sprow G, Afarideh M, Dan J, et al. Bullous systemic lupus erythematosus in females. Int J Womens Dermatol 2022;8(3):e034.

36. Sunthonpalin PB, Maguire HC. Blister fluid in bullous systemic lupus erythematosus. Br J Dermatol 1970; 82(2):125–8.

37. Camisa C, Sharma HM. Vesiculobullous systemic lupus erythematosus. Report of two cases and a review of the literature. J Am Acad Dermatol 1983; 9(6):924–33.

38. Duan L, Chen L, Zhong S, et al. Treatment of Bullous Systemic Lupus Erythematosus. J Immunol Res 2015;2015:1–6.

39. Torres Saavedra FA, Campo LR, Mendez MV, et al. Bullous lupus as the first manifestation of systemic lupus erythematosus in the pediatric population: A diagnostic challenge in daily practice. Lupus 2020; 29(14):1937–42.

40. Hasbún ZMT, Rollan MP, Chaparro RX, et al. Lupus eritematoso sistémico buloso: Una manifestación infrecuente en población pediátrica. Andes Pediatrica 2021;92(3):428.

41. Contestable JJ, Edhegard KD, Meyerle JH. Bullous Systemic Lupus Erythematosus: A Review and Update to Diagnosis and Treatment. Am J Clin Dermatol 2014;15(6):517–24.

42. Qiao L, Zhang B, Zheng W, et al. Clusters of clinical and immunologic features in patients with bullous systemic lupus erythematosus: experience from a single-center cohort study in China. Orphanet J Rare Dis 2022;17(1):290.

43. Grabell DA, Matthews LA, Yancey KB, et al. Detection of Type VII Collagen Autoantibodies Before the Onset of Bullous Systemic Lupus Erythematosus. JAMA Dermatol 2015;151(5):539.

44. Keshavamurthy C, Fibeger E, Virata A, et al. Successful treatment of bullous lupus with corticosteroids and belimumab: A case report. Mod Rheumatol Case Rep 2023;7(1):52–6.

45. de Risi-Pugliese T, Cohen Aubart F, Haroche J, et al. Clinical, histological, immunological presentations and outcomes of bullous systemic lupus erythematosus: 10 New cases and a literature review of 118 cases. Semin Arthritis Rheum 2018;48(1):83–9.

46. Sebaratnam DF, Murrell DF. Bullous Systemic Lupus Erythematosus. Dermatol Clin 2011;29(4):649–53.

47. Grover C, Khurana A, Sharma S, et al. Bullous systemic lupus erythematosus. Indian J Dermatol 2013;58(6):492.

48. Anyanwu CO, Ang CC, Werth VP. Oral mucosal involvement of Bullous Systemic Lupus Erythematosus. Arthritis Rheum 2013.

49. Jira M, Elqatni M, Sekkach Y, et al. Étude de trois cas de lupus érythémateux bulleux. Ann Dermatol Venereol 2013;140(12):778–83.

50. Hsieh FN, Yu-Yun Lee J. Leukocytoclastic Vasculitis Concurrent With Bullous Systemic Lupus Erythematosus Manifesting Striking Wood-Grain and Wi-Fi Sign-like Purpuric Lesions. J Clin Rheumatol 2019; 25(7):e104–5.

51. Robinson ES, Payne AS, Pappas-Taffer L, et al. The incidence of herpes zoster in cutaneous lupus erythematosus (CLE), dermatomyositis (DM), pemphigus vulgaris (PV), and bullous pemphigoid (BP). J Am Acad Dermatol 2016;75(1):42–8.

52. Aringer M, Costenbader K, Daikh D, et al. European League Against Rheumatism/American College of Rheumatology Classification Criteria for Systemic Lupus Erythematosus. Arthritis Rheumatol 2019; 71(9):1400–12.

53. Rutnin S, Chanprapaph K. Vesiculobullous diseases in relation to lupus erythematosus. Clin Cosmet Investig Dermatol 2019;12:653–67.

54. Vishwajeet V, Chatterjee D, Saikia UN, et al. Bullous lesions in patients with cutaneous lupus erythematosus: A clinicopathologic study. J Am Acad Dermatol 2021;85(6):1641–3.

55. Yang J, Li J, Shi L. Successful remission with tofacitinib in a patient with refractory bullous systemic lupus erythematosus. Rheumatology 2022;61(11):e341–3.

Generalized Pustular Psoriasis, Acute Generalized Exanthematous Pustulosis, and Other Pustular Reactions: A Clinical Review

Elisabeth Gössinger, MD[a], Roni Dodiuk-Gad, MD[b,c], Beda Mühleisen, MD[a], Hazel H. Oon, MD[b,d], Choon Chiat Oh, MD[e,f], Julia-Tatjana Maul, MD[g], Alexander A. Navarini, MD, PhD[a,h,i,j],*

KEYWORDS

- Generalized pustular psoriasis • Acute generalized exanthematous pustulosis
- Pustular skin eruptions • IL-36 pathway • Genetic mutations • Drug-induced reactions
- Biologic therapies

KEY POINTS

- Few skin conditions are as impressive as generalized pustular psoriasis (GPP), acute generalized exanthematous pustulosis, and other pustular reactions.
- However, they also pose important diagnostic and treatment challenges. All of these diseases produce disseminated and rapidly evolving pustules, usually coupled with systemic symptoms and inflammation.
- GPP is defined by sterile, macroscopically visible, non-acral pustules. It can be associated with plaque-type psoriasis and often produces systemic inflammation.

INTRODUCTION

Few skin conditions are as distinctively memorable as generalized pustular psoriasis (GPP), acute generalized exanthematous pustulosis (AGEP), and other pustular reactions.[1,2] However, they also pose important diagnostic and treatment challenges. All of these diseases produce disseminated and rapidly evolving pustules, usually coupled with systemic symptoms and inflammation. GPP is defined by sterile, macroscopically visible, non-acral pustules. It can be associated with plaquetype psoriasis and often produces systemic inflammation.[3,4] Initially considered a subtype of psoriasis, it is now understood that GPP has unique genetic and clinical features that distinguish it from common plaque psoriasis (PV). Flares of GPP are not usually associated with specific situations, but triggers have been described, among them drugs, infections, or sudden withdrawal of systemic glucocorticoids.[5,6] The rapid clinical progression

[a] Department of Dermatology, University Hospital of Basel, Burgfelderstrasse 101, Basel 4055, Switzerland; [b] Department of Dermatology, Emek Medical Center, Bruce Rappaport Faculty of Medicine, Technion Institute of Technology, Haifa, 3525433 Israel; [c] Division of Dermatology, Department of Medicine, University of Toronto, Toronto, Ontario M5S 1A1, Canada; [d] National Skin Centre and Skin Research Institute of Singapore (SRIS), 1 Mandalay Road, Singapore 308205, Singapore; [e] Department of Dermatology, Singapore General Hospital, Singapore, Singapore; [f] Duke-NUS Medical School, 8 College Road, Singapore 169857, Singapore; [g] Department of Dermatology, University Hospital of Zurich and Faculty of Medicine, Zurich 8091/8006, Switzerland; [h] Department of Biomedical Research, University of Basel, Allschwil 4123, Switzerland; [i] Department of Biomedical Engineering, University of Basel, Allschwil 4123, Switzerland; [j] Department of Clinical Research, University of Basel, Allschwil 4123, Switzerland
* Corresponding author.
E-mail address: alexander.navarini@usb.ch

Dermatol Clin 42 (2024) 317–328
https://doi.org/10.1016/j.det.2024.01.001
0733-8635/24/© 2024 Elsevier Inc. All rights reserved.

and severity of the disease require a timely and accurate diagnosis. The diagnosis of GPP should be made with accordance to the widely used criteria, namely the European Rare and Severe Psoriasis Expert Network (ERASPEN) criteria.[7] Due to the large clinical overlap with AGEP, a working diagnosis of "putative GPP/AGEP" should be used until a persistence of greater than 3 months or a relapse of pustules is confirmed.[7] This working diagnosis may also justify systemic treatments for GPP in cases of severe disease.

AGEP[1] belongs to the severe cutaneous adverse reactions (SCARs). It is almost always drug-induced.[8–10] Patients present with multiple sterile, nonfollicular, small pustules on erythematous skin. Upon stopping the offending drug, AGEP usually resolves spontaneously in most clinical situations. Severe cases may require systemic treatment. The rapid progression and potential for systemic involvement require early confirmation of the diagnosis and oftentimes inpatient treatment.

Other pustular drug reactions include drug reaction with systemic symptoms (DRESS), pustular forms of erythema exsudativum multiforme (EEM) and Stevens-Johnson syndrome/toxic epidermal necrolysis (SJS/TEN). The key to managing these reactions is prompt identification and discontinuation of the offending drug, as well as initiating immunosuppression medications in some cases. The prevalence of these conditions is not well-defined, partly due to their rarity and the overlap in clinical features that may lead to misdiagnosis. The morbidity associated with these pustular eruptions, the potential for systemic involvement, and the challenges posed in the differential diagnosis underscore the need for a keen understanding of their pathophysiology.

Lastly, we will discuss the clinical differential diagnosis of nondrug-induced pustular reactions such as subcorneal pustulosis, pustular Sweet syndrome, amicrobial pustulosis of the folds, as well as infectious folliculitis.

The aim of this article is to discuss these complex pustular dermatoses, specifically their etiology, pathophysiology, clinical presentation, diagnostic challenges, and therapeutic strategies. A summary of these conditions is presented in **Table 1**.

PATHOPHYSIOLOGY, TRIGGERS

The pathogenesis of GPP is closely linked to dysregulation of the immune system, in particular the interleukin (IL)-36 pathway, a member of the IL-1 cytokine family.[11] This has identified it as an auto-inflammatory disease, which means it produces unprompted inflammation without an identifiable antigen. The link has been proven by the highly significant association of GPP with damaging homozygous mutations in the *IL36RN* gene.[12,13] The gene product is the IL-36 receptor antagonist. When this protein is dysfunctional, unopposed IL-36 signaling has been observed, leading to increased keratinocyte proliferation and the neutrophilic infiltration characteristic of GPP lesions. This prompted the name *deficiency of interleukin-36 receptor antagonist* (DITRA) for this condition.[13] This unrestrained cytokine activity drives not only pustular formation but also systemic inflammation, which can lead to the severe systemic symptoms seen in GPP. Recent genetic analyses have elucidated a triad of mutations in addition to *IL36RN*, namely *CARD14*,[14,15] *MPO*,[16] *AP1S3*,[17–19] SERPINA3/A1,[20] BTN3A3,[21] TGFBR2, all of which are implicated in the pathogenesis of GPP, albeit accounting for only a subset of cases. The *IL36RN* mutation is notable for its role in disrupting IL-36 signaling, a pathway essential for innate immune responses and inflammation. *CARD14* mutations have been implicated in the activation of the NF-kB pathway, which is central to the proinflammatory cascade. The *AP1S3* mutation has been linked to autophagy and endosomal trafficking pathways, which are critical for cell homeostasis and may influence the inflammatory milieu. The fact that these mutations are not universally present in all cases of GPP suggests a polygenic etiology and perhaps an interaction with environmental triggers. Damaging mutations in the *MPO* gene, which encodes the major neutrophil protein myeloperoxidase, have been directly linked to the pustular reaction. A novel deletion and 3 missense mutations in the *SERPINA3* gene were found to impede or reduce activity of alpha-1-antichymotrypsin on cathepsin G in pediatric-onset GPP in Asians.[22]

AGEP has a multifactorial etiology involving not only drugs but also infections, vaccinations, iodinated contrast, food such as shiitake mushroom, environmental factors such as spider bite, and, probably, a genetic predisposition.[1] Epidemiologically, AGEP has an incidence of 1 to 5 cases per million per year and is more common in women (60%). The age of onset is typically 50 to 60 years, but cases can occur at any age. Despite its acute presentation, AGEP usually resolves favorably within 2 weeks of cessation of the offending agent and appropriate treatment, although a mortality rate of 3% has been reported, mainly due to multi-organ failure or superinfection. Genetic predisposition to AGEP is evidenced by findings such as *IL36RN* mutations, which are found in 4% of AGEP cases.[23] The occurrence of the disease in different ethnic groups, with a noted predominance in certain groups, underlines the role of genetics in

Table 1
Comparison of etiology, clinical presentation, pathogenesis, chronicity, histopathology and treatments of various pustular rashes.

Feature	GPP	AGEP	DRESS, Anticonvulsant Hypersensitivity Syndrome	Sneddon-Wilkinson	EEM, TEN/SJS	Sweet Syndrome	Infectious Folliculitis	Amicrobial Pustulosis of the Folds	Other Pustular Rashes
Etiology	Genetic predisposition, triggers like infections and medication withdrawal	Drug-induced, often antibiotics, hydroxychloroquine, and others	Drug-induced, including anticonvulsants	Unknown, possibly immune-mediated	Drug-induced or idiopathic	Idiopathic, respiratory tract infections, hematologic disease, rheumatologic, gastrointestinal disease, or drug-induced	Bacterial, fungal, or viral infections	Often associated with autoimmune diseases; sterile pustules	Various, including genetic, autoimmune, and inflammatory causes
Clinical presentation	Rapid onset of widespread nonfollicular pustules, often systemic symptoms	Rapid onset of widespread nonfollicular pustules, often fever	Rapid onset of follicular pustules, fever, often drug-specific symptoms	Recurrent superficial nonfollicular pustules, annular or serpiginous patterns	Targetoid lesions, mucosal involvement in severe forms	Painful, erythematous, edematous plaques and nodules, occasionally vesiculopustular	Follicular-based erythematous pustules	Chronic recurrent eruptions of sterile pustules, primarily in skin folds	Varies
Pathogenesis	Genetic mutations (eg, *IL36RN, CARD14*)	Immune-mediated response to drugs	Immune-mediated response to drugs, including specific syndromes like anticonvulsant hypersensitivity	Unclear, potentially immune-related	Immune-mediated response, often to drugs	Immune-mediated, often neutrophilic infiltration	Infection-driven	Unknown, possibly immune-related	Depending on the condition
Chronicity	Often chronic and relapsing	Self-limiting upon drug withdrawal	Self-limiting upon drug withdrawal	Chronic, relapsing	Acute and self-limiting	Acute, may recur in some cases	Resolves with treatment of the infection	Chronic and recurrent	Varies
Histopathology	Sterile spongiform pustules of Kogoj, neutrophils in the stratum corneum, parakeratosis, psoriasiform epidermal hyperplasia, no significant papillary dermal edema, scarce or no eosinophils. Dilated, tortuous blood vessels in the papillary dermis.	Eosinophils usually present, papillary dermal edema, spongiosis, necrotic keratinocytes, mixed interstitial and mid-dermal perivascular infiltrate, usually no dilated blood vessels in the papillary dermis.	Dense perivascular lymphocyte infiltration in the dermis, and atypical lymphocytes, often interface dermatitis.	Subcorneal neutrophilic pustules without eosinophils, no spongiosis, acanthosis, or significant dermal signs of inflammation.	EEM: Several necrotic keratinocytes throughout the epidermis with surrounding lymphocytic exocytosis, mild to moderate edema and perivascular lymphocytic inflammation with occasional eosinophils/ lymphocytes. TEN/SJS: Extensive necrosis of keratinocytes, leading to full-thickness epidermal necrosis, mild inflammatory infiltrate.	Dense neutrophilic infiltrate without vasculitis, lack of epidermal involvement, edematous papillary dermis.	Follicular pustules and (peri-)folliculitis with a neutrophilic or lymphocytic infiltrate, detection of organisms with special staining.	Sterile epidermal pustulation, neutrophilic infiltrate in the dermis, diagnosis dependent on clinical setting and association with autoimmune conditions.	Variable

(continued on next page)

Table 1
(continued)

Feature	GPP	DRESS, Anticonvulsant Hypersensitivity Syndrome	AGEP	Sneddon-Wilkinson	EEM, TEN/SJS	Sweet Syndrome	Infectious Folliculitis	Amicrobial Pustulosis of the Folds	Other Pustular Rashes
Treatment	Systemic agents, biologics targeting specific inflammatory pathways	Prompt identification and discontinuation of the offending drug, immunosuppressive drugs	Prompt withdrawal of the offending drug, supportive care	Topical corticosteroids, dapsone, or systemic corticosteroids	Withdrawal of the offending drug, systemic corticosteroids	Corticosteroids, dapsone	Antibacterial, antifungal, or antiviral agents, depending on the cause	Topical steroids, tacrolimus, systemic agents in severe cases	Dependent on the specific condition, may include immunosuppressants

AGEP. Various drugs have been reported to induce AGEP.[1] The most common drug triggers are antibiotics, particularly beta-lactams (18%–41% of cases), macrolides, and quinolones, together with other drugs such as hydroxychloroquine (13%), antineoplastics (12%), nonsteroidal anti-inflammatory drugs (5%), anticonvulsants (4%), and calcium channel blockers. Additional drugs include antiviral, antifungal, antiparasitic, anticoagulants, antiarrhythmics, antihypertensives, antipsychotics, diabetes therapy, hormonal therapy, opioids, and even topical agents.[1] The latency period between drug exposure and the onset of AGEP generally ranges from 1 to 13 days,[1] with a mean of 3 to 9 days, indicating the rapid onset of this hypersensitivity reaction. The pathogenesis is thought to begin with the generation of drug-specific T cells. Upon exposure to the drug, these T cells are activated and release a cascade of cytokines, in particular IL-8, which is chemotactic for neutrophils.[1] In contrast, recent work has identified a T cell-independent pattern recognition receptor-dependent triggered monocyte in AGEP.[24] The massive influx of neutrophils into the epidermis leads to the formation of the characteristic nonfollicular sterile pustules. The rapid resolution of AGEP after drug withdrawal supports the hypothesis that ongoing drug exposure is required to maintain the pathogenic process.

Apart from AGEP, there is a poorly defined group of other pustular drug reactions. This is a broad category that includes other SCARs that rarely present with pustules, namely DRESS, fixed toxic drug reaction, and SJS/TEN. In most of these cases, the detailed pathophysiology remains unknown.

CLINICAL FEATURES AND DIFFERENTIATION

Accurate diagnosis and differentiation between GPP, AGEP, and various other pustular reactions, including DRESS/anticonvulsant hypersensitivity syndrome, are both critical and challenging. These conditions, although distinct in pathophysiology and etiology, often present with overlapping clinical features, making their accurate identification and management difficult.[25,26]

Generalized Pustular Psoriasis

This condition presents with a diverse clinical picture, characterized by its distinct pustular eruptions[27] on various body parts, often accompanied by systemic symptoms. The ERASPEN criteria[7] were established to facilitate the diagnosis of GPP, acrodermatitis continua of Hallopeau, and palmoplantar pustulosis. GPP is characterized by the presence of widespread, visible, noninfectious pustules on the skin, typically outside of the acral extremities, and is not limited to existing psoriatic lesions (**Fig. 1**). This condition may present alongside systemic inflammatory symptoms, with or without concomitant PV, and can manifest as either recurring episodes or as a prolonged skin eruption lasting more than 3 months.

Since the publication of these criteria, new data have become available from several GPP cohorts. The ERASPEN criteria, but also newer consensus papers,[28] state that GPP produces innumerable nonfollicular pustules on the trunk, extremities, and head. Many cases demonstrate particularly intertriginous involvement. Clusters of pustules often coalesce to form larger areas of pus-filled "lakes of pus."[29–33] 76.0% the skin lesions are recurrent and do not clearly follow a flare pattern.[31] Annular GPP tends to have fewer fevers and relapses.[34] There is no clear gender predilection in GPP; a Turkish study and others found a female predominance,[33,35,36] a Korean cohort was evenly split between men and women,[31] and in a Portuguese study 61% were male, especially subjects with liver problems.[29] GPP typically starts in middle age, that is, 38.1 to 45.6 years.[31,33] Skin and joint pain are common, affecting 62.1% and 26.2% of GPP patients, respectively.[37] Lastly,

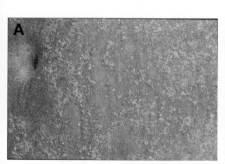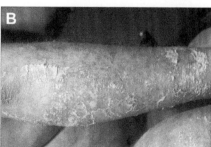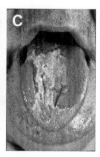

Fig. 1. Generalized pustular psoriasis (GPP) with (*A*) disseminated pustules, (*B*) lakes of pus and desquamation, and (*C*) lingua geographica that occurs in some populations, more frequently in genetically driven deficiency of interleukin-36 receptor antagonist (DITRA) with the c.115+6T > C/p.Arg10ArgfsX1 mutation.[65]

GPP can have severe consequences including miscarriages, sepsis, and death.[29,35,38]

GPP flares mostly occur without any discernible triggers. In the minority of cases, the patients report intake of certain medications such as lithium, sudden steroid withdrawal, upper respiratory infections, and pregnancy.[33,35,36] GPP is not just a skin disease but a systemic condition of intense inflammation. This is demonstrated by the elevation of C-reactive protein and leukocytosis in most patients, as well as internal manifestations that is, gastrointestinal problems.[39] Almost half of a Portuguese study group had liver enzyme abnormalities unrelated to previous medication, suggesting a direct link to GPP.[29] This study also found high white blood cell counts and a link between neutrophil levels and bilirubin, suggesting an interaction between inflammation and liver stress.[29] A recent paper stratified 416 Chinese GPP patients into 3 age groups, namely juvenile (9.5 years), middle aged (35.4 years), and seniors (62.6 years). A higher odds of a plaque-type psoriasis association was present in nonjuvenile patients. Also, juveniles had a lower incidence of comorbidities. As to the localization of lesions, juveniles had more facial, scalp, neck, and perineal lesions.[34] GPP patients without a history of psoriasis vulgaris tended to have more severe symptoms[34] and an earlier onset of disease.[36] In another Chinese study, infection and drugs were identified as presumable triggers for GPP,[36] which as confirmed in another cohort of 102 adult-onset GPP patients with systemic steroids, infections, and pregnancy as triggers.[38] In 2 studies from Malaysia, dyslipidaemia (26%), hypertension (26%), obesity (43%), and diabetes (24%) were common in pustular psoriasis (PP) patients, suggesting a link with metabolic syndrome.[32,38]

Acute Generalized Exanthematous Pustulosis

Comparatively, there are fewer data on AGEP patients. The largest study looked at 340 people, while another had 96.[40,41] Most AGEP patients are women, 56% to 68%.[40,41] The majority are white (60.6%) and non-Hispanic (70.3%), with an average age of 57.8 to 60 years.[40,41] Common symptoms include fever in 75% of patients and skin peeling in 64.7%.[40,41] AGEP produces innumerable small sterile and nonfollicular pustules that can are often focused on the intertriginous regions (**Fig. 2**). The pustules are often on edematous skin and the rash is accompanied by itch. Subsequently, desquamation follows. Medication is often the cause of AGEP, with different drugs implicated.[1,8] The latency can be as low as 24 hours, but some drugs such as hydroxychloroquine can take up to 3 weeks until the induction of AGEP. Infections were suspected triggers in a small number of cases. Liver and kidney function derangement have occurred in some cases. Treatment usually involves corticosteroids and other medications, and most patients improve. The 30-day mortality rate was 3.5%.[42] Some atypical forms of AGEP include targetoid lesion and blisters,[1] as well as a form that produces fewer but larger pustules up to 5 mm surrounded by an erythematous anulus (Navarini, personal communication). Apart from GPP and AGEP, there are also even more rare pustular reactions that must be considered. These also typically present with a rapid onset of pustules on erythematous skin.

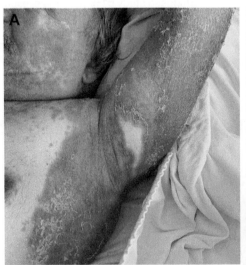
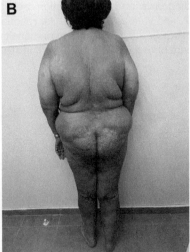

Fig. 2. Acute generalized exanthematous pustulosis (AGEP) (*A*) with disseminated pustules and (*B*) in resolution.

This similarity in initial presentation often leads to diagnostic confusion. A helpful diagnostic clue is that anticonvulsant hypersensitivity syndrome[43] (a form of DRESS) produces a follicular pustular reaction, which can help distinguish it from AGEP and GPP, as they are 2 otherwise closely related conditions. Systemic symptoms such as fever and malaise are common, further complicating the clinical picture. It is important to note that there have been cases of AGEP and DRESS overlap and AGEP and SJS/TEN overlap reported.[26,44] Diagnosis of AGEP is based on clinical and histologic criteria. A validated diagnostic scoring system for AGEP based on 3 major factors—morphology, clinical course, and histology—was published by the EuroSCAR study group.[45]

Other Pustular Conditions

Subcorneal pustulosis, or Sneddon-Wilkinson disease,[46,47] is a rare pustular dermatosis that presents with recurrent, flaccid, hypopyon-like superficial, nonfollicular pustule (**Fig. 3**), typically distributed symmetrically on the trunk, intertriginous areas, and flexures. The pustules are often arranged in annular or serpiginous patterns and can coalesce to form larger plaques. Histologically, it is characterized by subcorneal pustules filled with neutrophils without involvement of the epidermis, differentiating it from other neutrophilic

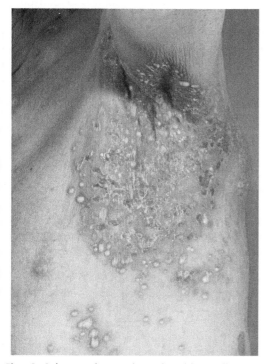

Fig. 3. Subcorneal pustulosis (Sneddon-Wilkinson). Note the "hypopyon" sign in some larger pustules.

dermatoses (PMID: 371657). In the ERASPEN consensus, it was grouped with GPP, and prospective data will hopefully show clearly whether it should be differentiated from GPP or not.

EEM and SCARs such as SJS and TEN can also exhibit pustular lesions. There are also overlaps between AGEP and EEM.[48] These conditions are acute and often drug-induced, characterized by targetoid erythematous lesions that in severe cases progress to large-surface epidermal detachment. In TEN/SJS, the involvement of mucosal surfaces is expected.

Sweet syndrome (acute febrile neutrophilic dermatosis) is characterized by the abrupt onset of painful, erythematous, and edematous plaques and nodules, which can evolve into vesiculopustular lesions. The face, neck, and upper extremities are commonly involved. Sweet syndrome is often associated with systemic symptoms like fever and leukocytosis and can be idiopathic, drug-induced, or associated with malignancies and other systemic diseases. It can be associated with generalized pustulosis.[49,50]

Amicrobial pustulosis of the folds,[51] first described by Crickx, is another important differential that must be considered. In a study of 63 cases, a significant majority (90%) were women, with an average age of 30. In most cases, it was associated with systemic lupus erythematosus and other conditions. The condition typically presents as pustules on an erythematous (reddened) background, often eroding and predominantly affecting areas like skinfolds, the anogenital region, scalp, ears, and umbilicus. Histologically, it is characterized by a spongiform layer of subcorneal pustules and a mixed inflammatory response in the dermis.

Infectious folliculitis produce pustules arising from hair follicles and are primarily caused by bacterial, fungal, or viral agents. The lesions are typically follicular-based, erythematous, and can be pruritic or tender. Common bacterial causes include *Staphylococcus aureus* and *Pseudomonas aeruginosa*, whereas fungal folliculitis can be caused by dermatophytes or yeasts such as *Candida* species.

A detailed patient history, particularly of recent medication use, is essential in identifying potential drug-induced reactions. Skin biopsies can provide valuable information. Features such as spongiform pustules of Kogoj are indicative of GPP, whereas a dense neutrophilic and/or eosinophilic infiltrate is characteristic of AGEP. In cases of suspected drug reactions, it is important to assess the likelihood that a drug is the culprit. This involves analyzing the timing of drug administration relative to symptom onset and understanding the typical reaction profiles of the drugs involved. For GPP, genetic testing may be helpful, especially in equivocal cases, to identify specific gene mutations associated with the disease.

DERMATOPATHOLOGY

As GPP and AGEP may not be differentiated clearly by their clinical features, a biopsy and clinical-pathologic correlations[52] are often performed. In the Japanese guideline for GPP, the presence of certain histologic features necessitating a biopsy is mandatory.[53] The histologic features of GPP include sterile spongiform pustules of Kogoj, which are defined as neutrophilic granulocytes accumulating within the stratum spinosum. Also, neutrophils are found more diffusely distributed in the stratum corneum (Munro abscesses) and in the upper dermis, and parakeratosis is expected. No significant papillary dermal edema is found. In addition, psoriasiform epidermal hyperplasia, hypogranulosis, suprapapillary plate thinning and tortuous, and dilated blood vessels in the stratum papillare may be seen especially in long-standing lesions.[52] It remains to be investigated if the later histologic changes are predominantly present in GPP patients with concomitant plaquetype psoriasis. Histology of GPP typically shows only scarce or no eosinophils. In general, in AGEP, eosinophils are typically more abundant. The first description of AGEP demonstrated 4 patients with predominantly eosinophilic pustules.[54] Other important histologic criteria that distinguish AGEP from GPP are keratinocyte necroses and a dermal edema, both of which are usually missing or only mild in GPP.[52,55] The neutrophil pustules in both GPP and AGEP are nonfollicular.[54] EEM shows necrotic keratinocytes within and above the basal layer surrounded by intraepidermal lymphocytes, a mild to moderate edema, and perivascular lymphocytes in the superficial dermis but normally no interface dermatitis. Eosinophils may be present, but they are not a diagnostic feature.[56] DRESS shows a denser perivascular lymphocytic infiltration in the dermis, as well as eosinophils and atypical lymphocytes. Often, there is an interface dermatitis present. The defining feature of TEN/SJS is extensive necrosis of keratinocytes, leading to full-thickness epidermal necrosis. The inflammatory infiltrate can be very mild, whilst interface changes defined by lymphocyte-mediated damage of the basal keratinocytes can be present. Sweet syndrome shows a dense neutrophilic infiltrate without vasculitis, a lack of epidermal involvement, whilst the papillary dermis is edematous. Subcorneal pustulosis, or Sneddon-Wilkinson disease, demonstrates subcorneal neutrophilic pustules without eosinophils. No spongiosis, acanthosis, or significant dermal signs of inflammation are expected in this condition.[57] In amicrobial pustulosis of the folds, there are sterile epidermal pustulation and a neutrophilic infiltrate in the dermis. This pattern is not distinctive and the diagnosis is dependent on the clinical setting, especially the association with autoimmune conditions. Lastly, infectious folliculitis demonstrate follicular pustules and (peri-)folliculitis with a neutrophilic or lymphocytic infiltrate, depending on the offending organisms that can be detected with special stainings.

TREATMENT

Accurately distinguishing between the various pustular conditions is important for several reasons. Specific treatments vary between these conditions. In addition, in drug-induced reactions, identification of the causative agent is essential to prevent relapses. The variety of treatments for GPP, with 17 different options identified by Noe and colleagues (2022),[37] reflects the wide range of options that were tried to control this condition. Primary options include acitretin, cyclosporine, methotrexate, and infliximab, each contributing to symptom relief and disease control. Acitretin, an oral retinoid, is a traditionally used drug for GPP[38] but is slow-acting and requires several years of contraception for women of childbearing age. Methotrexate, valued for its inflammation-reducing effects, has been beneficial in numerous GPP cases, according to retrospective studies.[38] Cyclosporine is an effective immunosuppressant but has numerous side effects when used on a long-term basis. Apremilast increases cyclic adenosine monophosphate levels intracellularly and has been shown to be useful against neutrophilic infiltrates. Monoclonal antibodies like infliximab, a TNF-alpha blocker, are effective therapies. IL-17 blockers such as secukinumab and ixekizumab are gaining attention, particularly secukinumab for its effectiveness in easing symptoms during clinical trials. Brodalumab, targeting the IL-17 receptor, has shown positive results in clinical remission and improvement. IL-23 blockers, like guselkumab, also demonstrate effectiveness, underscoring this pathway's role in GPP. Indeed, guselkumab has been registered in Japan for the treatment of GPP. However, in a retrospective study in Italy, IL-23 antagonists demonstrated inferiority to IL-17 blockers in PP.[58] The newest therapies focus on the IL-36 pathway, such as spesolimab and imsidolimab. Interestingly, they are proving effective in patients with or without *IL36RN* mutations.[59,60] After 1 week of spesoliumab, 54% of GPP patients had no more pustules, in contrast to 6% of placebo patients. A large study involving 123 patients in 60 hospitals and clinics showed that high-dose spesolimab greatly lowers the risk and frequency of GPP flares over 48 weeks compared to a placebo. This finding underscores spesolimab's role in preventing GPP flares.[61]

For AGEP and pustular drug reactions, the main approach is to discontinue the offending drug. The first critical step is identifying and stopping the trigger medication. Alongside supportive treatments like topical steroids, control of fluid intake and fever are crucial. In more severe instances, treatments might include systemic steroids or immunosuppressants/biologics. A study by Yanes found cyclosporine as effective as systemic glucocorticoids in halting pustule formation and helping with erythema resolution, without significant side effects.[62]

INTERNATIONAL RARE AND SEVERE PSORIASIS EXPERT NETWORK PROSPECTIVE REGISTRY AND FUTURE QUESTIONS TO BE ADDRESSED

Since the rarity of GPP makes research efforts difficult, the typical clinical course and the effects of pharmacologic treatments under real-world conditions remain poorly understood. Investigational endeavors are further complicated by varying geographic prevalence.[63] Therefore, international cooperation is essential to collect sufficient samples for comprehensive analysis. Historically, the lack of clear consensus criteria and heterogeneous patient populations for GPP and other PP subtypes have impeded targeted research efforts. To address this issue, ERASPEN was established in 2012 as a cross-sectional investigation of clinical phenotypes and genotypes of PP, which resulted in a consensus[7] defining the currently established diagnostic criteria for GPP. As these criteria were not chosen based on prospective data but rather on the opinion of experts, the decision to collect such data was made. Building on this collaborative effort, the ongoing, prospective International Rare and Severe Psoriasis Expert Network (IRASPEN) registry was created in 2020. By longitudinally following patients worldwide over a period of 5 years, several unanswered questions regarding PP subtypes will be addressed, including what overlapping phenotypes exist, the actual severity and frequency of flares, as well as the effect of established treatments such as systemic steroids that are (perhaps falsely) accused of triggering GPP flares. Naturally, emerging treatments will also be evaluated with real-world evidence in this noninterventional registry. Observation of the natural course of the disease allows further phenotypic characterization by considering the evolution of clinical features. A better clinical and pathophysiological understanding can be achieved by studying the short-term and long-term responses to therapeutic interventions. In addition, biological sampling including serologic deoxyribonucleic acid , ribonucleic acid, and proteomic analyses, as well as transcriptomics of lesional and unaffected skin samples, will be used to further characterize GPP and its inflammatory pattern at the molecular level. Since the underlying mutations have mainly been analyzed in sporadic cases or large pedigrees, systematic genetic profiling of patients and their first-degree and second-degree relatives will provide new insights. Currently, 8 centers in 7 different countries on 2 continents are participating in the registry, with more to be initiated soon to join the global cooperation.[64] The authors anticipate this collaborative registry will help address current and future clinical unmet needs of GPP (apply on iraspen.org).

Taken together, the authors have delved into the complexities of diagnosing and managing GPP, AGEP, and other pustular skin reactions. These conditions, while distinctive in their pathophysiology and triggers, present significant diagnostic challenges due to overlapping clinical features. GPP is characterized by widespread sterile pustular lesions, often associated with systemic inflammation, and can be triggered by various factors including drugs, infections, or steroid withdrawal. Its pathogenesis is closely linked to immune dysregulation, notably involving the IL-36 pathway and mutations in several genes. AGEP, commonly drug-induced, presents with multiple sterile pustules and is driven by T cell and monocyte activation.[65] The key to effective management is a precise diagnosis, which hinges on patient history, skin biopsies, and understanding the nuances of each condition. Treatment strategies differ: GPP often requires systemic agents and targeted biologics, while AGEP primarily involves withdrawing the offending drug and providing supportive care. Prospective registries and clinical studies will enable greatly improved treatment strategies for these neglected conditions.

CLINICS CARE POINTS

- In patients with disseminated non-follicular pustules think about GPP and AGEP. In severe cases, a working diagnosis of GPP/AGEP can be justified for systemic treatment, until the GPP diagnosis can be confirmed.
- Patients without systemic inflammation can still have GPP or AGEP.

- Patients without plaque-type psoriasis can still have GPP.
- Withdrawal of corticosteroids might not be a frequent cause of GPP.

ACKNOWLEDGEMENTS

This manuscript was funded by University of Basel. AAN declares being a consultant and advisor and/or receiving speaking fees and/or grants and/or served as an investigator in clinical trials for AbbVie, Almirall, Amgen, Biomed, BMS, Boehringer Ingelheim, Celgene, Eli Lilly, Galderma, GSK, LEO Pharma, Janssen-Cilag, MSD, Novartis, Pfizer, Pierre Fabre Pharma, Regeneron, Sandoz, Sanofi, and UCB.

DISCLOSURE

None.

REFERENCES

1. Parisi R, Shah H, Navarini AA, et al. Acute generalized exanthematous pustulosis: clinical features, differential diagnosis, and management. Am J Clin Dermatol 2023;24:557–75.
2. Fujita H, Gooderham M, Romiti R. Diagnosis of generalized pustular psoriasis. Am J Clin Dermatol 2022;23:31–8.
3. Boehner A, Navarini AA, Eyerich K. Generalized pustular psoriasis - a model disease for specific targeted immunotherapy, systematic review. Exp Dermatol 2018;27:1067–77.
4. Puig L, Choon SE, Gottlieb AB, et al. Generalized pustular psoriasis: A global Delphi consensus on clinical course, diagnosis, treatment goals and disease management. J Eur Acad Dermatol Venereol 2023;37:737–52.
5. Gregoire ARF, DeRuyter BK, Stratman EJ. Psoriasis flares following systemic glucocorticoid exposure in patients with a history of psoriasis. JAMA Dermatol 2021;157:198–201.
6. Zema CL, Valdecantos WC, Weiss J, et al. Understanding flares in patients with generalized pustular psoriasis documented in us electronic health records. JAMA Dermatol 2022;158:1142–8.
7. Navarini AA, Burden AD, Capon F, et al. European consensus statement on phenotypes of pustular psoriasis. J Eur Acad Dermatol Venereol 2017;31:1792–9.
8. Oh DAQ, Yeo YW, Choo KJL, et al. Acute generalized exanthematous pustulosis: Epidemiology, clinical course, and treatment outcomes of patients treated in an Asian academic medical center. JAAD Int 2021;3:1–6.

9. Vallejo-Yague E, Martinez-De la Torre A, Mohamad OS, et al. Drug triggers and clinic of acute generalized exanthematous pustulosis (AGEP): a literature case series of 297 patients. J Clin Med 2022;11.
10. Martinez-De la Torre A, van Weenen E, Kraus M, et al. A network analysis of drug combinations associated with acute generalized exanthematous pustulosis (AGEP). J Clin Med 2021;10.
11. Dinarello CA. Overview of the interleukin-1 family of ligands and receptors. Semin Immunol 2013;25:389–93.
12. Onoufriadis A, Simpson MA, Pink AE, et al. Mutations in IL36RN/IL1F5 are associated with the severe episodic inflammatory skin disease known as generalized pustular psoriasis. Am J Hum Genet 2011;89:432–7.
13. Marrakchi S, Guigue P, Renshaw BR, et al. Interleukin-36-receptor antagonist deficiency and generalized pustular psoriasis. N Engl J Med 2011;365:620–8.
14. Qin P, Zhang Q, Chen M, et al. Variant analysis of CARD14 in a Chinese Han population with psoriasis vulgaris and generalized pustular psoriasis. J Invest Dermatol 2014;134:2994–6.
15. Berki DM, Liu L, Choon SE, et al. Activating CARD14 mutations are associated with generalized pustular psoriasis but rarely account for familial recurrence in psoriasis vulgaris. J Invest Dermatol 2015;135:2964–70.
16. Onitsuka M, Farooq M, Iqbal MN, et al. A homozygous loss-of-function variant in the MPO gene is associated with generalized pustular psoriasis. J Dermatol 2023;50:664–71.
17. Setta-Kaffetzi N, Simpson MA, Navarini AA, et al. AP1S3 mutations are associated with pustular psoriasis and impaired Toll-like receptor 3 trafficking. Am J Hum Genet 2014;94:790–7.
18. Kantaputra PN, Chuamanochan M, Kiratikanon S, et al. A truncating variant in SERPINA3, skin pustules and adult-onset immunodeficiency. J. Dermatol 2021;48:e370–1. https://doi.org/10.1111/1346-8138.15942 [PubMed] [CrossRef] [Google Scholar].
19. Kantaputra P, Chaowattanapanit S, Kiratikanon S, et al. SERPINA1, generalized pustular psoriasis, and adult-onset immunodeficiency. J. Dermatol 2021;48:1597–601. https://doi.org/10.1111/1346-8138.16081 [PubMed] [CrossRef] [Google Scholar].
20. Zhang Q, Shi P, Wang Z, et al. Identification of the BTN3A3 gene as a molecule implicated in generalized pustular psoriasis in a Chinese population. J. Investig. Dermatol 2023. https://doi.org/10.1016/j.jid.2023.01.023 [PubMed] [CrossRef] [Google Scholar].
21. Kantaputra P, Daroontum T, Chuamanochan M, et al. Loss of Function TGFBR2 Variant as a Contributing Factor in Generalized Pustular Psoriasis and Adult-

Onset Immunodeficiency. Genes 2022;14:103. https://doi.org/10.3390/genes14010103 [PMC free article] [PubMed] [CrossRef] [Google Scholar].

22. Liu Y, Li H, Meng S, et al. Newly revealed variants of SERPINA3 in generalized pustular psoriasis attenuate inhibition of ACT on cathepsin G. J Hum Genet 2023;68:419–25.

23. Navarini AA, Valeyrie-Allanore L, Setta-Kaffetzi N, et al. Rare variations in IL36RN in severe adverse drug reactions manifesting as acute generalized exanthematous pustulosis. J Invest Dermatol 2013;133:1904–7.

24. Meier-Schiesser B, Feldmeyer L, Jankovic D, et al. Culprit drugs induce specific il-36 overexpression in acute generalized exanthematous pustulosis. J Invest Dermatol 2019;139:848–58.

25. Girijala RL, Siddiqi I, Kwak Y, et al. Pustular DRESS syndrome secondary to hydroxychloroquine with EBV reactivation. J Drugs Dermatol 2019;18:207–9.

26. Chowdhury TA, Talib KA, Patricia J, et al. Rare and complicated overlap of stevens-johnson syndrome and acute generalized exanthematous pustulosis. Cureus 2021;13:e15921.

27. Twelves S, Mostafa A, Dand N, et al. Clinical and genetic differences between pustular psoriasis subtypes. J Allergy Clin Immunol 2019;143:1021–6.

28. Armstrong AW, Elston CA, Elewski BE, et al. Generalized pustular psoriasis: a consensus statement from the national psoriasis foundation. J Am Acad Dermatol 2023.

29. Borges-Costa J, Silva R, Gonçalves L, et al. Clinical and laboratory features in acute generalized pustular psoriasis: a retrospective study of 34 patients. Am J Clin Dermatol 2011;12:271–6.

30. Chao JP, Tsai TF. Elderly-onset generalized pustular psoriasis: a case series. Clin Exp Dermatol 2022;47:1567–70.

31. Jin H, Cho HH, Kim WJ, et al. Clinical features and course of generalized pustular psoriasis in Korea. J Dermatol 2015;42:674–8.

32. Teoh XY, Suganthy R, Voo SYM, et al. Pustular psoriasis in malaysia: a review of the malaysian psoriasis registry 2007-2018. Exp Dermatol 2023;32:1253–62.

33. Tosukhowong T, Kiratikanon S, Wonglamsam P, et al. Epidemiology and clinical features of pustular psoriasis: A 15-year retrospective cohort. J Dermatol 2021;48:1931–5.

34. Xu Z, Liu Y, Qu H, et al. Clinical characteristics and heterogeneity of generalized pustular psoriasis: A comparative study in a large retrospective cohort. Exp Dermatol 2023.

35. Kara Polat A, Alpsoy E, Kalkan G, et al. Sociodemographic, clinical, laboratory, treatment and prognostic characteristics of 156 generalized pustular psoriasis patients in Turkey: a multicentre case

series. J Eur Acad Dermatol Venereol 2022;36:1256–65.

36. Wu X, Li Y. [Clinical analysis of 82 cases of generalized pustular psoriasis]. Zhong Nan Da Xue Xue Bao Yi Xue Ban 2017;42:173–8.

37. Noe MH, Wan MT, Mostaghimi A, et al. Evaluation of a Case Series of Patients With Generalized Pustular Psoriasis in the United States. JAMA Dermatol 2022;158:73–8.

38. Choon SE, Lai NM, Mohammad NA, et al. Clinical profile, morbidity, and outcome of adult-onset generalized pustular psoriasis: analysis of 102 cases seen in a tertiary hospital in Johor, Malaysia. Int J Dermatol 2014;53:676–84.

39. Lim LY, Oon HH. Gastrointestinal and hepatic manifestations in patients with generalised pustular psoriasis. Exp Dermatol 2023;32:1246–52.

40. Creadore A, Desai S, Alloo A, et al. Clinical Characteristics, Disease Course, and Outcomes of Patients With Acute Generalized Exanthematous Pustulosis in the US. JAMA Dermatol 2022;158:176–83.

41. Navarini AA, Simpson MA, Borradori L, et al. Homozygous missense mutation in IL36RN in generalized pustular dermatosis with intraoral involvement compatible with both AGEP and generalized pustular psoriasis. JAMA Dermatol 2015;151:452–3.

42. O'Brian M, Carr CL, Thomas C, et al. Clinical characteristics and management of acute generalized exanthematous pustulosis with haemodynamic instability. Skin Health Dis 2021;1:e74.

43. Kleier RS, Breneman DL, Boiko S. Generalized pustulation as a manifestation of the anticonvulsant hypersensitivity syndrome. Arch Dermatol 1991;127:1361–4.

44. Gey A, Milpied B, Dutriaux C, et al. Severe cutaneous adverse reaction associated with vemurafenib: DRESS, AGEP or overlap reaction? J Eur Acad Dermatol Venereol 2016;30:178–9.

45. Sidoroff A, Halevy S, Bavinck JN, et al. Acute generalized exanthematous pustulosis (AGEP)–a clinical reaction pattern. J Cutan Pathol 2001;28:113–9.

46. Barlow RJ, Schulz EJ. Chronic subcorneal pustulosis with vasculitis: a variant of generalized pustular psoriasis in black South Africans. Br J Dermatol 1991;124:470–4.

47. Lutz ME, Daoud MS, McEvoy MT, et al. Subcorneal pustular dermatosis: a clinical study of ten patients. Cutis 1998;61:203–8.

48. Lin JH, Sheu HM, Lee JY. Acute generalized exanthematous pustulosis with erythema multiforme-like lesions. Eur J Dermatol 2002;12:475–8.

49. Marzolf G, Lenormand C, Schissler C, et al. [Acute generalized pustular bacterid followed by Sweet's

syndrome and erythema nodosum]. Ann Dermatol Venereol 2020;147:298–302.

50. Vashisht P, Goyal A, Hearth Holmes MP. Sweet syndrome. StatPearls. Treasure Island (FL): StatPearls Publishing; 2023.

51. Schissler C, Velter C, Lipsker D. Amicrobial pustulosis of the folds: Where have we gone 25years after its original description? Ann Dermatol Venereol 2017;144:169–75.

52. Kardaun SH, Kuiper H, Fidler V, et al. The histopathological spectrum of acute generalized exanthematous pustulosis (AGEP) and its differentiation from generalized pustular psoriasis. J Cutan Pathol 2010;37:1220–9.

53. Fujita H, Terui T, Hayama K, et al. Japanese guidelines for the management and treatment of generalized pustular psoriasis: The new pathogenesis and treatment of GPP. J Dermatol 2018; 45:1235–70.

54. Beylot C, Bioulac P, Doutre MS. [Acute generalized exanthematic pustuloses (four cases) (author's transl)]. Ann Dermatol Venereol 1980;107: 37–48.

55. Halevy S, Kardaun SH, Davidovici B, et al. The spectrum of histopathological features in acute generalized exanthematous pustulosis: a study of 102 cases. Br J Dermatol 2010;163:1245–52.

56. Rzany B, Hering O, Mockenhaupt M, et al. Histopathological and epidemiological characteristics of patients with erythema exudativum multiforme major, Stevens-Johnson syndrome and toxic epidermal necrolysis. Br J Dermatol 1996;135: 6–11.

57. Sneddon IB, Wilkinson DS. Subcorneal pustular dermatosis. Br J Dermatol 1979;100:61–8.

58. Avallone G, Maronese CA, Murgia G, et al. Interleukin-17 vs. Interleukin-23 Inhibitors in Pustular and Erythrodermic Psoriasis: A Retrospective, Multicentre Cohort Study. J Clin Med 2023;12.

59. Bachelez H, Choon SE, Marrakchi S, et al. Trial of Spesolimab for Generalized Pustular Psoriasis. N Engl J Med 2021;385:2431–40.

60. Warren RB, Reich A, Kaszuba A, et al. Imsidolimab, an anti-interleukin-36 receptor monoclonal antibody, for the treatment of generalized pustular psoriasis: results from the phase II GALLOP trial. Br J Dermatol 2023;189:161–9.

61. Morita A, Strober B, Burden AD, et al. Efficacy and safety of subcutaneous spesolimab for the prevention of generalised pustular psoriasis flares (Effisayil 2): an international, multicentre, randomised, placebo-controlled trial. Lancet 2023;402: 1541–51.

62. Yanes D, Nguyen E, Imadojemu S, et al. Cyclosporine for treatment of acute generalized exanthematous pustulosis: A retrospective analysis. J Am Acad Dermatol 2020;83:263–5.

63. Feng JN, Guo JZ, Zhang Q, et al. Higher prevalence of generalized pustular psoriasis in asia? a population-based study using claim data in china and a systematic review. Dermatology 2023;239: 195–205.

64. Navarini AA, Maul JT. International Rare And Severe Psoriasis Expert Network (IRASPEN) Internet. 2023. Clinicaltrials.gov entry. https://clinicaltrials.gov/study/NCT04359394.

65. Liang J, Huang P, Li H, et al. Mutations in IL36RN are associated with geographic tongue. Hum Genet 2017;136:241–52.

Quality of Life with Neutrophilic Dermatoses

Ashley N. Gray, MD[a,b], Rohan Mital, BS[a,b], Abena Minta, BS[a,b], Margo Waters, BS[b], Farah Almhana, BA[b], Jourdan Hydol-Smith, BA[c], Benjamin H. Kaffenberger, MD, MS[a,*]

KEYWORDS

- Neutrophilic dermatoses • Quality of life • Assessment • Pyoderma gangrenosum
- Behçet's disease • Sweet syndrome

KEY POINTS

- Physicians should personalize therapeutic approaches to address impacts on quality of life (QoL) unique to individual neutrophilic dermatoses (NDs).
- Prompt recognition and early intervention are crucial to limit impacts of NDs on QoL.
- Disease-specific QoL assessments should be developed for chronic, relapsing–remitting NDs, whereas informal assessment of factors impacting QoL in transient, rapidly-resolving NDs is appropriate.

INTRODUCTION

Neutrophilic Dermatoses

Neutrophilic dermatoses (NDs) are a heterogenous group of disorders characterized by sterile neutrophilic infiltrates in the epidermis, dermis, or hypodermis in the absence of infection, sometimes accompanied by vasculitis.[1] Most NDs have systemic disease associations with accompanying extracutaneous manifestations. The NDs can be subdivided into chronic, relapsing–remitting disorders and transient, rapidly resolving conditions. Significant variability in morphology, severity, and disease course exists for this group of diseases, and consequentially, quality of life (QoL) differs between diseases.

Although extracutaneous manifestations can have a profound impact on QoL, the cutaneous processes involving neutrophilic infiltration often lead to swelling, fevers, and eventually painful ulcerations. For some NDs, their nature is so transient and predictable, studies on QoL are unnecessary. However, chronic, relapsing–remitting conditions require additional research and specialized QoL scoring systems to accurately assess their disease burden. Importantly, these rare diseases are discussed to highlight current research and inform physicians of what to expect when counseling patients. This information may help in managing pain regimens and aid in prognostic counseling and ancillary service allocation for patients.

In NDs, prompt recognition and treatment arrest disease progression and can produce complete resolution in certain cases. To address extracutaneous manifestations that may also be contributing to QoL, multidisciplinary approaches are often necessary. In this review, the authors address the burden that NDs have on QoL based on existing literature. To our knowledge, there are no current comprehensive reviews of QoL in NDs. The authors discuss aspects of QoL specific to individual NDs and how the current literature should guide patient care and potential development of disease-specific QoL assessment tools.

Quality of Life Assessment in Dermatology

In recent decades, assessment of QoL in dermatology has emerged as a necessary research topic. Currently available QoL assessments used

Funding sources: None.
[a] Department of Dermatology, Ohio State University Wexner Medical Center, 2012 Kenny Road, 2nd Floor, Columbus, OH 43221, USA; [b] The Ohio State University College of Medicine, 2012 Kenny Road, 2nd Floor, Columbus, OH 43221, USA; [c] Texas A&M University School of Medicine, 8447 Riverside Pkwy, Bryan, TX 77807, USA
* Corresponding author. OSU Dermatology, 2012 Kenny Road 2nd Floor, Columbus, OH 43221.
E-mail address: Benjamin.Kaffenberger@osumc.edu

Dermatol Clin 42 (2024) 329–338
https://doi.org/10.1016/j.det.2023.08.011
0733-8635/24/

in dermatology include Dermatology Life Quality Index (DLQI), Skindex-29, 36-Item Short Form Survey (SF-36), Health-related Quality of Life Assessment (HRQoL), and World Health Organization Quality of Life Assessment-Brief (WHOQOL-BREF).[2–6] The most widely used generic adult QoL assessments include SF-36 and EuroQoL 5-Dimension, whereas the most widely used dermatology-specific QoL assessments include the DLQI and Skindex-29.[7,8] A 2007 systematic review assessed QoL assessment tools and found that combination of SF-36 and Skindex-29 were the best dermatology QoL screening tools, when considering factors such as reliability, validity, and administrative burden; additionally, Skindex-17 and WHOQOL form were identified as promising new tools.[8] Despite these currently available instruments, many disease-specific analyses of NDs are not available.

Pyoderma gangrenosum

Pyoderma gangrenosum (PG) is a rare ND that is classically characterized by rapidly evolving painful ulcers, with undermined borders and peripheral erythema.[9] Patients typically present with erythematous edematous papules, plaques, nodules, or sterile pustules, and the secondary eruptions can include blisters, ulcers, and abscesses.[10] PG can arise as a solitary lesion usually at a site of minor trauma (ie, pathergy) or as several lesions. The disease course can be chronic or relapsing–remitting, and PG is often associated with autoimmune and immune-mediated diseases such as inflammatory bowel disease (IBD), rheumatoid arthritis (RA), and hematologic malignancies.[10] There are several subtypes of PG including classic, ulcerative, bullous, pustular, vegetative, peristomal, and postoperative.[10] The mainstays of PG treatment are immunosuppressive therapy and wound care.

Currently, QoL is rarely qualitatively or quantitatively assessed in PG studies, with multiple reviews identifying a need for a validated QoL assessment tool.[11,12] Multicenter studies emphasize the need for a disease-specific QoL measure.[12,13] Impacts on QoL can be quite severe, with considerable disability and mortality risk, multiple comorbid health disorders, and cost burden to patients.[14] Most of the current literature assesses QoL in PG by using the DLQI, a validated questionnaire designed to specifically measure the health-related QoL of adult patients suffering from a skin disease. Other studies attempt to characterize the effect of PG on patients through identifying interview themes, assessing patients' satisfaction with wound care, local therapy, and pain management, for identification of comorbid conditions, such as depression and anxiety.[15–17]

Factors that influence patients' satisfaction in PG treatment and perceived QoL include pain severity, extent of wounds, and impact of comorbid conditions that arise due to PG, such as anxiety and depression.[13] One study interviewed patients with PG to analyze health-related domains of QoL and detailed the multifaceted impact on physical, psychological, and social functioning of patients.[16] Emerging themes were pain, disease course, and wound care, with resulting negative impact on self-image and mental health.[16] From this study, general satisfaction was present with current systemic treatments for PG, but pain and comorbid anxiety and depression continue to be primary challenges in PG treatment.

PG is consistently one of the most painful skin diseases based on currently available QoL measures in dermatology.[10,18] Maverakis and colleagues found that DLQI scores of PG patients are higher than those of many other dermatologic conditions, largely attributable to pain scores.[10] Furthermore, adequacy of pain control significantly impacts the severity of depression and comorbid mental health conditions. A multicenter study demonstrated this finding by using the SATMED-Q (treatment SATisfaction with MEDicines), a validated, multidimensional generic questionnaire for chronic disease, to assess satisfaction with systemic therapies, wound care, care, and pain management as well as QoL by the DLQI.[13]

To accommodate the unmet needs for QoL improvements in PG, multiple groups indicate the development of a PG-specific QoL measure[10–13]; Gerard and colleagues emphasize that formal evaluation of QoL, specifically in PG clinical trials, is necessary to assess the holistic impact of emerging PG therapies.[11] Combining quantitative validated measures with subjective global QoL measures could lead to the development of a useful PG-specific tool, with a note to also consider feelings of stigma, specific pain ratings, effects of lesion odor, mood changes including depression and anxiety, feelings of isolation, presence of a support system, patient interest in and utilization of psychological support, occupational distress, self-perception, self-acceptance, and interference in daily living due to time spent on wound care.[11]

Although few studies have examined QoL in patients with PG, limitations in utility of these findings exist due to the absence of a QoL instrument that encompasses all the nuances experienced by PG patients. There is a need for a validated disease-specific QoL instrument, likely incorporating both quantitative and qualitative parameters. Overall, many factors influence QoL with PG, including individual patient factors, adequacy of pain management, and contribution to mental health. Identification of these effects combined with appropriate and prompt treatment is essential to improve the QoL of patients with PG.

Sweet syndrome (classical, histiocytoid, neutrophilic dermatosis of the dorsal hands)

Acute febrile ND (Sweet syndrome) is a relatively rare inflammatory disorder affecting the skin. It is characterized by sudden onset of painful and erythematous papules, plaques, or nodules with characteristic neutrophilic infiltrate of the dermis. Although Sweet syndrome classically affects the skin, systemic involvement is common and may manifest as fever, leukocytosis, or other organ involvement.

Sweet syndrome has a variety of etiologies, dividing the disorder into three main subtypes. Classical Sweet syndrome, also known as idiopathic Sweet syndrome, is the most common subtype and is associated with pregnancy, infections, and IBD.[19] Sweet syndrome may also occur as a malignancy-associated subtype, classically occurring with hematologic malignancies as well as a drug-induced subtype.

Histiocytoid Sweet syndrome is a variant of Sweet syndrome and is differentiated by infiltration within the dermis of histiocyte-like immature myeloid cells rather than the neutrophilic infiltrate seen in classical Sweet syndrome.[20] Diagnosis of this variant may be difficult as histiocytoid Sweet syndrome may present similarly to leukemia cutis.[21]

An additional distributional variant of Sweet syndrome is ND of the dorsal hands (NDDH), characterized by dense dermal neutrophilic infiltrates with upper dermal edema on histopathology.[22] Misdiagnosis is also common in NDDH, as the tender, violaceous inflammatory papules mimic infection.

Characterization and study of QoL in patients with Sweet syndrome is sparse, and there is an active need for research in this area. Although no studies, per our review, have directly assessed QoL in a validated manner in patients with Sweet syndrome, several studies have described the effect of this disease on patients.

Manifestations of Sweet syndrome can be debilitating to patients. A cohort study of 25 patients with Sweet syndrome showed that the most common associated symptoms were pain (88%), fever (76%), and cough (44%), with the most common presentation being nodules on the lower legs.[23] Additional case reports were also found in the literature detailing a variety of symptoms that may affect patient QoL. In one case, a patient with interferon-beta-induced Sweet syndrome was unable to walk due to severe pain from lesions affecting the legs.[24] Other case reports detail further extracutaneous manifestations including severe recurrent jaw pain and myalgia,[25] and conjunctivitis and splenomegaly mimicking an infectious process.[26]

Importantly, appropriate treatment for Sweet syndrome with corticosteroids has been shown in multiple studies to result in prompt resolution of symptoms. In one cohort of 52 patients with Sweet syndrome, most of the patients showed rapid improvement after steroid therapy initiation. Importantly, this improvement did not persist in patients with malignancy-associated Sweet syndrome until adequate treatment for the malignancy was achieved.[27] Symptoms may differ in patients with the histiocytoid variant of Sweet syndrome, which may affect patient QoL and outcomes. Although classical Sweet syndrome will often heal with little to no scarring, one case report was found detailing residual hypertrophic scar formation following treatment of histiocytoid Sweet syndrome. Interestingly, resolution in this patient was complicated due to limited response to steroid treatment.[28] Further reports detail additional potentially debilitating symptoms such as uveitis,[29] which may further complicate treatment in these patients. In NDDH, average time to clinical improvement after correct treatment initiation was 5 days.[30] In addition, early disease recognition may facilitate appropriate workup to exclude associated diseases, especially malignancies for patients with NDDH.[22,31–33] Owing to the rapid resolution that may be achieved when appropriate treatment is initiated, it is important that diagnosis and treatment are prompt to minimize effects on patient QoL.

Although no direct studies have been conducted examining QoL in patients with Sweet syndrome, the severe presentation and rapid resolution with appropriate treatment suggest that prompt identification and treatment may limit effects of this disease on patient QoL.

CLINICS CARE POINTS

- Symptoms of Sweet syndrome may be debilitating to patients and can affect activities of daily living (ADLs) such as walking and eating.
- Although cutaneous manifestations are common, extracutaneous manifestations may present with Sweet syndrome and clinicians must be aware of these potential effects.

Palisading Neutrophilic Granulomatous Dermatitis

Palisading neutrophilic granulomatous dermatitis (PNGD) is an inflammatory ND that may present with erythematous papules, nodules, and plaques with ulceration and crusting.[34] Histopathologically, PNGD is a leukocytoclastic vasculitis with dense neutrophilic infiltrates, focal degeneration of collagen, and palisading granulomas.[34] To date, the specific etiology of PNGD is unknown.[35] However, PNGD commonly presents in female patients with concurrent connective tissue diseases such systemic lupus erythematosus (SLE), inflammatory arthritis, and hematology disorders.[35] Symptoms range from asymptomatic dermatoses to diffuse, painful lesions, thus corroborating the potential impact of PNGD on patient QoL.[36,37]

Awareness of the association of PNGD with autoimmune and inflammatory disease may facilitate early recognition of dermatologic manifestations and subsequent treatment initiation.[38] There is a paucity of literature assessing the impact of PNGD on the QoL of patients. The focus of current literature is primarily regarding dermatologic presentation and associated systemic disease; detailed characterization of the QoL of patients with PNGD is needed.

CLINICS CARE POINTS

- The QoL burden of PNGD is unknown; thus, clinicians should broadly survey patients to determine if various QoL domains are affected and require more targeted treatments.

Bowel Bypass Syndrome (Bowel-Associated Dermatitis–Arthritis Syndrome)

Bowel bypass syndrome, also known as bowel-associated dermatitis–arthritis syndrome (BADAS), is an ND caused by bacterial overgrowth in the bowel facilitating inflammation and immune complex deposition.[39] Histopathologic evaluation of early lesions is remarkable for neutrophilic and perivascular mononuclear infiltrates, and late lesions show edema leading to vesicle followed by pustule formation.[40] Prior jejunoileal bypass surgery, IBD, diverticulitis, and peptic ulcer disease are common concurrent conditions associated with BADAS.[41]

BADAS commonly presents with symptoms of panniculitis, pustular vasculitis, polyarthritis, diarrhea, and malabsorption which may complicate disease course or surgical recovery, thus corroborating the potential impact of BADAS on patient QoL.[40] One case described polyarthralgia and dermatitis following jejunoileal anastomosis with complications such as depression and cognitive changes consequent of surgically induced vitamin deficiencies.[42] Otherwise, current literature focus is primarily regarding time of onset of BADAS, symptoms, and associated systemic diseases.[43]

There is limited literature evaluating the impact of BADAS on patient QoL, particularly as a complication of surgery and comorbidity with IBD. There is a need for more detailed characterization of the QoL of patients with BADAS using dermatologic measures.

CLINICS CARE POINTS

- The QoL burden of BADAS is unknown and thus clinicians should broadly survey their patients to facilitate early diagnosis and personalize treatments.

Behçet's Disease

Behçet's disease (BD) is a chronic, systemic vasculitis of unknown etiology that commonly presents with mucocutaneous and joint involvement. Ocular, vascular, gastrointestinal, and neurologic involvement may cause significant morbidity and mortality in patients with BD. The relapsing-remitting, multisystemic inflammatory manifestations associated with BD are often progressive, which may impact physical and mental functions and contribute to impairments of patient QoL.[44]

Previous literature has found QoL impairment in BD to be strongly associated with disease activity and severity. A cross-sectional study using the Short Form-36 QoL Scale (SF-36) found that the overall QoL score and subset domain scores including general health, mental health, and physical health were significantly lower in BD patients compared with the control group ($P < .05$).[44]

These findings are corroborated by several studies of disease activity by the BD Current Activity Form, where QoL domains including physical health and psychological health are inversely correlated with disease activity.[45,46] Further, clinical symptoms including genital ulcers, ocular, and central nervous system involvement are often the main factors negatively affecting QoL in BD.[44,45,47,48] Among patients with BD, early disease onset and prolonged disease duration (>5 years) are associated with lower general health score.[47] In addition, previous literature correlates disease onset and severity with patient lifestyle factors. Multivariable regression modeling identified sleep quality as the single most important factor associated with self-rated wellness and health status in patients with BD.[43]

Although elucidation of the etiology of BD is still underway, previous literature suggests that lifestyle factors such as physical activity, smoking, and sleep patterns may mitigate impact on disease course and symptom severity. Clinicians should counsel that lifestyle modifications such as smoking cessation and sleep hygiene may improve QoL and reduce health care burden.[43] There is a plethora of literature evaluating the impact of BD on patient QoL, particularly in relation to disease severity measured by the BD Current Activity Form. Other common QoL assessment tools include SF-36 QoL Scale and the WHOQOL-BREF.[49] Identifying the etiology of BD may facilitate the development of novel therapeutic agents to improve the standard of care for patients. The relapsing–remitting course of BD renders assessment of effective therapy difficult. Treatment of mucocutaneous BD should be tailored to the patient's QoL needs and concerns based on European Alliance of Associations for Rheumatology recommendations.

CLINICS CARE POINTS

- BD is a multisystemic inflammatory vasculitis; thus, optimal management involves multidisciplinary collaboration.

Neutrophilic Eccrine Hidradenitis

Neutrophilic eccrine hidradenitis (NEH) is a rare disorder affecting the eccrine glands, leading to eccrine unit necrosis. It is characterized by the sudden onset of painful and edematous plaques. Although NEH classically affects the skin, systemic involvement is common, including an acute onset of fever due to the reactive nature of the disease. The etiology of NEH is not completely known; however, it is classically associated with cytotoxic agents in chemotherapy[50] and heat damage of the eccrine glands in pediatric patients.[51]

Characterization and study of QoL in patients with NEH is sparse, and there is an active need for research in this area. Although no studies per our review have directly assessed QoL in patients with NEH, some studies have characterized the effect of this disease on patients. Patients with NEH most commonly presented with symptoms of pain and fever, with the most common presentation being highly painful edematous plaques on the hands and feet.[50] In one case, a patient with chemotherapy-induced NEH developed tender and painful erythematous nodules, and a fever that disappeared after a high dose of corticosteroid therapy.[52] Although NEH usually resolves, it can recur and is characteristically painful.

Although there is no widely accepted treatment for NEH, symptomatic management of fever and pain is encouraged. Most lesions will resolve spontaneously, but supportive treatment is important to minimize the effects on patient QoL.

Although no direct studies have been conducted examining QoL in patients with NEH, the severe presentation and successful treatments suggest that prompt identification and treatment may limit the effects of this disease on patient QoL.

CLINICS CARE POINTS

- Symptoms of NEH may be debilitating to patients and can potentially affect ADLs.
- Systemic corticosteroids and nonsteroidal anti-inflammatory drugs (NSAIDs) have been shown to reduce pain and fever.

Neutrophilic Urticarial Dermatosis

Neutrophilic urticarial dermatosis (NUD) is a rare form of dermatosis that presents as an urticarial rash. It is characterized by pink-to-red plaques or macules, with characteristic neutrophilic infiltration of the dermis. NUD often occurs in the setting of an underlying systemic condition, such as Schnitzler syndrome or SLE.[53]

Patients with NUD often present with symptoms of fever and joint or muscle pain and, in some cases, thoracic or abdominal pain and neurologic manifestations such as vertigo and delirium.[54] In one case, a patient experienced a 10-month history of polyarthralgia, fever, and fatigue in addition to her painful skin eruption before treatment.[55]

In patients in whom NUD occurs concomitantly with SLE, neutrophil migration inhibitors such as colchicine must be initiated. In patients in whom NUD occurs concomitantly with Schnitzler syndrome, the most effective treatments are interleukin-1 (IL-1) antagonists.[56]

Although no direct studies have been conducted examining QoL in patients with NUD, the severe presentation and successful treatments suggest that prompt identification and treatment may limit the effects of this disease on patient QoL.

CLINICS CARE POINTS

- Clinicians should be aware that treatment of NUD is highly dependent on underlying etiology, so treatment of pain may also be highly variable.

SUMMARY

The heterogeneity among NDs limits the development of a unified assessment instrument. For chronic relapsing–remitting disorders, including necrotizing NDs and BD, specific QoL instruments are necessary. Many aspects of these conditions, including both cutaneous and extracutaneous manifestations, are not properly assessed in the existing literature or available dermatologic QoL instruments. To adequately manage important aspects of patient care, including pain, mental health, barriers to activities and occupation, sexual health, and cost to patients, we must develop and advocate for disease-specific QoL instruments for individual chronic NDs. The efficacy of emerging therapies and utility of existing therapies in these conditions cannot be properly assessed without a thorough appreciation of the significant potential impacts on QoL.

Although some of the more transient, rapidly evolving NDs do not necessitate a specific disease QoL measure, physicians should be aware of potential impacts on QoL so that proper care, ancillary services, and prognostic guidance can be elicited. Particularly, transient NDs can be exquisitely painful, and physicians have an obligation to adequately treat pain. Physicians should maintain a high index of suspicion for these disorders, as they often resolve rapidly with early diagnosis and appropriate immunosuppressant treatment.

Interestingly, no NDs have their own specialized scoring systems, aside from BD. Although BD was evaluated using a disease-specific QoL assessment, only a generic dermatology QoL assessment was used to assess PG, which failed to fully encompass many of the disease-specific impacts on QoL. Based on the currently available QoL assessment validation studies, Skindex-29 and SF-36 should be the first-line assessments for chronic NDs.[8]

Further, specific dermatology QoL tools already exist for many individual conditions, including acne, atopic dermatitis, psoriasis, and chronic urticaria. The HRQoL has also been deemed relevant for use in dermatology and may be even more beneficial for diseases with prominent extracutaneous manifestations.[57] It is particularly useful for patients with chronic skin diseases; some groups call for Skindex-29 to be first choice for dermatology. A 2007 systematic review assessed QoL assessment tools and found that the combination of SF-36 and Skindex-29 was superior to others while identifying Skindex-17 and WHOQOL as promising new tools.[8]

Despite these current tools, the chronic NDs with a relapsing–remitting course such as PG require disease-specific QoL measurement tools, as many disease aspects simply cannot be captured in a generic dermatology QoL form. Particularly, the impact of odor and drainage, stigma of wound appearance, and barriers to occupational and ADLs are not applicable to other dermatologic conditions, especially to the extent that they are in PG. Other NDs that likely warrant disease-specific QoL indices are BD that has already been developed and BADAS due to their chronic nature and unique symptoms. Other NDs likely do not warrant disease-specific QoL assessment or formal QoL assessment of any kind, but our review highlights important symptoms that physicians should be aware of. Many of the acute NDs are mild if diagnosed early, so physicians should maintain a high index of suspicion for erythematous, edematous papules, and plaques, especially that appear in patients with associated systemic manifestations. Full summaries of QoL literature review and clinical recommendations are provided (**Table 1**).

Future directions should also assess whether QoL varies based on proximity to academic medical centers capable of multidisciplinary approaches for complex diseases with cutaneous and extracutaneous manifestations.

CLINICS CARE POINTS

- Prompt therapy to arrest disease activity and wound care are essential to limit effects on quality of life (QoL).
- Understand that pyoderma gangrenosum (PG) is an extremely painful condition, often requiring narcotic management.
- Acknowledge and address additional QoL measures including impact of pain, mental health, stigma related to odor and appearance, and sexual health.

Table 1
Summary of quality of life in neutrophilic dermatoses

	Disease Course	Systemic Associations + Comorbidities	Quality of Life Assessments Used	Physical Manifestations	Mental and Psychosocial Manifestations	Care Points
Pyoderma gangrenosum	Chronic	IBD, RA, hematologic malignancies	DLQI	Pain	Depression, anxiety, stigma, isolation, impact of odor, drainage, barriers to activities, occupational and sexual health	• Early diagnosis to arrest disease progression • Treat pain adequately • Screen for depression/anxiety • Counsel family on the extreme pain of condition
Sweet syndrome (classical, histiocytoid, NDDH)	Acute	IBD, RA, infections, malignancy, pregnancy, drug-induced	None	Pain, fever, cough	None identified	• Find and treat underlying etiology • Early, accurate diagnosis critical • Initiate corticosteroid therapy early in treatment
Palisading neutrophilic granulomatous dermatitis	Chronic	CTD, SLE, RA, inflammatory arthritis, hematologic disorders	None	Pain, arthralgia, fever, fatigue	None identified	• Early, accurate diagnosis critical
Behçet's disease	Chronic	Genital, ocular, and gastrointestinal ulcers	SF-36, BD Current Activity Form, WHOQOL-BREF	Pain, ocular, gastrointestinal, neurologic, genital ulcers	Mental health	• Optimize of lifestyle factors is (ie, physical activity, smoking, sleep) • Coordinate multidisciplinary collaboration

(continued on next page)

Table 1
(continued)

	Disease Course	Systemic Associations + Comorbidities	Quality of Life Assessments Used	Physical Manifestations	Mental and Psychosocial Manifestations	Care Points
Bowel-associated dermatitis–arthritis-syndrome (BADAS)	Chronic	Prior jejunal bypass surgery, IBD, diverticulitis, PUD	None	Pain, panniculitis, pustular vasculitis, polyarthritis, diarrhea/malabsorption, malaise, joint effusions	Depression, cognitive changes	• Screen patients following bypass surgery and/or IBD diagnosis
Neutrophilic eccrine hidradenitis	Acute	Chemotherapy-associated	None	Pain, fever	None identified	• Corticosteroids and NSAIDs best to control symptoms
Neutrophilic urticarial dermatosis	Acute	SLE, Schnitzler syndrome	None	Pain, fever, arthralgias, myalgias, fatigue	None identified	• Colchicine if SLE associated • IL-1 antagonist for Schnitzler syndrome

Abbreviations: CTD, connective tissue disease; DLQI, dermatology life quality index; IBD, inflammatory bowel disease; NDDH, neutrophilic dermatosis of the dorsal hand; PUD, peptic ulcer disease; RA, rheumatoid arthritis; SF-36, short form-36; SLE, systemic lupus erythematosus; WHOQOL-BREF, World Health Organization QoL Assessment-Brief.

CONFLICT OF INTEREST

None declared.

REFERENCES

1. Nelson CA, Stephen S, Ashchyan HJ, et al. Neutrophilic dermatoses: Pathogenesis, Sweet syndrome, neutrophilic eccrine hidradenitis, and Behçet disease. J Am Acad Dermatol 2018;79(6):987–1006.

2. Finlay AY, Khan GK. Dermatology Life Quality Index (DLQI)–a simple practical measure for routine clinical use. Clin Exp Dermatol 1994;19(3):210–6.

3. Chren MM. The Skindex instruments to measure the effects of skin disease on quality of life. Dermatol Clin 2012;30(2):231–6, xiii.

4. Ware JE, Sherbourne CD. The MOS 36-item short-form health survey (SF-36). I. Conceptual framework and item selection. Med Care 1992;30(6):473–83.

5. Yin S, Njai R, Barker L, et al. Summarizing health-related quality of life (HRQOL): development and testing of a one-factor model. Popul Health Metr 2016;14:22.

6. The WHOQOL Group. Development of the World Health Organization WHOQOL-BREF Quality of Life Assessment. Psychol Med 1998;28(3):551–8.

7. Devlin NJ, Brooks R. EQ-5D and the EuroQol Group: Past, Present and Future. Appl Health Econ Health Policy 2017;15(2):127–37.

8. Both H, Essink-Bot ML, Busschbach J, et al. Critical review of generic and dermatology-specific health-related quality of life instruments. J Invest Dermatol 2007;127(12):2726–39.

9. Wang EA, Maverakis E. The rapidly evolving lesions of ulcerative pyoderma gangrenosum: a timeline. Int J Dermatol 2018;57(8):983–4.

10. Maverakis E, Marzano AV, Le ST, et al. Pyoderma gangrenosum. Nat Rev Dis Primer 2020;6(1):81.

11. Gerard AJ, Feldman SR, Strowd L. Quality of Life of Patients With Pyoderma Gangrenosum and Hidradenitis Suppurativa. J Cutan Med Surg 2015;19(4):391–6.

12. Ighani A, Al-Mutairi D, Rahmani A, et al. Pyoderma gangrenosum and its impact on quality of life: a multicentre, prospective study. Br J Dermatol 2019;180(3):672–3.

13. Hobbs MM, Byler R, Latour E, et al. Treatment of pyoderma gangrenosum: A multicenter survey-based study assessing satisfaction and quality of life. Dermatol Ther 2021;34(2):e14736.

14. Narla S, Silverberg JI. The inpatient burden and co-morbidities of pyoderma gangrenosum in adults in the United States. Arch Dermatol Res 2021;313(4):245–53.

15. Hobbs MM, Byler R, Latour E, et al. Treatment of pyoderma gangrenosum: A multicenter survey-based study assessing satisfaction and quality of life. Dermatol Ther 2021;34(2). https://doi.org/10.1111/dth.14736.

16. Nusbaum KB, Ortega-Loayza AG, Kaffenberger BH. Health-related domains of quality of life in pyoderma gangrenosum: A qualitative analysis. J Am Acad Dermatol 2022;86(6):1382–5.

17. McPhie ML, Fletcher J, Machado MO, et al. A Systematic Review of Depression and Anxiety in Adults with Pyoderma Gangrenosum. Adv Skin Wound Care 2021;34(8):432–6.

18. Beiteke U, Bigge S, Reichenberger C, et al. Pain and pain management in dermatology. J Dtsch Dermatol Ges J Ger Soc Dermatol JDDG 2015;13(10):967–87.

19. Cohen PR. Sweet's syndrome–a comprehensive review of an acute febrile neutrophilic dermatosis. Orphanet J Rare Dis 2007;2:34.

20. Requena L, Kutzner H, Palmedo G, et al. Histiocytoid Sweet syndrome: a dermal infiltration of immature neutrophilic granulocytes. Arch Dermatol 2005;141(7):834–42.

21. Chavan RN, Cappel MA, Ketterling RP, et al. Histiocytoid Sweet syndrome may indicate leukemia cutis: a novel application of fluorescence in situ hybridization. J Am Acad Dermatol 2014;70(6):1021–7.

22. Micallef D, Bonnici M, Pisani D, et al. Neutrophilic Dermatosis of the Dorsal Hands: A Review of 123 Cases. J Am Acad Dermatol 2019. https://doi.org/10.1016/j.jaad.2019.08.070. S0190962219326787.

23. Dan H, Yanmei L, Yue X, et al. Sweet syndrome associated with malignancies: A retrospective analysis of 25 patients from West China hospital. Dermatol Ther 2020;33(4):e13588.

24. Rodriguez-Lojo R, Castiñeiras I, Juarez Y, et al. Sweet syndrome associated with interferon. Dermatol Online J 2014;21(2):13030. qt2006n4sp.

25. Limdiwala PG, Parikh SJ, Shah JS. Sweet's syndrome. Indian J Dent Res Off Publ Indian Soc Dent Res 2014;25(3):401–5.

26. Polimeni G, Cardillo R, Garaffo E, et al. Allopurinol-induced Sweet's syndrome. Int J Immunopathol Pharmacol 2016;29(2):329–32.

27. Jung EH, Park JH, Hwan Kim K, et al. Characteristics of Sweet syndrome in patients with or without malignancy. Ann Hematol 2022;101(7):1499–508.

28. Lee KP, Tschen JA, Koshelev MV. Histiocytoid Sweet syndrome recalcitrant to prednisone causing severe scarring. JAAD Case Rep 2019;5(11):937–9.

29. Kato K, Namiki T, Tokoro S, et al. Histiocytoid Sweet syndrome with ophthalmologic involvements: A novel association with uveitis. J Dermatol 2017;44(2):216–7.

30. Wolf R, Tüzün Y. Acral manifestations of Sweet syndrome (neutrophilic dermatosis of the hands). Clin Dermatol 2017;35(1):81–4.

31. King BJ, Montagnon CM, Brough K, et al. Neutrophilic dermatosis of the dorsal hands is commonly associated with underlying hematologic malignancy

and pulmonary disease: A single-center retrospective case series study. J Am Acad Dermatol 2023; 88(2):444–6.

32. Fustà-Novell X, Bermejo S, Creus-Vila L. Neutrophilic dermatosis of the dorsal hands. Rev Clínica Esp Engl Ed 2021;221(9):553–4.

33. Gloor AD, Feldmeyer L, Borradori L. Neutrophilic dermatosis of the dorsal hands triggered by mechanical trauma. J Eur Acad Dermatol Venereol 2021;35(1). https://doi.org/10.1111/jdv.16750.

34. Lora V, Cerroni L, Cota C. Skin manifestations of rheumatoid arthritis. Ital J Dermatol Venereol 2018; 153(2). https://doi.org/10.23736/S0392-0488.18. 05872-8.

35. Rosenbach M, English JC. Reactive Granulomatous Dermatitis. Dermatol Clin 2015;33(3):373–87.

36. Kawakami T, Obara W, Soma Y, et al. Palisading Neutrophilic Granulomatous Dermatitis in a Japanese Patient with Wegener's Granulomatosis. J Dermatol 2005;32(6):487–92.

37. Zabihi-pour D, Bahrani B, Assaad D, et al. Palisaded neutrophilic and granulomatous dermatitis following a long-standing monoclonal gammopathy: A case report. SAGE Open Med Case Rep 2021;9. https:// doi.org/10.1177/2050313X20979560. 2050313X2097956.

38. Chua-Aguilera CJ, Möller B, Yawalkar N. Skin Manifestations of Rheumatoid Arthritis, Juvenile Idiopathic Arthritis, and Spondyloarthritides. Clin Rev Allergy Immunol 2017;53(3):371–93.

39. Hassold N, Jelin G, Palazzo E, et al. Bowel-associated dermatosis arthritis syndrome: A case report with first positron emission tomography analysis. JAAD Case Rep 2019;5(2):140–3.

40. Alavi A, Sajic D, Cerci FB, et al. Neutrophilic Dermatoses: An Update. Am J Clin Dermatol 2014;15(5): 413–23.

41. Rosen JD, Stojadinovic O, McBride JD, et al. Bowel-associated dermatosis-arthritis syndrome (BADAS) in a patient with cystic fibrosis. JAAD Case Rep 2019;5(1):37–9.

42. Bowen RC, Shepel L. Physical and psychological complications after intestinal bypass for obesity. Can Med Assoc J 1977;116(8):871–5.

43. Khabbazi A, Ebrahimzadeh Attari V, Asghari Jafarabadi M, et al. Quality of Life in Patients With Behçet Disease and Its Relation With Clinical Symptoms and Disease Activity. Reumatol Clínica 2021; 17(1):1–6.

44. Masoumi M, Tabaraii R, Shakiba S, et al. Association of lifestyle elements with self-rated wellness and health status in patients with Behcet's disease. BMC Rheumatol 2020;4(1):49.

45. Fabiani C, Vitale A, Orlando I, et al. Quality of life impairment in Behçet's disease and relationship with disease activity: a prospective study. Intern Emerg Med 2017;12(7):947–55.

46. Aflaki E, Farahangiz S, Salehi A. Quality of Life Assessment in Patients with Behçet's Disease using the Persian Version of the Leeds BD-QoL Questionnaire. Iran J Med Sci 2020;45(5). https://doi.org/10. 30476/ijms.2020.72634.0.

47. Melikoğlu M, Melikoglu MA. What affects the quality of life in patients with Behçet's disease? Acta Reumatol Port 2014;39(1):46–53.

48. Bodur H, Borman P, Özdemir Y, et al. Quality of life and life satisfaction in patients with Behçet's disease: relationship with disease activity. Clin Rheumatol 2006;25(3):329–33.

49. Uğuz F, Dursun R, Kaya N, et al. Quality of life in patients with Behçet's disease: the impact of major depression. Gen Hosp Psychiatry 2007;29(1):21–4.

50. Denny GO, Cohen BA. Reactive erythema. In: Pediatric dermatology. Philadelphia, PA: Elsevier; 2022. p. 180–226.

51. Harrist TJ, Fine JD, Berman RS, et al. Neutrophilic Eccrine Hidradenitis: A Distinctive Type of Neutrophilic Dermatosis Associated With Myelogenous Leukemia and Chemotherapy. Arch Dermatol 1982; 118(4):263.

52. Nikkels AF, Hansen I, Collignon J, et al. Neutrophilic Eccrine Hidradenitis. A Case Report. Acta Clin Belg 1993;48(6):397–400.

53. Gusdorf L, Lipsker D. Neutrophilic urticarial dermatosis: A review. Ann Dermatol Vénéréologie 2018; 145(12):735–40.

54. Tolkachjov SN, Wetter DA. Schnitzler Syndrome With Delirium and Vertigo: The Utility of Neurologic Manifestations in Diagnosis. J Drugs Dermatol JDD 2017; 16(6):625–7.

55. Sode T, Uzoma B, Vandergriff T, et al. Urticaria and a rare mutation: An unusual case of neutrophilic urticarial dermatosis. JAAD Case Rep 2020;6(6):543–5.

56. Lipsker D. The Schnitzler syndrome. Orphanet J Rare Dis 2010;5(1):38.

57. van Cranenburgh OD, Prinsen CaC, Sprangers MaG, et al. Health-related quality-of-life assessment in dermatologic practice: relevance and application. Dermatol Clin 2012;30(2):323–32.

Moving?

Make sure your subscription moves with you!

To notify us of your new address, find your **Clinics Account Number** (located on your mailing label above your name), and contact customer service at:

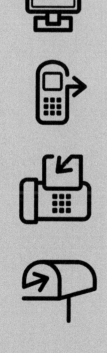

Email: journalscustomerservice-usa@elsevier.com

800-654-2452 (subscribers in the U.S. & Canada)
314-447-8871 (subscribers outside of the U.S. & Canada)

Fax number: 314-447-8029

Elsevier Health Sciences Division
Subscription Customer Service
3251 Riverport Lane
Maryland Heights, MO 63043

*To ensure uninterrupted delivery of your subscription, please notify us at least 4 weeks in advance of move.